ISSUES OF CANCER SURVIVORSHIP

AN INTERDISCIPLINARY
TEAM APPROACH TO CARE

ISSUES OF CANCER SURVIVORSHIP

AN INTERDISCIPLINARY
TEAM APPROACH TO CARE

EDITORS

Debra Kantor, PhD, APRN, BC
Associate Professor
Molloy College
Division of Nursing
Rockville Centre, New York

Zelda Suzan, MA, RN, CNE
Associate Professor / Course Coordinator
Phillips Beth Israel School of Nursing
New York, New York

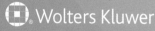

Philadelphia · Baltimore · New York · London
Buenos Aires · Hong Kong · Sydney · Tokyo

Executive Editor: Shannon W. Magee
Product Development Editor: Maria M. McAvey
Senior Marketing Manager: Mark Wiragh
Senior Production Project Manager: Cynthia Rudy
Design Coordinator: Holly Reid McLaughlin
Manufacturing Coordinator: Kathleen Brown
Prepress Vendor: Aptara, Inc.

9 8 7 6 5 4 3 2

Printed in the U.S.A.

ISBN: 978-1-45119-438-8
Library of Congress Cataloging-in-Publication Data available upon request from the Publisher.

DEDICATION

To my son Gregory, whose presence in my life is proof that dreams do come true. And to my husband Jerry. Through his 13 years of survivorship, I became more aware of the tremendous burden a diagnosis of cancer places on the individual and the family and how much difference an informed, caring nurse can make.

Debra Kantor, PhD, APRN, BC

To my family and friends who have experienced the continuum of cancer survivorship and shown me how it could be done. Thank you. To my husband, Edward, and my daughter, Rebecca, your love and support are priceless.

Zelda Suzan, MA, RN, CNE

ABOUT THE EDITORS

Debra P. Kantor, PhD, APRN, BC

Debra P. Kantor has been a nurse for over 40 years and a nurse educator since 1987. She has taught in both associate and undergraduate nursing programs and currently is a faculty member at Molloy College in Rockville Centre, New York, where she teaches a medical/surgical nursing course for students who have prior undergraduate degrees. Originally a graduate from a diploma program, she earned her bachelor's degree from New Jersey City University, her Master's degree from Hunter College, and her doctoral degree from Adelphi University. Through her professional and personal experiences she developed an interest in addressing the psychosocial needs of oncology patients and recognized that nursing students as well as graduates would benefit from learning about the needs of oncology patients in order to improve their nursing practice.

Zelda Suzan, MA, RN, CNE

Zelda Suzan has been a nurse for 40 years and a nurse educator for 36 years. She is a faculty member at the Phillips Beth Israel School of Nursing, where she teaches and coordinates the maternal-child course. She received her Master's in Nursing from New York University and is currently a doctoral candidate at Walden University. Since 1978, she has been actively involved at the American Cancer Society and has encouraged her students to participate in activities such as Making Strides Against Breast Cancer.

CONTRIBUTORS

Heidi Bentos-Pereira, MSN, MBA, RN, OCN
Clinical Nurse Specialist, Department of
    Nursing Education
St. Francis Hospital
Infusion Unit of the Cancer Institute at
    St. Francis Hospital
Roslyn, New York

Maryellen Brisbois, PhD, RN, APHN-BC
Assistant Professor at College
    of Nursing
Community Department
University of Massachusetts,
    Dartmouth
Dartmouth, Massachusetts

Maureen Cardoza, PhD, RN, CDP
Assistant Professor of Nursing
New York Institute of Technology
Department of Nursing
Old Westbury, New York

Elizabeth Danells Chin, PhD, RN, ANP
Assistant Professor
College of Nursing
University of Massachusetts,
    Dartmouth
Dartmouth, Massachusetts

Joyce Davis, BS, RN
Nurse Navigator
North Huntington Hospital
Huntington, New York

Rabbi Stephanie Dickstein, LMSW
Spiritual Care Coordinator
Shira Ruskay Center/Jewish Board of
    Family and Children's Services
New York, New York

Akhtar Ebrahimi Ghassemi, PhD, MHC, MSN, RN
Assistant Professor
Mental Health Counselor/Educator
Adelphi University, College of Nursing &
    Public Health
Mental Health, Family, & Community
    Systems Department
Garden City, New York

Susan Glodstein, PMHNP-BC, PMHCNS-BC
Clinical Instructor
Stony Brook School of Nursing, Graduate
    Studies
Stony Brook, New York

Nona Holmes, DNP, APRN-BC, NP Psychiatry
Assistant Professor
Psychiatric Nurse Practitioner Coordinator,
    Clinical Nurse Practitioner
Molloy College
Division of Nursing
Rockville Centre, New York

Eun-Ok Im, PhD, MPH, RN, CNS, FAAN
Professor and Marjorie O. Rendell
    Endowed Professor
School of Nursing
University of Pennsylvania
Philadelphia, Pennsylvania

Yaelim Lee, MSN, RN, PhD(c)
School of Nursing
University of Pennsylvania
Philadelphia, Pennsylvania

Paula Lester, MD, FACP
Associate Fellowship Program Director,
    Geriatric Medicine
Winthrop University Hospital, Mineola,
    New York
Associate Medical Director for Palliative
    Care
Highfield Gardens Care Center Nursing
    Home, Great Neck, New York
Division Member, Division of Palliative
    Medicine and Bioethics
Winthrop University Hospital, Mineola,
    New York
Assistant Professor of Clinical Medicine
Stony Brook University Medical Center,
    Stony Brook, New York

**Ann Marie Paraszczuk, EdD, RNC,
IBCLC**
Associate Professor
Molloy College
Division of Nursing
Rockville Centre, New York

Kathleen Pelc, MS, RN, OCN
Centers of Excellence Nurse Manager,
    Oncology
Visiting Nurse Service of New York
New York, New York

Rebecca Perez, RN, BSN, CCM
President/Owner
Carative Health Solutions, LLC
High Ridge, Missouri

**Rabbi/Chaplain Abraham
Rabinowich, MA, CPE**
Chaplain
Chaplaincy Services
Huntington Hospital
Huntington, New York

Mary E. Rzeszut, MSW, LCSW
Social Worker
North Shore/LIJ
Department of Kidney Diseases
Great Neck, New York

Michelle Schaefer, RN, BSN, CPON
Registered Nurse, Pediatrics
Winthrop University Hospital
Mineola, New York

Judith A. Schreiber, PhD, RN
Assistant Professor
University of Louisville
School of Nursing
Louisville, Kentucky

Kristen Sethares, PhD, RN, CNE
Professor of Nursing
Adult and Child Nursing
University of Massachusetts
Dartmouth, Massachusetts

Alaine Stadelman, MSN, RN
Adjunct Instructor
Molloy College
Division of Nursing
Rockville Centre, New York

**Jessica Weinberger, MS, FNP,
ACHPN**
Coordinator, Palliative Care Services
Division of Palliative Medicine and
    Bioethics
Winthrop University Hospital
Mineola, New York

INTRODUCTION

Reform can be accomplished only when attitudes are changed.
—*Lillian Wald*

The word "cancer" is derived from the Latin word *cancri*, which literally means "crab." Cancer has been referred to as evil, malignant, and a scourge. Despite the improvement in survival rates, the prevailing view of cancer remains one of negativity and death. Adding to the negative perception is the oftentimes presence of lingering effects of the treatments. While some effects are visible, others are apparent only to the individual diagnosed with the disease; some effects are physical, others are psychological in nature.

Historically, the care of the patient with cancer focused on the medical and surgical treatments necessary to prolong life and to achieve the benchmark of the 5-year goal. Today, millions of individuals diagnosed with cancer are able to achieve this goal and beyond, which has resulted in an increased awareness that life after a diagnosis of cancer is different from what it was before. There is a new normal. Although patients treated for cancer go on with their lives, many report they feel as if the Sword of Damocles is hanging over their head. Others report that the long-lasting or late effects of the treatments they received impact their activities of daily living or interfere with their quality of life.

In 2008, the Institute of Medicine (IOM) recommended that all cancer patients receive adequate and appropriate care addressing psychological needs. The expectation is that the care of psychosocial issues of cancer survivorship will be addressed from the moment of diagnosis. In addition, concerned about the lack of appropriate psychological care, the IOM recommended the provision of funds to educate healthcare practitioners about the need for psychological care of cancer patients.

While previously cancer was an acute illness for many individuals, the disease has now taken on the characteristics of a chronic illness, in terms of lingering effects from a wide array of cancer treatments. Cancer survivorship is a personal journey, yet others feel the impact. The purpose of this textbook is to emphasize the psychosocial issues of cancer survivorship in order to assist nurses in understanding these issues and to improve the nursing care of patients. That this topic needed dialogue is exemplified by a nursing student's comments after completing a course on the issues of cancer survivorship: "Just being able to finally openly discuss what was going on with my family really just relieved so much stress and emotions I have kept to myself for a long time. Like I mentioned in class, it is hard because I cannot talk about it with my siblings. They are clueless to the extent of my father's illness, and as for my mom, I am trying stay strong for her. I am just really grateful for you and your class and being able to discuss everything."

Organization of the Text

The idea for this book originated from personal experience and observations as well as the reports of limited attention given to the psychosocial needs of patients diagnosed with cancer by nurses in various oncology settings. The literature reports two reasons for the omission of care directed at psychosocial issues: nurses not recognizing the importance of addressing these issues and not knowing how, or not feeling comfortable enough, to discuss sensitive issues. Furthermore, the search for a textbook to use in teaching a course to undergraduate nursing students on the psychosocial issues of cancer survivors was unsuccessful. Topics related to the psychosocial needs of cancer patients frequently appear in end-of-life publications, but not every patient with cancer is dying. In order to improve nursing practice, we focused on what nurses "need to know" to provide more holistic care. Hence, such topics are included in this book.

Because patients with cancer may be treated in various clinical settings anywhere along the disease trajectory and can develop other health concerns, this book is targeted not only to nursing students but also to new nurses, nurses who care for cancer patients who are not necessarily on oncology units, oncology nurses, and advanced practice nurses.

The textbook is divided into eight sections. Section I gives a brief historical perspective of cancer and the factors that have contributed to the increased number of individuals living with cancer and the increase in their longevity. Additional topics include the phases of cancer survivorship, a survivorship care plan, the role of the Institute of Medicine, and the roles of specific healthcare team members.

Section II discusses the potential consequences of cancer management. The first chapter discusses clinical manifestations such as nausea, vomiting, and fatigue, as well as anxiety and depression. The next chapter explains the phenomenon of psychological distress.

Section III discusses psychosocial issues related to cancer survivorship. The purpose of this section is to broaden the reader's understanding of the impact that a diagnosis of cancer may have on family relationships, social support, fear of recurrence, and finances. Also included in this section is a discussion of the impact that cancer may have on an individual's spirituality.

Section IV presents the issues related to children diagnosed with cancer and their survivorship. This includes not only what the patient may be experiencing, but also the impact of the cancer on the immediate family. The developmental differences of pediatric patients are addressed, as are the long-term effects of cancer treatments.

Section V presents five middle range nursing theories to assist the reader in understanding the experience of cancer survivorship. Middle range theories provide structure for research on a given topic or phenomenon and can also be used in nursing practice to ultimately benefit the patient. The selected theories span the continuum of survivorship. The purpose of this section is not to give a detailed explanation of each theory, but to give an overview to increase the reader's awareness of middle range theories developed by nurses in the context of cancer survivorship.

Section VI contains four chapters, each chapter discussing a specific nursing role in the care of patients with cancer. The roles discussed are the oncology clinical nurse specialist, the oncology nurse navigator, the oncology case manager, and the mental health nurse.

In Section VII, the reader is provided the opportunity to learn about specific members of the healthcare team who collaborate to provide psychosocial care. The roles of the social worker, the clergy, and the pain and palliative care team are discussed.

Section VIII presents issues related to life after cancer treatment and the fear of recurrence.

Each section in this book contains key words, learning objectives, references, and case studies with critical thinking questions to assist the reader in understanding the material presented in the chapter. The appendix includes a glossary of terms and a list of valuable resources for nurses to use when caring for patients along the cancer care trajectory.

Our hope is that this book will serve as a catalyst for increasing awareness of cancer survivorship issues and that the reader will be able to incorporate the information into the plan of care of patients and families adjusting to life after a diagnosis of cancer.

Debra Kantor, PhD, APRN, BC
Zelda Suzan, MA, RN, CNE

ACKNOWLEDGMENTS

While the origins of this book came from personal observations and professional experiences, the inspiration to publish this book emanated from the desire to improve nursing practice by improving the understanding of what the challenges are after a cancer diagnosis. As with any project, a heartfelt "thank you" goes to a cast of many.

First and foremost to Shannon W. Magee, Executive Editor at Wolters Kluwer. Thank you for understanding and recognizing the value of this project. To Maria McAvey, Product Development Editor at Wolters Kluwer, and Joanna Hatzopoulos, Development Editor, for their assistance and guidance. Thank you to the National Comprehensive Cancer Network (NCCN) and particularly to Kimberly Brydges, Business Development Specialist, and Elyse Becker, Business Development Coordinator, for their support and assistance in including the NCCN, a valuable resource in understanding cancer survivorship for professionals, patients, and their caretakers.

Thank you also to the contributors, whose expertise in their respective fields is collectively focused on the challenges faced by individuals diagnosed with cancer. Thank you for responding to the emails and phone calls and for your willingness to share what you know and what you do.

CONTENTS

Section VIII   Life After Cancer Treatment   231

Chapter 19•When the Cloud Returns   232
Maureen Cardoza, PhD, RN, CDP

SECTION I
UNDERSTANDING SURVIVORSHIP

CHAPTER 1
SURVIVORSHIP

This chapter explores cancer survivorship, the advances that led to the view of cancer as a chronic disease, and the challenges of living with this chronic disease during diagnosis, treatment, and beyond.

Key Terms

survivor • cancer survivor • survivorship care plan • psychological distress

Upon completing this chapter, you will be able to do the following:

1. Define cancer survivorship.
2. Identify factors influencing longer cancer survival.
3. Describe the stages of cancer survivorship.
4. Discuss the IOM's recommendations for the care of cancer survivors.

The scenarios presented in this chapter demonstrate the experiences of a cancer patient in 1983 and 2013. This 30-year timespan experienced earlier cancer diagnoses secondary to improved screening, the development of national consensus guidelines for cancer surveillance in the normal adult population, and advances in the treatment of cancer that changed the journey of many cancer patients. Improved treatment outcomes and long-term survival are a reality today; many cancers are now considered chronic diseases, and nurses who care for patients with cancer are keenly positioned to advocate for patients experiencing a "new normal" with survivorship care and support.

1983

B. J. is a 39-year-old admitted to the inpatient oncology unit with complaints of shortness of breath upon exertion, fatigue, and red rash on her extremities and torso. A complete blood count reveals below normal counts with dangerously low white blood count and platelet count. The rash is petechiae resulting from thrombocytopenia. A bone marrow biopsy indicates acute myeloid leukemia (AML). It is theorized that the AML is a secondary cancer resulting from high doses of the alkylating agent cyclophosphamide during breast cancer adjuvant chemotherapy completed 18 months ago. She received 12 courses of adjuvant chemotherapy with cyclophosphamide, methotrexate, and 5-fluorouracil every 3 weeks.

B. J. receives AML induction chemotherapy with cytarabine for 7 days along with daunorubicin for 3 days. She fails to achieve remission and receives re-induction chemotherapy with no success. B. J. remains hospitalized secondary to sepsis and bleeding, and expires 6 weeks after her diagnosis.

2013

B. J. is a 39-year-old who received adjuvant cyclophosphamide, methotrexate, and 5-fluorouracil every 3 weeks for six cycles as an outpatient for stage I breast cancer diagnosed 18 months ago following a right mastectomy. At the end of her six cycles of chemotherapy, scans indicate that she is free of disease. She follows up with her oncologist 1 month after her last treatment, and she receives a survivorship care plan from her physician (Fig. 1.1). This plan outlines a summary of her treatments, a cancer surveillance plan, routine cancer surveillance plan for the normal adult population, psychosocial guidance, and nutrition guidance. She receives psychosocial support to address her fear of recurrence, mild anxiety, and fears related to her return to the workforce. The nutritionist meets with her after successful remission to guide B. J. in managing her weight gain of 15 pounds during chemotherapy treatment. B. J. will follow up with her oncologist every 3 months for 1 year, every 6 months for the next year, and then yearly. B. J. has participated in a postremission breast cancer support group since her remission. Her 18-month physician follow-up visit and surveillance testing indicate that she continues to be in remission.

Cancer Survivors

The estimated number of cancer survivors in the United States as of January 1, 2014, was 14,483,830 according to the Data Modeling Branch, Division of Cancer Control and Population Sciences of the National Cancer Institute. The population of cancer survivors is expected to reach 19 million by January 1, 2024 (DeSantis et al., 2014). These numbers are staggering and should be cause for celebration; however, cancer survivors often experience fear and anxiety as they enter the after-treatment survivorship phases. They enter a new normal world that presents new issues, problems, and challenges. Long-term side effects, fear of recurrence, difficulty with return to the workforce, and personal role changes are several examples of the challenges that cancer survivors face. How did cancer become a chronic disease? The historical overview that follows will illustrate advances in science and technology that have changed the journey of millions of patients with cancer across the United States.

Historical Overview and Factors Influencing Longer Cancer Survival

Cancer has afflicted human beings for thousands of years, and the fight to eradicate cancer has been a journey over hundreds of years. The terms carcinos and carcinoma

Summary of Breast Cancer Treatment and Recommendations for Survivorship Plan

Name: BJ
DOB: 1/21/75
Diagnosis: Stage 1 breast cancer
Diagnosis Date: 2/15/13
Medical Oncologist: Dr. Oncology
Primary Care Provider: Dr. PCP
Breast Surgeon: Dr. Surgery
Radiation Oncologist: NA

Date Issued to Survivor: 8/1/13

Genetic Testing: None.

Telephone: 516 555-1111
Telephone: 516 555-2222
Telephone: 516 555-3333
Telephone: NA

BREAST SURGERY

Date	Procedure
2/15/13	Right Mastectomy with sentinel node biopsy

CHEMOTHERAPY/BIOTHERAPY TREATMENT SUMMARY

DRUG	DATES To — From	Schedule of Treatment (Total dose of Anthracycline received- if applicable)
Cyclophosphamide	3/25/13 through 7/10/13	Every three weeks x 6 months
Methotrexate	3/25/13 through 7/10/13	Every three weeks x 6 months
5-Fluorouracil	3/25/13 through 7/10/13	Every three weeks x 6 months

ONGOING TREATMENT

DRUG	DIRECTIONS
NA	

FOLLOW UP PLAN: THE FOLLOWING IS YOUR PLAN FOR CARE FOLLOWING THE COMPLETION OF ACTIVE TREATMENT FOR CANCER. PLEASE REFER TO THESE SUGGESTIONS AND UPDATE AS NEEDED.

FOLLOW UP	FREQUENCY	SPECIFICS	OTHER
Medical Oncologist	Every 3 months for one year, every six months for one year and then yearly		
Surgeon:	FOLLOW UP TO BE DETERMINED BY YOUR SURGEON		
Radiation Oncologist: FOLLOW UP TO BE DETERMINED BY YOUR RADIATION ONCOLOGIST	NA		
Gynecologist	Yearly		
Primary Physician	Yearly and as needed		
Lab Work	Each oncologist visit		
Osteoporosis screening with Bone Densitometry *For patients at risk for osteoporosis	Every 2 years—can be directed by gynecologist		
Breast Self Exam	monthly		
OTHER TESTING	As needed		

ROUTINE CANCER SCREENING	TEST	PHYSICIAN
Colorectal	Colonoscopy as directed by your Medical Oncologist: every 5 years	GASTROENTEROLOGIST
Cervical		AS DIRECTED BY YOUR GYNOCOLOGIST
Skin		AS DIRECTED BY YOUR DERMATOLOGIST
Other	Mammography every 6 months	Oncologist

HEALTH BEHAVIOR RECOMMENDATIONS

X   Osteoporosis screening with Bone Densitometry <u>Frequency</u> = every 2 years   X   Remain tobacco free
X   Weight control   ☐   Annual cholesterol screening
X   Regular sun protection with sunscreen   ☐   Annual influenza vaccination
NA   Stop smoking   ☐   Moderate physical exercise
X   OTHER: is invited to Path Wellness Survivorship Program. Call Dana J. LMSW @ 516-555-4444

X   Psychological-Emotional Support: _____ CALL SOCIAL WORK @ 515 555-4444
X   Nutrition & Wellness Counseling: _____ is invited to come in for Healthy Diet Lifestyle Counseling. Amy K. MS.RD.CDN @ 516-555-5555   Weight Control Program—contact Sylvia C. 516 555-5551

OTHER SYMPTOM MANAGEMENT
Please follow up with the following physician for management of other symptoms

Symptom Related to Cancer or Treatment	Physician:	Telephone:
Call with any concerning symptoms or questions		

IMPORTANT SYMPTOMS TO REPORT TO THE ONCOLOGIST: NEW LUMPS, BONE PAIN, CHEST PAIN, SHORTNESS OF BREATH, DIFFICULTY BREATHING, ABDOMINAL PAIN, PERSISTENT HEADACHES, INCREASE IN FATIGUE.—*Call your medical oncologist with any concerns, especially if you have a new or persistent problem. Be sure to see your local primary physician annually or as needed, as well.*

Approved by Oncologist: Signature/Date: _____

Patient Signature: _____

Copy to Patient, PCP, Surgeon, Gynecologist

Figure 1.1 • Summary of breast cancer treatment and recommendations for survivorship plan.

were first used by Hippocrates in the third century BC to describe tumors. Brilliant men and women such as William Halstead, Wilhelm Conrad Roentgen, Marie Curie, and Sidney Farber pioneered the journey that has resulted in the three major approaches to cancer treatment: surgery, radiation, and chemotherapy (American Cancer Society, 2012).

Cancer surgeries have been performed since ancient times, but early physicians noted that even with surgical removal of tumors, the cancer returned. The use of anesthesia occurred in 1846, and this contributed to the rapid developments in surgical procedures over the next century. Despite radical surgeries, such as the radical mastectomy for breast cancer, tumors returned or developed in other organs. Hence, the theories of spread of cancer, via the blood and lymph nodes, became an accepted belief in the medical communities. Less radical surgeries are performed today due to better surgical techniques, as well as the combination treatment modalities used today. Surgery is often combined with radiation and/or chemotherapy in order to target microscopic disease not observed during surgical procedures (American Cancer Society, 2012).

Radiation techniques have evolved over the past century secondary to advances in radiation physics and computer technology. New techniques have enabled physicians to visualize tumors in three dimensions, allow more control in the protection of normal tissue near the focus site, allow large doses of radiation to small tumors (stereotactic surgery), deliver radiation during surgery, and deliver therapies that increase the tumor's sensitivity to radiation (American Cancer Society, 2012).

A chemical weapon of war used in the First and Second World Wars led to the use of chemotherapeutic agents to halt tumor cell proliferation that was out of control. The chemical weapon was mustard gas, and the exposure of military personnel to this chemical resulted in toxic changes to the bone marrow. Nitrogen mustard was studied and found to be effective in the treatment of Hodgkin lymphoma. This discovery led to the investigation of other chemicals that proved to be effective in the treatment of other tumors, solid and hematological. The use of chemotherapeutic agents is considered systemic therapy, that is, the agent is given via various routes (intravenously, intramuscularly, intra-arterially, subcutaneously, or orally), and travels throughout the body. These agents target cells undergoing rapid proliferation. Since certain normal tissues are composed of rapidly proliferating cells, patients experience side effects related to the normal cells that are affected. Normal cells repair and resume their functions after a certain time, but cancer cells cannot recover from the onslaught of these drugs. Combination therapy allows several drugs with different side effects to be utilized, thus resulting in enhanced effect against tumor growth without fatal toxicities (American Cancer Society, 2012).

Agents that decrease side effects have lead to less patient decisions regarding stopping therapies found to be intolerable. Potential curative treatments can now be completed and thus result in successful cures. Biotherapies that resemble the natural signals that control cell growth can now be manufactured and delivered to the patient to enhance normal immunological signals and improve patient outcomes. Biological response modifiers are also used to manage side effects of chemotherapy such as anemia and neutropenia.

Scientists continue to investigate improved methods to cure or control cancer. Today, new drugs that target certain cell receptors are the focus of research. These drugs bind with receptors on the surface of the cell, and these receptors allow the drugs to enter the cell. The drug then alters signaling pathways for cell proliferation resulting in cell death, known as apoptosis. However, normal cells may also have the same targeted receptors on their surfaces, and it is the binding of such receptors that lead to the particular side effects of these therapies. These side effects are different from those resulting from chemotherapy, but can be devastating for the patients, and may lead to the discontinuation of therapy.

The advances in cancer treatments are possible today because of continued research to detect cancer in the early stages; new therapies, focused on cancer cure or the amelioration of side effects, have led to improved patient outcomes, and the designation of cancer as a curable or chronic disease. These advances have made survivorship a reality, and this has left professional caregivers with the awesome charge of developing methods to follow and care for cancer survivors throughout longer life spans, and living with a new normal. Advances in cancer treatments have led to cancers that are now considered "curable." These cancers include, but are not limited to, acute lymphocytic leukemia (ALL), Hodgkin lymphoma, testicular cancer, and early stage breast cancer. ALL and Hodgkin lymphoma are highlighted in relation to long-term side effects (DeSantis et al., 2014).

Acute lymphoblastic leukemia in young children has a favorable prognosis of an 85% cure rate; however, treatment usually results in long-term side effects. These long-term effects of treatment can include growth and development issues, secondary cancers, cardiac problems, pulmonary problems, learning issues, and emotional and psychosocial issues (Dana-Farber.org; DeSantis et al., 2014). Hodgkin lymphoma is an example of cancer that manifests in early adulthood. It is considered one of the most curable diseases, with an 80% to 90% response rate. Clinical trials that have contributed to evidence-based practice and have resulted in the utilization of different chemotherapy regimens, reduced doses of chemotherapy, and refined radiation therapy techniques and technologies have increased long-term survival in these populations. Patients with Hodgkin lymphoma who experience long-term survival also experience the long-term side effects of therapy, and they are known to experience higher morbidity and mortality than other people of the same age. The long-term side effects are physical, emotional, and psychosocial in nature. Physical side effects can include cardiovascular morbidities, lung diseases, endocrine abnormalities, fertility problems, and secondary malignancies. Survivors may develop leukemias, non-Hodgkin lymphomas, myelodysplastic disorders, lung cancers, and breast cancers (Gotti et al., 2013). Emotional and psychosocial side effects include, but are not limited to, anger, fear of recurrence, anxiety, guilt, and posttraumatic syndrome disorder. Adler and Page (2008) remarked that "the remarkable advances in biomedical care for cancer have not been matched by achievements in providing high-quality care for the psychological and social effects of cancer" (p. 23). This remark prefaced the report, *Cancer Care for the Whole Patient: Meeting Psychological Needs;* this report was requested of the Institute of Medicine (IOM) by the National Institutes of Health in order to develop a plan of action for healthcare disciplines, so that the psychological and social stresses of cancer can be better understood in healthcare communities (Adler & Page, 2008). In 2012, the National Comprehensive Cancer Network (2012) defined distress as "a multifactorial unpleasant emotional experience of a psychological, social and/or spiritual nature that may interfere with the ability to cope effectively with cancer, its physical symptoms and its treatments" (p. 2). The evaluation of psychosocial distress will become a mandated standard of care for Commission on Cancer accreditation in 2015. The Commission on Cancer STANDARD 3.2 Psychosocial Distress Screening specifies "The cancer committee develops and implements a process to integrate and monitor on-site psychosocial distress screening and referral for the provision of psychosocial care" (p. 76). This standard represents the value this accrediting body places on psychosocial issues and the holistic approach to patient care. Healthcare organizations must meet this standard for future accreditation (Commission on Cancer, 2012). Oncology nurses are uniquely positioned to define and implement methods to ensure the appropriate and timely assessment of psychological distress and to educate patients. They can lead the programs that effectively utilize methods that address the vital needs of patients facing cancer, treatment, and the long-term effects of a cancer survivorship (Hammelef, Friese, Breslin, Riba, & Schneider, 2014).

Phases of Cancer Survivorship

Fitzhugh Mullen, a physician who was diagnosed with cancer at age 32, wrote about his experiences with his illness and its consequences in the *New England Journal of Medicine* in 1985. Mullen states, "It was survival—an absolutely predictable but ill-defined condition that all cancer patients pass through as they struggle with their illness" (p. 271). Mullen ruminated about cure, victory over illness, and survival statistics, but realized that the literature did not address the individual who may be cured, or one who may live with incurable cancer. He wrote that survivor was a more useful term because it could be used for anyone diagnosed with cancer without regard to the course of the disease for a particular individual. He felt that all patients went through predictable stages of survival, although individual journeys may differ (Mullen, 1985).

Mullen identified three seasons of survival. They are acute survival, extended survival, and permanent survival. Acute survival begins with diagnosis, and it encompasses both diagnostic and medical procedures to cure, control, or palliate the disease. The patient's physical well-being and mental well-being are impacted by pain, anxiety, and fear; these distresses are present because the disease and the treatment side effects can be uncomfortable, painful, and emotionally debilitating. Patients and families are in need of support from friends and their communities as they face the realities of active treatment. Extended survival starts when active treatment ends. The patient faces fear of recurrence, side effect recovery, and emotional stress or distress as he/she steps back into the healthy world forced to face a new normal. Unfortunately, the support of the professional caregivers diminishes as the patient moves away from the acute stage. In reality, the support is needed more now when the patient and family engage in readjusting to the world around them. Permanent survival is cure; the patient moves to a time when it is unlikely that the cancer will return. Mullen (1985) writes, "No matter how long we live, cancer patients are survivors—at once wary and relieved, bashful and proud" (p. 272). Survivors experience employment, insurance, legal, and health problems, and they often face discrimination in the workplace or when seeking employment. Mullen concluded that despite enormous efforts in discovering effective cancer treatments, very little has been done to address the needs of the cancer patient in transition to survivor and onward (Mullen, 1985).

Mullen's framework was adopted by the National Coalition for Cancer Survivorship, founded in 1986. The founders from 20 organizations pioneered work to change the perceptions of an individual with cancer as cancer victim to cancer survivor. The work of this coalition led to the publication of *Imperatives for Quality Cancer Care: Access, Advocacy, Action and Accountability,* and was the first examination of care from the perspective of a survivor (Doyle, 2008; Morgan, 2009).

Miller, Merry, and Miller (2008) proposed a modified model of Mullen's framework that would include new knowledge regarding cancer survivorship that occurred over the past 20 years. They wrote that cancer survivor experiences varied with the individual. The new model identified acute survivorship, transitional survivorship, extended survivorship, and permanent survivorship. Acute survivorship is the period of diagnosis and treatment as in 1986. Transitional survivorship may include those patients who experience watchful waiting, those on maintenance therapies such as trastuzumab for breast cancer, or those for whom there was no remission and living with the cancer is a reality. Extended survivorship includes those in remission without maintenance therapy, those who need ongoing treatment to stay in remission, and those with advanced disease that has become a chronic condition. Finally, permanent survival has four subgroups: (1) cancer-free and free of cancer; (2) cancer-free but not free of cancer (those who live with the physical and emotional scars of their cancer); (3) secondary cancers as a result of treatments; and (4) the other cancer survivors—family and caregivers. Understanding the journey of the cancer survivors enhances our ability to provide quality care. Each survivor is unique, and each deserves an individualized approach to ongoing care and surveillance (Miller et al., 2008).

Institute of Medicine: Wisdom and Guidance for Survivorship Care

The IOM published the book *From Cancer Patient to Cancer Survivor: Lost in Transition* in 2005. The IOM identified that a bridge was needed to close the gap that existed between care of the survivor and quality cancer survivorship care. There were many opportunities for healthcare providers, cancer patients and their advocates, insurance providers, researchers, and government officials to improve the delivery of cancer survivorship care. Ten recommendations were made:

1. Raise awareness of the needs of cancer survivors, and establish cancer survivorship as a unique phase of cancer care.
2. Primary cancer care providers should provide survivorship care plans after active treatment, and this service should be reimbursable.
3. Evidence-based guidelines should be developed to manage the late effects of cancer.
4. Develop quality of survivorship metrics.
5. Qualified organizations, such as the Centers for Medicare and Medicaid Services and the Department of Veterans Affairs, support demonstration projects that test survivorship care models.

6. The government should support the development of cancer control plans.

7. Professional and national organizations should provide educational programs to prepare healthcare professionals to address health issues and quality-of-life issues that face cancer survivors.

8. Community and government organizations should develop methods to eliminate discrimination in the workplace.

9. Policy should be developed to ensure cancer survivors' access to adequate insurance.

10. National organizations, government agencies, and insurance providers should support survivorship research.

These recommendations by the IOM formalized the immediate focus on the development of cancer survivorship initiatives that served to enhance the care and follow-up of cancer survivors (Institute of Medicine, 2005).

The Role of Healthcare Providers in Cancer Survivorship

Since the IOM's report in 2005, cancer care providers have moved to create awareness of the needs of the cancer survivors from diagnosis through end-of-life. The needs of survivors vary with the individual and the types of cancers. Patient concerns may be social, physical, psychosocial, and/or spiritual. Survivors may experience concerns in all domains or some domains, and the concerns can shift to different domains during survivorship. Therefore, the individual survivorship plan is not static, but it is a changing plan dedicated to the individual survivor and his/her changing needs.

The ability for healthcare providers to provide optimal care throughout survivorship is strongly dependent on the patient/caregiver relationship, a comprehensive care plan, and consistent follow-up at predetermined intervals. Unfortunately, patients continue to face challenges in education, access to care, insurance issues, employment bias, and primary care hand-off. Oncologists may believe that normal surveillance issues are addressed in the primary care setting, but often, the oncologist is considered the primary physician in the patient's eyes. The ability of the oncologist to meet the expectations of the survivor may be impossible, and the challenge to support the patient must be addressed in health care today. Primary care physicians need information and education regarding survivor needs and challenges. The successful hand-off to primary care depends heavily on the comfort this physician has to address and care for the survivor. Survivor adherence to plan of care is essential for long-term survival (Oncology Roundtable, 2011). The Oncology Roundtable (2011) identified essential survivorship care components: (1) patient education, (2) emotional support, (3) treatment summary and care plans, (4) surveillance care, (5) supportive care, (6) education for primary care providers, (7) management of late and long-term side effects, (8) psychosocial support, and, finally, (9) coordination with primary care providers.

These services would ideally sit in one comprehensive program, but this is rare in the present healthcare world. Nurse-Led programs, NP-Led Survivorship Clinic, Multidisciplinary Survivorship Clinic, and PCP-Led Survivorship Care are several models used in the United States today. Creativity is essential for the development of meaningful survivorship programs. Group appointments and the development of survivorship clinics need to be carefully analyzed for feasibility that addresses comprehensive care as well as reimbursement concerns. Judicious use of appropriate resources is the key to success (Oncology Roundtable, 2011). Ferrell, Virani, Smith, and Juarez (2003) conclude, "Oncology nurses are central to all aspects of survivorship for patient care and family support. Extensive support is needed to expand education and research to ensure quality care for the future" (p. E11).

Conclusion

The key to comprehensive cancer survivorship care is a clear understanding of the survivor's journey; education of the survivor and healthcare community; and a willingness to investigate and consider creative, dynamic, and ongoing models of survivorship care. Nurses serve in many roles, one of which is patient advocate. Nurses can lead this creative journey to enhance the patients' journey during survivorship and until end-of-life, and through the development of programs focused on optimum patient outcomes and patient experience, nurses are positioned to advance the care of cancer survivors.

• Critical Thinking **Questions**

1. What factors have influenced the survival time of cancer survivors?
2. What are the phases of cancer survivorship?
3. What role does the primary care provider play in cancer survivorship and what are some of the obstacles that might hinder the primary care provider's participation?
4. Discuss why survivorship care plans are essential to positive outcomes during cancer survival.
5. What are some of the recommendations that the IOM made in terms of quality care for individuals diagnosed with cancer?

References

Adler, N. E., & Page, A. E. K. (2008). *Cancer care for the whole patient: Meeting psychosocial needs.* Washington, DC: National Academic Press.

American Cancer Society. (2012). *Cancer treatment and survivorship facts & figures 2012–2013.* Atlanta, GA: American Cancer Society.

Commission on Cancer. (2012). *Cancer program standards 2012: Ensuring patient-centered care V1.2.1.* Chicago, IL: Commission on Cancer.

DeSantis, C. E., Lin, C. C., Mariotto, A. B., Siegel, R. L., Stein, K. D., Kramer, J. L., … Jemal, A. (2014). Cancer treatment and survivor statistics. *CA: A Cancer Journal for Clinicians, 64*(4), 252–271.

Doyle, N. (2008). Cancer survivorship: Evolutionary concept analysis. *Journal of Advanced Nursing, 62*(4), 499–509.

Ferrell, B. R., Virani, R., Smith, S., & Juarez, G. (2003). The role of oncology nursing to ensure quality care for survivors: A report commissioned by the National Cancer Policy Board and the Institute of Medicine. *Oncology Nursing Forum, 30*(1), E1–E11.

Gotti D, Danesi M, Calabresi A, Ferraresi A, Albini L, et al. (2013) Clinical characteristics, incidence, and risk factors of HIV-related Hodgkin lymphoma in the era of combination antiretroviral therapy. *AIDS Patient Care STDS, 27,* 259–265.

Hammelef, K. J., Friese, C. R., Breslin, T. M., Riba, M. & Schneider, S. M. (2014). Implementing distress management guidelines in ambulatory oncology: A quality improvement project. *Clinical Journal of Oncology Nursing, 18*(1), 31–36.

Institute of Medicine. (2005). *From cancer patient to cancer survivor: Lost in transition.* Washington, DC: The National Academic Press.

Miller, K, Merry, B., & Miller, J. (2008). Seasons of survivorship revisited. *The Cancer Journal, 14*(6), 369–373.

Morgan, M. A. (2009). Cancer survivorship: History, quality-of-life issues, and the evolving multidisciplinary approach to implementation of cancer survivorship care plans. *Oncology Nursing Forum, 36*(4), 429–436.

Mullen, F. (1985). Seasons of survival: Reflections of a physician and cancer. *New England Journal of Medicine, 313*, 270–273.

National Comprehensive Cancer Network®. (2012). *NCCN Clinical Practice Guidelines® in Oncology: Distress management (v.1.2012).* Retrieved from http://www.nccn.org/patients.guidelines/default.aspx

Oncology Roundtable: The Advisory Board. (2011). Delivering sustainable survivorship care: Lessons for program design and implementation. 3–56.

SECTION II

POTENTIAL CONSEQUENCES OF CANCER MANAGEMENT

CHAPTER 2
SYMPTOM MANAGEMENT

"I knew something was wrong by the symptoms I was having but I cannot believe this happened to me. Somehow I felt immune to illness myself and never expected to develop cancer. I see myself as a compassionate nurse and have been caring for the sick and infirm my whole life…that I would somehow be rewarded by a long and healthy life…not as a cancer patient."

—An oncology patient

Key Terms

anxiety · constipation · depression · diarrhea · fatigue · nausea · pain · sleep–wake disturbances · symptoms · vomiting

Upon completing this chapter, you will be able to do the following:

1. Discuss the significance of symptom management in patients diagnosed with cancer.
2. Describe available fatigue assessment tools.
3. Identify sleep–wake disturbances.
4. Identify at least three gastrointestinal symptoms.
5. Differentiate between anxiety and depression.
6. Discuss the role of nursing in symptom management.

Significance of Symptom Management

In this chapter, common symptoms that cancer patients experience throughout their survivorship journey will be explored. There are many physical and psychological symptoms associated with cancer. People are living longer from the time of cancer diagnosis in part from the advances in cancer screening, diagnosis, treatment, and posttreatment surveillance. The impact of cancer on the person and his/her family members, friends, and caregivers is an added dimension to survivors facing physical, psychological, social, spiritual, and financial challenges. Surviving cancer can lead to an array of acute and chronic symptoms that nurses are equipped to manage across patient care settings. Lingering somatic, cognitive, and emotional symptoms may be related to the cancer, surgery, and/or treatment modalities ultimately impacting functional ability and quality of life. The significance of symptom management for practitioners is evidenced by the number of cancer survivors in the United States that is expected to rise from the current 14.5 million to nearly 19 million by the year 2024. Currently more cancers are cured, more people are living longer with the disease, and people are living longer in general. The risk for developing cancer rises with age as does the reoccurrence or development of secondary cancers, thus increasing the number of cases and survivors that are expected to rise in the next decade. Two thirds of today's survivors were diagnosed at least 5 years ago and 15% were diagnosed 20 or more years ago. Approximately half of all cancer survivors are of age 70 or older and only 5% are under 40 years of age. Cancer survivors are at greater risk of second cancers and require frequent surveillance and monitoring for cancer recurrences and symptoms of prior treatment modalities (DeSantis et al., 2014).

The 2013 Institute of Medicine (IOM) report *Delivering High-Quality Cancer Care: Charting a New Course for a System in Crisis* key points included an adequately staffed, trained, and coordinated workforce and evidence-based cancer care. The IOM reports that the Goal 4 recommendation requires all individuals caring for cancer patients to have appropriate core competencies that address the quality of cancer care throughout the diagnosis, treatment, long-term survivorship, and end-of-life care trajectory (IOM, 2013; see Table 2.1). This report has implications for oncology nurses who play a vital role in the future design and delivery of cancer care. Nurses are frequently the steadying force as patients navigate the myriad of cancer treatments. Nurses guide patients through the treatment plan, administer therapeutics, manage symptoms, and provide supportive care and counseling to cancer survivors, utilizing the national and global guidelines of clinical and ethical standards of oncology nursing care. In response to the IOM report, the NCCN Clinical Practice Guidelines in Oncology, 2014 (NCCN Guidelines) website houses a virtual library of five cancer-related topics that include (1) guidelines for the treatment of cancer by site, (2) guidelines for detection, prevention, and risk reduction, (3) guidelines for supportive care, (4) age-related recommendations, and (5) comprehensive guidelines for patients (NCCN, 2014). Professional nursing practice and research demonstrate that nurses practicing with oncology patients must remain abreast of the current practices associated with oncology, which requires a commitment to

Table 2.1 • Institute of Medicine: Goal 4 (2013)

Institute of Medicine: Goal 4: All individuals caring for cancer patients should have appropriate core competencies.

Recommendation 4
- Professional organizations should define cancer core competencies.
- Cancer care delivery organizations should require cancer care teams to have cancer core competencies.
- Organizations responsible for accreditation, certification, and training of nononcology clinicians should promote the development of relevant cancer core competencies.
- HHS and others should fund demonstration projects to train family caregivers and direct care workers.

continuing education. One research study identified that the most common challenge for primary care providers to implement survivorship care plans (SCPs) was their insufficient knowledge of cancer survivor issues as a primary barrier to providing appropriate follow-up care (Dulko et al., 2013). The NCCN Guidelines educate nurses with algorithms, treatment strategies, and the latest evidence that improves the quality, effectiveness, and efficiency of cancer care.

Cancer Diagnosis

Cancer is nondiscriminatory. The initial shock of a cancer diagnosis may manifest as disbelief, anger, resentment, and fear of uncertainty and mortality that can result in stress-related symptoms associated with anxiety, depression, acute stress disorder (ASD), and posttraumatic stress disorder (PTSD). These behavioral health manifestations can last throughout life, permanently altering one's view of the world and self (Fleishman, 2012; Deimling, Kahana, Bowman, & Schaefer, 2002).

Survivorship underpinnings were initially described by Mullan (1983), a physician and cancer patient, as "seasons" named *acute survival*, *extended survival*, and *permanent survival*. *Acute survival* was the experience of diagnosis and treatment, where fear and anxiety were a constant element. The second season was *extended survival* that encompassed the rigorous course of treatment phase that was a period of physical limitations and somatic symptoms that were dealt with in the home, community, and workplace. This is a "watchful waiting" time with periodic examinations and/or intermittent therapy that is emotionally dominated by fear of recurrence and somatic symptoms until remission or termination occurs. The last season was *permanent survival*, synonymous with cure, but acknowledged that the person had been indelibly changed by the experience that included social problems such as finances and employment. The lasting and secondary effects of cancer treatment on the person's health are representative of cancer survivors at risk and include not only physical alterations but changes to their psychological, social, economic, and spiritual self (Mullan, 1983, 1985).

Today acute cancer survivorship remains a time of intense emotional and medical treatment that requires supportive nursing measures to aid and navigate the myriad of potential and experiential symptoms. Miller, Merry, and Miller (2008) proposed a modification to Mullan's "*seasons*" by the inclusion that after the intense initial therapy was completed the survivor entered a season called "transitional cancer survivorship," addressing numerous levels of survivorship. The levels are a journey from acute treatment to careful surveillance where emotional, social, and medical adaptation occurs for the survivor, family, and caregivers.

Transitional cancer survivorship is a term widely accepted today. Cancer survivors are in varying stages of therapy, experiencing different levels of side effect intensity and functional ability. Some of these side effects are visible reminders, such as surgical scars, burns, alopecia, and weight fluctuations, or invisible to others, such as peripheral neuropathy, altered taste, and "brain fog." Cancer survivorship often changes the daily function and role performances of the individual and the family structure, employment, and social interactions. Adaptation to a changing self-identity and confrontation with one's mortality may cause physical and emotional distress that compound the illness burden for the individual and their friends and family, leading to depression and anxiety. The growing population of cancer survivors and their significant others walk a fine line between illness and wellness, often vacillating between the challenges of everyday living and the future.

Navigating the cancer trajectory begins with the recognition by the patient of symptoms or dysfunction, with the sense that "something is wrong." In contemporary society, many people are exposed to an abundance of reading materials, television programming, and cinema that include cancer references and story lines; as a result it is unusual in the United States to encounter someone who is unfamiliar with cancer. The media often portray cancer experiences in sensationalized or romanticized ways, and inaccurately portray the individualized cancer experience. The fear and uncertainty of a cancer diagnosis can be intensified by the often time-consuming and painful radiographic, laboratory, and biopsy diagnostics. The confirmation of a cancer diagnosis conjures thoughts of debilitating and exhaustive treatment options of pain and suffering, leading to death; thus the diagnostic process can be a time of extreme anxiety, worry, and sleeplessness for patients. Oncology nurses provide education and psychological support to patients and families at all phases of oncology treatment, providing strategies of symptom management, treatment navigation, and end-of-life care.

Understanding Treatment Reactions

Oncology patients experience multiple symptoms associated with cancer disease and active treatment that can have a negative effect on quality of life and patient outcomes. The occurrence of multiple symptoms, referred to as symptom clusters, requires the clinician to screen, assess, and manage according to clinical practice guidelines.

Chemotherapy, radiation therapy, hormone therapy, biological response modifiers, and surgery are medical interventions for the treatment and palliation of cancer. These treatments often result in pain and suffering followed by periods of improvement specific to the treatment course (Jung-Eun, Dodd, Aouizerat, Jahan, & Miaskowski, 2009; Davis, 2014; NCCN, 2014). Cancer treatment options require an interdisciplinary coordinated approach that may result in symptoms and side effects that are experienced differently by each person. Treatment protocols are based on the cancer type, location, and stage, but the reaction to the treatment may result in unpleasant side effects with emotional and physical reactions. Treatment may occur daily, weekly, or monthly followed by a rest period, allowing the person to experience days of extreme, then waning suffering. Initial treatment may be followed by maintenance chemotherapy prolonging the symptoms of treatment. Symptoms associated with cancer treatments can be managed using prophylactic pharmaceuticals, complimentary alternative medicine (CAM) modalities, and self-empowerment strategies that support the person during the peri-oncology experience.

Fatigue

"I am so exhausted, especially the few days after my chemo. I can barely muster the strength to roll over in bed. My husband has to do all the house stuff and go to work. My children help me do everything except breathe and even that is exhausting. No child should have to wash, dress, and empty the commode for their mother. I don't even have the strength to cry."

—*A cancer survivor*

The growing groups of cancer survivors are leading a life that balances between the everyday challenges of "regular life" and the "ups and downs" of living with cancer and its treatment. Their family and caregivers are living in this same state with what one survivor describes as a "sense of fear and impermanence mixed with healthy denial, a focus on the present, and even confidence."

Fatigue is a very common symptom associated with cancer treatment and throughout the illness trajectory. According to a survey of 1569 cancer patients fatigue occurred in 80% of individuals receiving chemotherapy and/or radiotherapy and in 75% of individuals at the end-of-life stage (Berger, 2014; Denlinger et al., 2014). Fatigue can be caused by anemia, accumulation of cellular destruction waste products from radiation or chemotherapy treatments, protein and calorie malnutrition, sleep disturbances, chronic pain, anxiety, depression, and the stress of coping with cancer. Fatigue may be an initial symptom that leads to a cancer diagnosis or a response from the effect of active or postoncology treatment, or experienced in the advanced stages of the disease and at the end of life. Regardless of the occurrence along the trajectory patients struggling with fatigue suffer immeasurably.

The NCCN Guidelines for Cancer-Related Fatigue define fatigue as "a distressing, persistent, subjective sense of physical, emotional and/or cognitive tiredness or exhaustion related to cancer or cancer treatment that is not proportional to recent activity and interferes with usual functioning" (Berger, 2014, p. FT-1). The prevalence of fatigue is well represented in the literature with the recommendation that the assessment of fatigue should be consistently assessed based on the patient's self-report occurring throughout the illness and treatment course. Screening for fatigue includes the degree of intensity assessment as well as evaluation for cluster symptoms associated with fatigue such as pain, worry, depression, anxiety, and sleep disturbances. Cluster symptoms are the presence of three or more co-occurring symptoms. Based upon the clinicians' focused disease status and treatment evaluation of the patient and review of his/her treatment plan the NCCN Guidelines for Cancer-Related Fatigue recommendations and interventions include patient/family education and counseling that are correlated with the patient's clinical status as in the active treatment, posttreatment, or end-of-life illness trajectory. Based on the patient's clinical status the National Comprehensive Cancer Network (Berger, 2014) algorithm identifies general strategies for management of fatigue that include nonpharmacologic and pharmacologic interventions.

Fatigue Assessment

The literature supports the use of a number of valid and reliable fatigue assessment instruments that provide measures of symptoms and distress in oncology patients (see Table 2.2). One of the first and most popular is the *Symptom Distress Scale*, where patients' self-reported symptom distress are measured using a 1- to 5-point Likert scale where 1 denotes the least amount of distress and 5 means extreme distress (Jung-Eun et al., 2009; Aaronson et al., 1999; Lou, Yates, McCarthy, & Wang, 2013). Additional commonly used measures of fatigue include the Fatigue Scale and Fatigue Observation Checklist (Rhoten, 1982), Piper Fatigue Scale that has been used extensively in oncology patients (Piper et al., 1989), and the Visual Analog Scale for Fatigue (VAS-F) (Lee, Hicks, & Nino-Murcia, 1991).

Table 2.2 • **Sample Fatigue Instruments**

Research Instrument	Measures	Implementation
Symptom Distress Scale (McCorkle & Young, 1978)	Characterizations of fatigue and physical and cognitive consequences attributed to fatigue (i.e., fatigue, pain, insomnia, poor activity, concentration, mood, and altered appearance)	13-item self-report 1–5-point Likert type scale
The Fatigue Scale and Fatigue Observation Checklist (Rhoten, 1982)		
Multidimensional Assessment of Fatigue (MAF) (Tack, 1991) (Is a revision of the Piper Fatigue Scale)	Addresses aspects of fatigue and rates the degree of fatigue experienced in the last week	2-item subscales
Piper Fatigue Scale (Piper et al., 1989)	Assesses multiple characteristics of fatigue through identification subscales	Lengthy
Visual Analog Scale for Fatigue (VAS-F) (Lee, Hicks, & Nino-Murcia, 1991)	5-item energy subscale and 13-item fatigue subscale. Behavioral and characteristics of fatigue in current state	18-item scales

As with many oncology symptoms, fatigue is dynamic and ever changing particularly in advanced disease, thus requiring frequent reassessment by clinicians. When assessing illness fatigue one must consider the physical, psychological, and spiritual human components. As with pain assessment, fatigue is also measured in terms of being whatever the patient says it is. A focused history and physical includes a review of systems and laboratory tests that include hematology and metabolic profiles, and hormone levels that may be useful in determining if various organ systemic disease involvement are contributing to the fatigue. Weight and appetite fluctuations can contribute to anemia and hypoproteinemia; electrolyte and mineral imbalances can cause muscle wasting, listlessness, and fatigue. Assessment should include questioning that explores the meaning and dynamics of fatigue such as sleep *disturbances*, the *location* or where the body fatigue occurs such as muscle fatigue, emotional or mental fatigue. What is the level of *intensity or severity* of the fatigue and how does fatigue impact the enjoyment and activities of daily life? Evaluate the *duration* or how long the fatigue lasts in minutes, hours, or days. Chronic fatigue lasts more than 6 months and is there a *pattern* to the fatigue such as occurring in the evening or transient in nature? Determine the presence of *aggravating or alleviating factors*. Evaluation of the patients' *knowledge* and their assigned meaning of fatigue as well as *medication* use by the patients may symbolize a worsening of their condition or disease progression (Berger, 2014; Ferrell & Coyle, 2006; Nettina, 2014).

Fatigue management includes education and counseling, physical activity, psychosocial interventions, and pharmacologic treatments.

General Strategies of Fatigue Management

The practical nursing management for cancer-related fatigue begins with explanations of the complex nature of fatigue which through open communication with clinicians identifies the problem, helping to reduce the anxiety and explore the disease process and realistic expectations of treatment, promoting dignity and meaningful interactions.

General strategies include the following:

- Energy conservation such as setting priorities or one main activity per day
- Scheduling activities at peak energy levels
- Pacing activities
- Delegating tasks to others
- Postponing nonessential activities
- Using energy saving devices (i.e., wheelchairs, remote and motorized carts, commodes, motion- or voice-activated devices)
- Alternating periods of rest and activity
- Limiting naps to 1 hour and not near bedtime
- Setting sleep schedule (wake-up and bedtime)
- Using diversional activities such as TV, reading, music, crafts, journaling, hobbies, and socialization

Physical activity has improved functional status and fatigue in cancer patients. There is evidence to include an individualized exercise program for patients on chemotherapy and/or radiation therapy. Studies showed no adverse effects of exercise such as increased fatigue or falls (Mock et al., 2005; Kuchinski, Reading, & Lash, 2009; Mustian et al., 2007). Physical activity is necessary to maintain muscle and promote balance and physical stamina, and it contributes to mental well-being. Individualized physical activity is based on the dynamic state of the cancer patients and should include isometric, passive resistance, and active exercises individually or in group settings within the physical ability of the individual being receptive to the patients' pace and ability. Consultations with physical and occupational therapists are beneficial to evaluate the physical state and to develop realistic goals for cancer patients. Psychosocial support and activities that promote physical and mental stamina, which make life meaningful, should be encouraged in cancer patients. Before engaging in an exercise program caution should be used in the presence of bone metastases, blood dyscrasias or anemia, pulmonary/oxygen insufficiency, fever or infection, and limitations from metastases or other illnesses that would predispose the cancer patient to further distress.

Encourage physical activity, such as the following:

- Exercise equipment (e.g., recumbent stationary bicycle)
- Yoga
- Meditation
- Pilates
- Tai Chi
- Stretching with or without resistance bands. (Can be done on chair or bedside)
- Massage therapy
- Cinema and concerts
- Outdoor activities such as walking, swimming, gardening, fishing, sitting, and bird watching.

- Car and/or boat rides
- Travel

  Psychosocial activities include the following:

- Meditation and mindfulness cognition exercises
- Spending time with friends and family
- Journaling and legacy building activities (videos, travel log)
- Gaming: poker, mahjong, solitaire

Pharmacologic interventions for the symptom management of fatigue include identifying the cause of the fatigue and prescribing indicated medications. Medications such as corticosterioids (methylprednisone), methylphenidate stimulants (Concerta, Methylin, Ritalin, Equasym XL), and Epoetin alfa have been useful in improving the anemia, appetite, fatigue, cognition, and pain associated with cancer treatments, advanced cancer, and cancer pain. Research study results vary but supporting data exist for the use of pharmacologic agents for the treatment of physical and cognitive fatigue in cancer patients (Lasheen et al., 2010; Davis, Ahlberg, Berk, Ashley, & Khasraw, 2013).

Cancer patients frequently associate fatigue and sleep disturbances that interfere with the enjoyment of life events as problematic. Therefore clinicians screening for fatigue should also include the evaluation of sleep perception and patterns of cancer patients.

Sleep–Wake Disturbances

"I never feel rested. My dreams are vivid and I usually wake up with my heart pounding and a feeling that something is gonna happen. I try not to nap but I don't have the strength to get through the day without a lie down or two."

—*A cancer patient*

Chronic insomnia affects approximately half of all cancer patients, increasing their fatigue, and they are reluctant to discuss it with their clinicians. Sleep disturbances have been associated with fatigue, psychological distress, and diminished quality of life. Flynn et al. (2010) found that in 10 focus groups patients reported cancer and its treatment disturbed the wake–sleep functioning. Multiple sleep disturbances included pain and restless legs, abnormal dreams, cancer diagnosis and recurrence anxiety, night sweats, problems with sleep and sleep positioning. Other precipitated insomnia distressing factors included nausea, hot flashes, incontinence and diarrhea, delirium, draining lesions, pruritis, and respiratory difficulty. Lifestyle choices such as caffeine and nicotine use may cause insomnia. Physiologic syndromes such as paraneoplastic affect sleep patterns associated with cortisone and melatonin hormone secretions. Many cancer patients felt that the sleep problems reduced their productivity, concentration, social interactions, and overall quality of life (Davidson, Fledman-Stewart, Brennenstuhl, & Ram, 2007; Vena et al., 2006). The efficacy of pharmacologic agents for sleep disturbances in cancer patients such as sedative–hypnotic drugs (benzodiazepines) is limited despite its widespread use. The benefit of somnolence drug use versus the harm in cancer patients is unknown and some clinicians believe it should be used only when behavioral and cognitive approaches have been exhausted (Davidson, MacLean,

Brundage, & Schulze, 2002; Langford, Lee, & Miaskowski, 2012; Berger, 2009; Crump-Woodward, 2011).

Sleep strategies: clinician:

- Assess and screen for sleep–wake disturbances
- Provide sleep–wake information to patient and family
  - Education brochures, videos, online treatments, and self-help strategies
  - Referral to sleep center
- Clinician trained cognitive behavior therapy
- Tailor education and interventions to individual patient needs and disease state

Pharmacologic treatments:

- Clinician review of currently prescribed and self-administered over-the-counter medication and herbal drugs
- Trial use of over-the-counter sleep aids such as Sleepeez and antihistamines (diphenhydramine) and are also used for the treatment of pruritis
- Prescriptive SSIs used for the treatment of depression and anticonvulsants (amitriptyline, gabapentin, pregabalin) for the treatment of neuropathic pain and seizures have a somnolent effect
- Oxygen therapy and/or CPAP for dyspnea and apnea

Self-help strategies:

- Maintain sleep–wake patterns
  - Dedicate bed and bedroom for sleeping
  - Consistent bedtime and rising
  - Use pillows and wedges to promote comfort
  - Limit the length and frequency of daytime naps
  - Avoid caffeine products (tea, coffee, chocolate) and greasy or high-sugar products 4 to 6 hours before bedtime
  - Eat a healthy diet with light snack before bedtime
  - Avoid alcohol
  - Avoid excess fluid intake before bedtime
  - Avoid disturbing TV or discussion prior to bedtime
  - Sleep only as necessary; get out of bed when rested
- Environment
  - Comfortable temperature
  - Adequate air circulation (fan, air conditioner)
  - Light control (room darkening curtains, night light, "Clapper")
  - Noise control (ear plugs, headphones, white noise device)
  - Frequently used items placed within reach (TV and air conditioner remotes, tissues, blanket, phone)
  - Assistance call device (bell, buzzer) within reach
- Complementary medicine
  - Yoga, guided imagery, and meditation techniques
  - Music (soothing, instrumental, nature)
  - Massage therapy
  - Aromatherapy

○ Commercially prepared compact discs (CDs), electronic device downloadable applications for relaxation or breathing techniques

(Strategies adapted from Crump-Woodward, 2011; Kwekkeboom, Cherwin; Lee & Wanta, 2010; Foley, Baillie, Huxter, Price, & Sinclair, 2010; Anderson & Taylor, 2012).

Pain

"I have been pain free for 2 years. Now that doesn't mean I haven't had a headache or sore muscles once in a while. I mean to say that the non-stop pain from surgery, chemo and radiation was just excruciating. The happy drugs helped … but they made me stupid and I couldn't think straight."

—*A cancer survivor*

Pain in patients with cancer can occur at any point along the illness trajectory from diagnosis as a cardinal symptom of dysfunction, during and after therapeutic interventions, a signal of the disease reoccurrence, or in the advanced and end-of-life phase. The NCCN Guidelines define pain (Swarm et al., 2014) as an unpleasant, multidimensional, sensory, and emotional experience associated with actual or potential tissue damage, or described in relation to such damage.

There are a plethora of multiprofessional research studies, journal articles, national and global guidelines, and books written that demonstrate cancer pain interferes with function, activities of daily living, and social interactions that diminish the quality of life for cancer survivors and caregivers. Acute and chronic cancer pain affects mood and psychological functioning, thus increasing the risk of anger, depression, anxiety, and suicidal ideation expressions.

Management of Oncology Pain

The physiology and pharmacokinetics of oncology pain are beyond the scope of this chapter but the management of oncology pain will be discussed. Nurses are often tasked with the prescriptive and administrative management of oncology pain. Cancer pain is very complex and can be subdivided into acute and chronic pain syndromes that are often the result of tumor pressure or invasion of surrounding tissue, nerves, and bone; disruption in organ function; or associated with therapeutic treatment and procedures. Acute pain is self-limiting in that once the underlying cause, such as a diagnostic puncture, surgery, or a fracture, is healed the associated pain dissipates in a few days or up to 3 months. Chronic pain syndromes may worsen in intensity and time often lasting months and years. Acute pain is believed to leave an imprint on the central nervous system and that if it is poorly controlled can precipitate chronic pain syndromes therefore it is essential for nurses to recognize and treat the underlying cause of acute pain. Pain can further be categorized as nociceptive often referred to as somatic or visceral affecting internal tissues or organs, causing pain by direct tumor involvement or sensory receptors in cutaneous or deep tissues, resulting in abnormal activation of pain pathways. Neuropathic pain results from dysfunction to the peripheral or central nervous system as a result of abnormal nerve lesions, nerve compression, and damage to the nerve signaling pathway. The nerve path results in chaotic altered pain signal activity and transmission. Neuropathic pain is associated with limb amputations or disease and treatment-associated neuralgias where the pain can be initiated by nonpainful stimuli (i.e., touch) or hyperexaggerated. Neuropathic pain is often characterized as tingling, burning, icy cold, pins and needles, shooting, or electric sensations.

Chronic pain syndromes in cancer patients are generally associated with tumors or related to treatment and may occur within months or long after completing cancer treatment. Chronic pain syndromes may be identified as bone pain syndrome, visceral pain syndrome, neuropathic pain syndrome, or treatment-related pain syndromes. Chronic pain may be indicative of stable cancer disease, compression, or infiltration of surrounding structures such as bone, nerves, or viscera. Chronic pain may also be due to disease recurrence or unrelated to the cancer such as arthritis. Treatment-related chronic pain syndromes occur postchemotherapy and may include neuropathy, avascular necrosis, hormone treatment such as gynecomastia, and exacerbation of joint pain postbreast or prostate cancer treatment. Postsurgical pain syndromes occur commonly after mastectomy, thoracotomy, amputation, and pelvic surgery. Contributors to chronic postradiation pain syndromes include peripheral nerve tumors, brachial and lumbosacral plexopathies, radiation myelopathy, osteoradionecrosis, and chronic radiation enteritis and proctitis. Continued pain assessment is vital to the management of cancer-related pain in addition to the pharmacologic and nonpharmacologic pain management strategies.

Clinician Pain Assessment Strategies

Pain assessment is referred to as the fifth vital sign and a priori patient assessment. The goal of a comprehensive pain assessment is to identify the cause and characteristics of pain, and administer optimal analgesia to alleviate suffering. The NCCN Guidelines (2014) recommend using two comprehensive pain intensity rating scales that include a numerical, verbal, and written scale as well as faces rating scales. Initial pain assessment incorporates reviewing the patients' past and present medical and surgical history including exploring the patients' prior pain management interventions. Physical dependence and tolerance to analgesics commonly occur with protracted pain, requiring escalating doses or adjuvant medications to control pain.

Numerous pain assessment instruments are available for clinicians, which include multidimensional factors such as the Short Form McGill Pain Questionnaire (SF-MPQ) and the Brief Pain Inventory (BPI). One-dimensional pain measuring instruments include the Pain Thermometer and the Wong-Baker Faces Scale. Pain dynamics can be measured numerically using the (NRS 0–10) rating scale where patients rate their current pain or pain from the last week at a low of "0" meaning no pain to a high of "10" meaning the worst pain imaginable (NCCN, 2014; Swann, 2010; Herr, Spratt, Garand, & Li, 2007).

Neuropathic pain has specific characteristic and there are a number of studies attesting to the efficacy of using scales that measure neuropathic pain characteristics. Various neuropathic pain scales include the Douleur Neuropathique en Questions (DN4), PainDetect, Leeds Assessment of Neuropathic Symptoms and Signs (LANSS), and the Neuropathic Pain Questionnaire (NPQ) (Swann, 2010; Bisaga, Dorazil, Dobrogowski, & Wordliezek, 2010; Tyson & Brow, 2014). The measurement of neuropathic pain helps practitioners to identify neuropathic symptom characteristics and provide appropriate analgesic medications that interfere with the oncology patient's function to improve his/her quality of life. Individualized pain treatment is based on the characteristics, causes, and the patient's clinical condition in collaboration with the patient-centered care goals.

General nursing assessment and identification of pain:

- All patients must be screened for pain at each contact for:
  - type and etiology of pain utilizing established pain assessment instruments
  - intensity and anatomical radiation of pain
  - quality and duration
  - exacerbating factors—what make pain better or worse
  - relieving factors—medication, positioning, comfort devices, and diversion
  - effect on physical and cognitive functional state, activity, and well-being

Pain assessment of nonverbal patients, due to cognitive or physiological barriers, is an opportunity for nurses to utilize their observation and deduction skills. In the absence of self-report, observations of patient behaviors may indicate increased levels of pain, suffering, and distress. Family or caregivers may give insight into patient behaviors, reactions, or verbal utterances that indicate pain or discomfort. A number of pain assessment instruments that measure behavioral indicators of pain for nonverbal patients include the Discomfort Scale for Dementia of the Alzheimer Type (DS-DAT) (Hurley, Volicer, Hanrahan, Houde, & Volicer, 1992), the checklist of nonverbal pain indicators (CNPIs) (Feldt, 2000; Feldt, Ryden, & Miles, 1998), and the Non-communicative Patient's Pain Assessment Instrument (NOPPAIN) (Snow et al., 2004) are a few that measure dimensions and parameters of pain for nonverbal or cognitively impaired adults with or without cancer.

General behavioral observations for nursing pain assessment of nonverbal patients:

- Utilizing established nonverbal pain assessment instruments
- Identifying behavioral responses to pain and discomfort that may include the following:
  - Changes in blood pressure, pulse, respirations, and breathing heavily
  - Guarding, splinting, or withdrawal from stimuli
  - Facial grimaces, frowns, wrinkling, sad or frightened look, furrowed brow, clenched jaw, or teeth grinding
  - Restlessness, agitation, rocking, shifting position, bracing, and massaging
  - Vocalizations such as moaning, groaning, crying, whining, oohing, screaming, and crying out
  - Changes in mental status such as confusion, disorientation, and distress
- Changes in activity and patterns or routines and personal interactions:
  - Diminished appetite
  - Sleep alterations
  - Changes in ambulation or immobility
  - Decreased socialization

(Adapted from Ferrell & Coyle, 2006; Herr, Bjoro, & Decker, 2006)

Management Approaches for Cancer Pain

The key to pain management for oncology patients is flexibility based on the diagnosis, disease stage, the clinician's careful assessment of the pain, and the patient's preference and responses to pain and interventions. Nursing principles guiding an individualized pain care plan include the following: Regularly ask the patient about their pain and believe the patient and families' report of pain. Ask the patient what symptoms are most distressing and what his/her preference of analgesic is. Administer the intervention in a timely and coordinated manner and enable the patient to control their pain management. Pain management strategies include pharmacologic and nonpharmacologic approaches either singly or in combination. Flexibility and trials of several interventions may identify combinations of pain management that meet the patients' individual comfort.

Pharmacologic Pain Management

Pharmacologic pain management includes analgesics that are given in doses and routes of administration based on the changing needs of the individual. Analgesic routes of administration include oral, buccal, sublingual, intranasal, rectal, subcutaneous, intravenous, and transdermal. Analgesics should be given at regular intervals considering the pain intensity using a pain assessment scale, considering the drug's therapeutic action, dose, and adverse effects in accordance to the individual's pain level and comfort. Drug use should be based on the symptom presentation by the patient and appropriate for a therapeutic effect. Classifications of drugs commonly used include acetaminophen and nonsteroidal anti-inflammatory drugs such as ibuprofen, naproxen, and aspirin that provide relief for mild-to-moderate pain without the effects of sedation, nausea and vomiting, or constipation. Opioid drugs are available in many different preparations depending on their action, duration (immediate or modified release), and routes of administration (subcutaneous, intravenous, liquid, buccal or sublingual forms, oral tablets or capsules, transdermal patches, and lollipops). Opioid drugs include morphine, codeine, fentanyl, hydrocodone, methadone, and oxycodone. Selective opioids can be readily titrated or bolused based on the changing condition and pain relief needed by the patient. Patients taking regular doses of opioids must be monitored for side effects that include sedation, nausea, constipation, and opioid toxicity. Intramuscular administration of opioids is discouraged and the alternative subcutaneous route is advised. Changing from one opioid to another or one route to another may be necessary and drug equivalence charts should be consulted when changing opioid drugs or doses.

Breakthrough pain is defined as a transient exacerbation of pain that occurs either spontaneously or in relation to a specific predictable or unpredictable trigger, despite relatively stable and adequately controlled background pain. Breakthrough pain is a combination of different conditions including the causation and/or invasion of surrounding tissues, disruption of neuromechanisms, and the clinical characteristics of the pain that include the patient's tolerance and interpretation of the pain exacerbation. In response to the exacerbation of pain rescue medication is taken as necessary rather than regularly scheduled analgesia. The use of a fixed dose, immediate release formulation of morphine is the opioid rescue primary drug of choice for breakthrough pain but is only one aspect of breakthrough pain management. Titration of the scheduled opioid analgesic is one strategy but often limited due to the adverse effects. Changing the type of opioid and/or route of administration can be effective as is the addition of adjuvant analgesics such as nonsteroidal anti-inflammatory drugs (NSAIDs), anticonvulsants, or antispasmodic medications (Davies, 2011).

The use of adjuvant drugs assists with the management of anxiety, depression, seizures, organ or muscular spasms, neuropathic pain that also includes bisphosphonates for bone pain, and calcium channel blockers for ischemic and neuropathic pain (see Table 2.3). Topical or local anesthetics such as EMLA (external use only) and Oraqix (oral use only) are lidocaine products that provide local anesthesia for puncture, dermal,

Table 2.3 • Adjuvant Analgesics

Type	Purpose
Tricyclic antidepressants	Treatment of neuropathic pain such as burning or electric pain and poor sleep
Anticonvulsants	Seizures, neuropathic pain such as shooting pain, breakthrough pain
Corticosteroids	Cerebral edema, spinal cord compression, bone pain, neuropathic pain, visceral pain
Local anesthetics	Local and neuropathic pain
Bisphosphonates	Osteolytic bone pain
Calcitonin	Neuropathic pain, bone pain
Capsaicin	Neuropathic pain
Baclofen	Neuropathic pain
Calcium channel blockers	Ischemic pain, neuropathic pain, smooth muscle spasms with pain
Nonsteroidal anti-inflammatory drugs (NSAIDs)	Breakthrough pain

Adapted from Valerand & Sanoski (2014).

oral procedures, and neuropathic pain. Adjuvant drug use in combination with analgesics contributes to the management of cancer distress when used routinely or PRN (as needed) based on the patient's state.

Nonpharmacologic Pain Management

Optimal pain control requires a combination of pharmacological and nonpharmacological approaches. Occupational therapy and physical therapy can reduce pain and improve the function and quality of life for cancer survivors. Interventions can include therapeutic exercises, purposeful activities, pacing activities, and assistive devices to conserve energy and promote muscle strength. Therapeutic use of transcutaneous electrical nerve stimulation (TENS), heat or cold treatments, and massage can promote comfort, relieve muscle strain, improve posture, and prevent exacerbations of musculoskeletal symptoms associated with illness and fatigue. Complementary and alternative medicine treatments as previously discussed in the fatigue self-help strategies section are applicable therapies as adjuvant to pharmacological treatment for cancer pain.

Nurses providing information, education, and management of procedural, surgical, disease components, pain and breakthrough pain symptom management are essential members of the pain management team for cancer survivors and their families throughout the cancer trajectory. Education promotes informed decision making and engagement that enables patients to be proactive in their symptom management and cancer care.

Gastrointestinal Symptoms

"It all started with a belly ache and vomiting that I thought was a stomach bug. For two days I didn't poop or pass gas. I was vomiting this brown stuff and finally went to the emergency room. Some young, Doogie Howser-looking doctor came in and said I probably have a tumor blocking my bowels and if so it is most likely cancer. What?"

—A colon cancer survivor

Gastrointestinal dysfunction encompasses a group of symptoms associated with cancer pathology and treatment that have acute and chronic implications for survivors. Surgical, chemotherapy, and radiation treatments for cancer affect the functioning of the gastrointestinal system that can manifest in a variety of symptoms.

Oral Cavity

Chemotherapy changes the reproduction of the taste buds that may produce an unpleasant taste so that favored foods and liquids lose their appeal whereby the cancer patients are at risk for diminished intake that interferes with the nutrition and the fluid and electrolyte imbalance. Oral symptoms as a result of cancer treatments may also include mucositis, stomatitis, dryness, or xerostomia (extreme dryness of the mouth from lack of normal secretions). Inflammation of the tongue and mouth including the lips and mucous membranes may cause oral pain when eating or drinking, which can result in halitosis, dysphagia, and malnutrition. Nursing management of oral pain includes assessment of the oral cavity for areas of redness, white patches, and ulcers that may require treatment with antifungal, antibacterial, or antiviral therapy. The use of local anesthetic combinations such as viscous lidocaine may provide symptomatic control and maintenance of oral intake. Encouragement of an oral hygiene routine includes tooth brushing two or three times a day with a soft nylon-bristled toothbrush with fluoride-containing toothpaste; the use of dental floss with frequent mild antiseptic mouth rinses promote oral cleanliness and dental health. If gum bleeding, infection, or loose teeth occur, a dentist should be consulted without delay. Advise patients to know the signs and symptoms of infection and report oral changes to their clinician and seek immediate treatment.

Patients with concurrent renal or hepatic disease are at greater risk for anorexia.

Constipation

Constipation is a distressing gastrointestinal symptom that may be transient or chronic experienced by cancer survivors. Constipation is the infrequent passage of stool or the sensation of bowel fullness. Cause of constipation may be disease related such as partial or complete bowel obstruction or from metabolic disturbances such as hypocalcemia or hypokalemia. Physical inactivity and/or neuropathic dysfunction can also result in decreased bowel motility. Constipation may also be related to improper diet, treatment, or medication (e.g., opioids) use. If constipation is present, bowel, abdominal, and rectal assessments are indicated to identify the cause and severity to rule out bowel impaction or obstruction. Preventive measures are the key to constipation management and include increasing fluids and dietary fiber and physical activity (see Table 2.4). The use of stimulant laxatives and stool softeners may promote nonforced bowel movements every 1 or

Table 2.4 • **Bowel Prophylaxis**

Stool Softener

Senna 2–3 tablets every night

Docusate 2–3 tablets every night

Laxatives

Polyethylene glycol 1 capful in 8 ounces of water

Lactulose 30–60 mL one or two times a day

Bisacodyl 1 rectal suppository daily

Sorbitol 30 mL every 2 hrs times three, then as needed

Magnesium hydroxide 30–60 mL once or twice daily

Magnesium citrate 8 ounces daily

Palliative Care

Methylnaltrexone for opioid-induced constipation 0.15 mg/kg SC every other day

Adapted from Valerand & Sanoski (2014).

2 days. Monitoring gastric symptoms and reassessment for treatment effectiveness and with acceptable symptom control reduce patient distress.

Diarrhea

Diarrhea is the frequent passage of nonformed stool that can result in fluid and electrolyte imbalance, skin breakdown, treatment delays, fatigue, malnutrition, and hospitalizations. Causes of diarrhea can be disease or treatment related, concurrent disease, or psychological. Approximately 90% of patients receiving chemotherapy, biologic, and radiation treatment regimes experience diarrhea. Diarrhea can be acute lasting a few days or chronic lasting 3 or more weeks. Diarrhea can be severe in human immunodeficiency virus (HIV) and bone marrow transplant patients from irradiation or graft-versus-host disease. The presence of diarrhea can be physically and socially isolating, increasing debilitation and depression. Nurses play a significant role in recognizing, educating, and managing diarrhea symptoms.

Diarrhea assessment requires a careful history that includes identifying the frequency and characteristics of the stool, and an abdominal and rectal examination. The National Cancer Institute Scale of Severity of diarrhea is a grading instrument from 0 to 4. Stools are rated by (1) the number of loose stools per day and (2) symptoms (see Table 2.5).

Medication, dietary, and supportive care are the combination of treatments for diarrhea. After determining the cause of the diarrhea, common drugs are prescribed and administered. Loperamide (Imodium) 2 to 4 mg once or twice a day is the usual management for diarrhea. Diphenoxylate (Lomotil 2.5 mg with atropine 0.025 mg) is given one or two tablets orally as needed for loose stools. Codeine as an opioid is useful in the reduction of diarrhea and Tincture of Opium decreases peristalsis. Absorbent agents such as pectin and methylcellulose add bulk and increase the consistency of the stool. Anticholinergic drugs reduce gastric secretions and decrease peristalsis that includes atropine, scopolamine, and sandostatin. Bismuth subsalicylate (Pepto-Bismol),

Table 2.5 • National Cancer Institute Scale of Severity of Diarrhea

	0	1	2	3	4
Increased number of loose stools/day	Norm	2–3	4–6	7–9	>10
Symptoms		None	Nocturnal stools and/or moderate cramping	Incontinence and severe cramping	Grossly bloody and/or need for parenteral support

aspirin, and indomethacin are useful for bacteria, radiotherapy, and prostaglandin-secreting tumors. Clonidine is useful for controlling watery diarrhea in bronchogenic cancer patients and Lactaid for malabsorption diarrheas.

Nonpharmacologocial interventions for diarrhea management include identifying foods that irritate the gastrointestinal system. Dietary contributors to diarrhea include milk and milk products, caffeine-containing foods and beverages, carbonated and acidic high-sugar, high-sorbitol juices, spicy foods, raw vegetables, sushi, and gas-producing fruits and vegetables that should be limited and avoided. Eliminating foods that are potential diarrhea-causing irritants including screening for herbal remedy use such as milk thistle, aloe, cayenne, and Lactobacillus acidophilus. Maintaining fluid intake is a vital part of diarrhea treatment. Cancer patients suffering with diarrhea should be encouraged to drink 3 to 4 L of varied fluids that include water, sports drinks, broth, decaffeinated teas, clear diluted juices, and gelatin. Cancer patient should avoid alcoholic, caffeinated, and high-sugar drinks (NCCN, 2014; Shaw & Taylor, 2012).

Persistent diarrhea can cause ostomy or peri-anal skin irritations that are both painful and potentially infectious. Patient and family education on the importance of cleansing the perineum gently with a mild solution to prevent skin breakdown is essential. Sitz baths provide cleansing comfort and skin barrier products such as Desitin protect sensitive skin. If the patient has an ostomy, the stoma should be assessed daily for ulceration and bleeding as the diarrheal gastric acids erode sensitive bowel mucosa. Skin surrounding the stoma should be monitored for redness irritation from diarrhea and reactions to ostomy products. Patient and family education includes the signs and symptoms that should be reported promptly to the clinicians that include excessive thirst, dizziness, fever, palpitations, rectal spasms, excessive cramping, water, or bloody stools. Early recognition of complications can prevent the sequelae of treatment complication that contribute to hospitalizations and mortality.

Gastrointestinal disturbances are an ongoing challenge for cancer survivors. Bowel and dietary assessments should be performed at the start and throughout treatment and recovery. Nutritional and fluid management along with pharmacologic measure help to manage diarrhea episodes, improving the quality of life for cancer survivors.

Nausea and Vomiting

Nausea and vomiting are common and significant symptoms associated with cancer surgery, chemotherapy, and radiation and maintenance chemotherapy treatments for cancer survivors. Nausea and vomiting create a disruption in daily activities, physical and psychological well-being of the cancer patient that increase the risk of hospitalization and failure to complete treatment.

Nausea and vomiting, although two distinct physiologic mechanisms, are often reported cojointly. Nausea and vomiting are caused by stimulation of the vagus nerve by serotonin releaser by cells in the upper gastrointestinal tract. The incidence of nausea and vomiting is dependent upon the chemotherapy agent, the dose and schedule of the agent and, if applicable, the radiation or surgical site. Prevention of chemotherapy-induced nausea and vomiting (CINV) can be managed effectively with appropriate antiemetic therapy. Oncology nurses when assessing and developing a treatment plan for CINV are instrumental in collaborating with oncologists and pharmacists to create an emetogenic plan that meets the patient needs and improves adherence to the chemotherapy regime and completion of treatment.

Pharmacologic Management of Nausea and Vomiting

Assessment and evaluation include the patterns and triggers of nausea and vomiting. Oncology nurses assess for the frequency, timing of the event, duration, and severity of nausea and vomiting episodes before and after treatment. There are generally three patterns of nausea and vomiting. First is anticipation—a conditioned response from repeated associations between therapy and vomiting that can be prevented with adequate antiemetic control. This can be initiated by cues including thoughts, smell, or sights. Second is the acute pattern that occurs 0 to 24 hours after chemotherapy is administered. Third is the delayed pattern that can occur 1 to 6 days after chemotherapy administration when nausea is often worse than vomiting. Patterns of nausea and vomiting may follow administration of certain drugs, movement, foods, or smells.

NCCN Guidelines for Antiemesis (AE-1) (Ettinger et al., 2014) recommend treating CINV based on the emetogenic potential of the antineoplastic agent including the CINV pattern. Antiemetic agents include 5-HT3 receptor antagonists, NK1 receptor antagonists, and corticosteroids as well as dopamine receptor antagonists, benzodiazepines, olanzapine, and cannabinoids. Current antiemetic control targets the peripheral, cortical, and brain's chemoreceptor trigger zone pathways.

Ondansetron was the first 5-HT3 receptor antagonists that was found effective for the patient's receiving cisplatin-based agents. There are currently four 5-HT3 receptor antagonists approved for use—ondansetron, granisetron, dolasetron, and palonosetron. These agents are believed to prevent CINV by antagonizing 5-HT3 receptors either peripherally or at vagal nerve terminals and/or centrally in the chemoreceptor zone and have a high rate of CINV prevention and tolerable side effects.

NK1 receptor antagonists inhibit substance P in peripheral and central emetic pathways. Aprepitant is administered orally with downward titrating doses in days postchemotherapy for the prevention of CINV in patients receiving high emetogenic drugs. The side effects include fatigue, headache, anorexia, diarrhea, hiccups, and increased transmainases. Aprepitant dose adjustment is required in patients receiving dexamethasone and warfarin. Fosaprepitant is administered intravenous before chemotherapy and only used on day 1 and has a comparable effect as the third day oral Aprepitant regime.

Corticosteroids have been found to be effective when used alone for prevention of CINV in low emetogenic chemotherapy. Dexamethasone is the recommended corticosteroid but the tolerability of any corticosteroid can be concerning as side effects include insomnia, agitation, weight gain, hyperglycemia, and epigastric discomfort.

Dopamine receptor antagonists are mostly used in the treatment of breakthrough emesis. The dopamine antagonists include the classification of phenothiazines (e.g., prochlorperazine), butyrophenones (e.g., haloperidol, droperidol), and benzamides (e.g., metoclopramide). Common side effects include extrapyramidal symptoms, dystonia, and drowsiness which are more suitable of breakthrough nausea rather than primary prophylaxis.

Benzodiazepines are adjunctive therapies to decrease treatment-related anxiety and treatment of anticipatory nausea and vomiting. Lorazepam and alprazolam are the primary agents with sedation being the most common adverse effect.

Olanzapine, the antipsychotic, has a multichemical antagonistic effects that are safe and effective, prevents acute, delayed, and breakthrough CINV for patients receiving moderately and highly emetogenic chemotherapy. Side effects include sedation, weight gain, orthostatic hypotension, hyperglycemia, and a black box warning for use in elderly patients with dementia-related psychosis.

Cannabinoids such as dronabinol and nabilone are approved for CINV in patients who have not responded adequately to conventional antiemetics. Cannabinoids may produce vertigo, euphoria, and somnolence that limit their use.

Oncology clinicians should assess and evaluate patients with CINV with each administration and consider changing antiemetic therapy to a higher-level primary treatment for the next cycles if there is inadequate patient antiemetic response. Currently most research focuses on treatment-induced nausea and vomiting in patients receiving chemotherapy for disease control with few clinical trials in patients with advanced disease or in palliative and end-of-life care (NCCN, 2014).

Nonpharmacologic Management of Nausea and Vomiting

Nonpharmacologic management of nausea and vomiting for cancer survivors involves simple self-care techniques. These self-care techniques are adaptive or behavioral interventions. These techniques may include relaxation, biofeedback, meditation, yoga, guided imagery, cognitive distraction, and systematic desensitization. Other therapies include acupuncture, acupressure, and music therapy. Behavioral interventions may be helpful in giving the patient a sense of control that decrease the sense of helplessness as active participants in their symptom management and serve as distractions from the nausea and vomiting sensation.

Strategies for nausea and vomiting management include the following:

- Have adequate antiemetic and pain medication control
- Decrease noxious odors
- Promptly remove foul-smelling body fluids, excrement, soiled dressings, and garbage from the patient area
- Use neutral-smelling room deodorizer
- Eat bland (dry crackers or pretzels) cold or room temperature foods
- Restrict fluids with meals
- Eat frequent small meals

- Avoid fatty, overly spicy, or sugary foods
- Wear loose fitting clothes
- Ventilate room with fresh air (open window, fan)
- Perform oral care after each emesis
- Apply cool cloth to neck, forehead, and wrists

Depression

"Most days since I found out…I can't get out of bed. My mind races to when I'm not here anymore, to the special family milestones I won't be around for. I know the battle is just beginning but I don't know if I have it in me."

—Cancer patient

Cancer is a dreaded and distressing disease. There are fewer life-altering words that elicit such fear and anguish in a person or family than hearing a diagnosis of cancer. The word "cancer" is perceived as synonymous with death and as such the recipient of such a diagnosis must don the armor of battle and wage a strenuous campaign to beat the enemy at all costs, for to do anything less would be to cowardly surrender to the invading enemy. The psychological effects of having cancer begin with the diagnosis that becomes a defining part of the person's identity. Survivors often refer to cancer as a life-defining marker and their life events are timeline referenced as "before I had cancer or after I had cancer." The psychological reaction and behavioral actions of the cancer patient and family are an uncharted course requiring the interprofessional healthcare team to meet the dynamic and evolving needs of patients and families affected by cancer. According to the American Cancer Society (ACS) (2014), 25% of patients nationally will display symptoms of anxiety and depression. Psychological challenges associated with cancer treatment require healthcare providers to remain attuned to the fluctuating emotional state of patients as their emotional status and previous response to adverse life events may be a protective factor.

The Diagnostic and Statistical Manual of Mental Disorders, fifth edition (2013), (DSM-V) of the American Psychiatric Association describes several categories of mood depression (major depression, minor depression, adjustment disorder with depressed mood, and dysthymia) mainly based on severity or length of illness. Major depression is present in approximately 16% of patients with cancer, with minor depression and dysthymia combined reported in almost 22% of patients, as confirmed by the meta-analysis of 94 interview-based studies (Mitchell et al., 2011). Depression overlaps with the other symptoms of cancer and treatments such as physical pain, fatigue, anorexia, insomnia, cognitive impairment, and the desire for a hastened death. The presence of depression in a cancer should not be dismissed as natural to the diagnosis but should always be treated to improve the function, adherence to a treatment plan, and quality of life for survivors.

Assessment of depression includes exploring situational factors and symptoms, previous psychiatric history, and other factors including the availability and utilization of social support networks and presence of pain or functional losses (Pasacreta, Minarik, & Neild-Anderson, 2006). Oniszczenko and Laskowska (2014) found that destructive coping style and high emotional reactivity were temperament traits that intensified cancer trauma symptoms in adult patients.

The primary care provider and cancer patient relationship is vital to the treatment care plan as prior therapeutic relationships contain psychosocial baseline information that is essential as a comparative reference point. Priest (2006) postulates that developing a therapeutic relationship with patients reduces psychological distress associated with illness. Clinical depression impairs function and causes great distress; additionally screenings for depression may evoke guarded or defensive behaviors. The clinician screening for depression must be sensitive to the stigma associated with depression and that some of the symptoms may also be attributed to the cancer and its treatment. Causes of depression may be disease related, psychological responses to adverse events, and medication-related effects. Symptoms of clinical depression or major depressive disorder that occur nearly every day and for 2 weeks or more require consultation with a qualified health or mental health professional.

Symptoms of clinical depression include the following:

- Unabated sadness, hopelessness, or a blunted mood most of the day, nearly every day
- Continued loss of interest or pleasure in most activities most of the day, nearly every day
- Weight gain or weight loss (when not dieting)
- Inertia or agitation nearly every day
- Enduring fatigue
- Insomnia, hypersomnia, or sleeplessness with early waking nearly every day
- Inability to focus, difficulty thinking, remembering, or decision making nearly every day
- Speech that is slow, halting, and anxious
- Feeling guilty, helpless, and worthless nearly every day
- Hopelessness about the future
- Recurrent invasive thoughts of death or suicidal ideation without a specific plan, or a suicide attempt, or a specific plan for committing suicide

Healthcare providers should assess patient and family adaptation and mental state for difficulties along the diagnosis, treatment, and long-term survival trajectory and implement stress management and social support services as part of the initial treatment plan from diagnosis and that continues throughout survivorship (see Table 2.6).

Many patients with cancer experience "emotional distress" particularly their quality of life. Madden asserts the continuum of distress for cancer patients ranges from feelings of vulnerability, grief, and worry to issues such as "depression, anxiety, panic, social isolation, and existential and spiritual crisis" (2006, p. 615). The Oncology Nursing Society's *Statement on the Scope and Standards of Oncology Nursing Practice* recommends that oncology nurses assess patient psychosocial issues such as distress monitoring, patient's coping, and comfort. Oncology nurses should refer patients exhibiting coping issues to mental health practitioners for pharmacotherapy and psychotherapy support (Brant & Wickham, 2004). Limited time may make assessing anxiety and depression difficult for practitioners but screening statements such as, "You seem worried today. Have you been feeling blue lately?" can begin discussion and provide a segue for advanced discussions with assessments. Table 2.7 presents sample assessment and screening tools.

Pharmacological Management of Depression

Patients with cancer and other chronic illnesses may exhibit transient depression throughout the illness trajectory. Depressive symptoms may be caused by the cancer

Table 2.6 • Difficulties Experienced by Patients During Cancer Diagnosis, Treatment, and Survivorship

Diagnosis	Treatment	Long-Term Survivorship
Behavior: • Anger • Anticipatory loss • Bodily exposure • Confusion • Death anxiety • Decisional conflict • Financial and work constraints • Relationship changes • Remorse over family life disruption • Test result scrutiny	Adaptation: • Altered sense of self • Emergent crises • Imposition on family • Ongoing interface with ambulatory practice, laboratory tests, and radiology • Out-of-pocket expenses • Partial reentry into normal life • Physical compromise • Threat of treatment-related sequelae • Toxicities • Trusting strangers	Integration of: • Family worry • Financial constraints • Full reentry into normal life • Insurance discrimination • Ongoing debilitation and long-term effects • Permanent altered sense of self • Recurrence anxiety • Relationship changes • Reminders of cancer threat • Response to anniversaries • Separation anxiety

Adapted from Boyle (2006).

Table 2.7 • Sample Assessment and Screening Tools

Research Instrument	Measures	Implementation
Hospital Anxiety and Depression Scale (Snaith, 2003)	Anxiety and depression	14-item questionnaire
The Beck Depression Inventory (Beck, Steer, & Brown, 2006)	Depression	21-item questionnaire
Zung Self-Rating Depression Scale (Dugan et al., 1998)	Depression	20-item questionnaire
Hamilton Anxiety Scale (Health Care Technology Systems, 2006)	Anxiety self-rating	14-item scale
Beck Anxiety Inventory (Beck, Epstein, Grown, & Steer, 1988)	Anxiety self-rating	21-item scale
The Brief Patient Health Questionnaire (Lowe, Kroenke, Herzog, & Grafe, 2004)	Anxiety and depression	34-question tool
The Distress Thermometer (Larouche & Edgar, 2004)	Anxiety and depression	Visual Analog in the word Scale 11-point visual analog scale 0 (none) to 10 (extreme distress)
Distress Management Assessment Tool (Beck, Steer, & Brown, 2006)	Distress subdivided into five categories of problems: physical, practical, emotional, spiritual and religious, family	35-item checklist The tool takes approximately 3 or 4 min to complete.

itself, or associated with therapeutic drugs or treatments, nonprescribed drugs or alcohol, or by illness markers that have been caused by psychosomatic changes such as worsening condition, cancer recurrence, or treatment futility. Further complicating depression management in older adults is their greater risk for adverse effects from pharmaceuticals due to absorption and metabolic changes that would require modifying prescribing regimes. Other guidelines include the following:

- Choosing medication with the least potential for drug interactions and adverse effects considering the patient's past mental health history, age, gender, stage of the cancer, system vulnerabilities (i.e., gut motility in colon cancer, hormone-producing and dependent cancers), cancer recurrence and/or metastasis, and the potential for improving depressive symptoms
- Weighing the risk of additional effects from antidepressant side effects and concurrent chemotherapeutic side effects
- Beginning with low dosages and increasing slowly based upon therapeutic response
- Regularly reevaluating dosages; assessing for therapeutic effect, adverse events, and depression abatement

Antidepressants are the primary classification of drugs used to treat depression and the prescribing regime modified to treat or manage symptoms. No one antidepressant medication is clearly more effective than another. Tricyclic antidepressants and Trazodon are the first-generation antidepressant having a broad spectrum action. These drugs often produce intolerable effects such as dry mouth, constipation, and orthostatic hypotension which are restrictive to oncology patients in addition to being cardiotoxic-producing clinical dysrhythmias and cardiomyopathy. In this class Amitriptyline is mainly used for oncological neuropathic pain. Trazodon is a second-generation nontricyclic antidepressant with a sedative effect useful in insomnia and palliative care.

The selective serotonin reuptake inhibitors (SSRIs) class (fluoxetine, fluvoxamine, paroxetine, sertaraline, citalopram, and escitalopram) have fewer long-term side effects than the tricyclic antidepressants and are usually the first antidepressant treatment. The nausea side effect, in the first weeks of treatment, can cause nonadherence to treatment. SSRIs have an antiaggregation activity and bleeding risk should be monitored in patients with hematological alterations, the elderly, and in the presence of other antiplatelet drugs. Treatment with SSRIs can cause tremor, bradykinesia, and emotional blunting but can reduce the hot flashes associated with chemotherapy, antiestrogen drugs (i.e., tamoxifen), or ovariectomy and hysterectomy.

Serotonin noradrenaline reuptake inhibitors (SNRIs) class (venlafazine, duloxetine, and milnacipran) are dual-acting antidepressants because they have a higher efficacy than SSRIs on residual and somatic symptoms of depression, particularly the painful physical symptom cluster (physical, emotional, cognitive).

Other dual-acting antidepressants are bupropion which is effective in treating fatigue and mirtazapine that is useful when depression and nausea are present during chemotherapeutic treatment but has an antihistamine effect that is favorable in patient requiring sedation such as anxiety or insomnia. Psychostimulants such as dextroamphetamine and methylphenidates have a rapid action and side effect clearance that are also useful in treating depression in medically ill patients (Torta & Ieraci, 2013; Lippincott, 2014).

The effectiveness of an antidepressant regime in oncology patients must be assessed routinely for effectiveness and the presence of undesired side effects. A combination of antidepressant medication and psychotherapy are often effective in treating depressive disorders. Patient education is essential to decrease nonadherence to medication regime to improve the cancer survivor's functional recovery, quality of life, coping strategies, and adaptation to change.

Psychotherapeutic Modalities

Psychosocial interventions are directed at improving the quality of life for those coping with cancer. The goals of such modalities are to lessen emotional distress and improve the morale, self-esteem, coping ability, sense of control and well-being, and problem-solving ability of cancer survivors (IOM, 2008). Education programs should use cognitive methods and problem-solving strategies that promote accurate understanding of medical terms and treatment processes clarifying medical misinformation and increasing trust in healthcare provider that alleviate fear and promote active decision making throughout the illness trajectory.

Additional therapeutic measures include the following:

- *Psychodynamic Therapy*—helps patients to become aware of unconscious anger directed toward the diagnosis and work through feeling to alleviate depression. Encourages discussion of loss associated with anger and aggression that inwardly leads to negative feelings about oneself leading to depression. This may include inpatient or outpatient treatment and medication stabilization programs.
- *Cognitive Therapy*—is the recommended therapeutic approach for depression. That includes identifying and challenging the accuracy of the patients' negative thought patterns and encourage behaviors designed to counteract depressive symptoms.
- *Family Education and Health Maintenance*—assists the patient and family in developing a sense of self that is separate from the family as a whole. Personal responsibility is encouraged while direct education and information is provided about the depression and the effect on the family system.
- *Support groups*—that provide cancer survivors with individual, spousal, and family interventions to strengthen coping and sense of hope through open, honest dialog exploring and validating each other's feelings (Lippincott, 2014).

A systematic review of psychosocial interventions as mediators for cancer patients by Moyer, Goldenberg, and Hall revealed that few studies included examination of potential mediator of change and that it is important to continue testing which psychosocial interventions are efficacious in improving the quality of life for cancer survivors (Moyer, Goldenberg, & Hall, 2012).

Beginning with the initial shock of the cancer diagnosis consideration should be given to the patients and family expectations. The success of cancer treatment that is measured by a cure can have an adverse effect on the patient's emotions and decision making. Realistic discussions should include the attainable goals of treatment and include the psychological fortitude necessary for transitional survivorship. Management for depression may include single or combinations of therapies. Nonpharmacologic interventions for depression include psychotherapy, support groups, grief counseling, or cognitive behavioral therapy. Strengthening coping and a sense of hope are strategic goals of therapeutic interventions. Pharmaceutical interventions are aimed at increasing serotonin and norepinephrine. Selective prescribed drugs may include the use of antidepressants, stimulants, nonbenzodiazepines, or steroids. Patients may use complementary and alternative treatments that include meditation, guided imagery, mindfulness, and yoga. The use of medicinal and nutritional supplements should be discussed with the clinician because of potential drug interactions.

Anxiety

"I feel like I could jump out of my skin! For no reason my heart starts to pound, I can't see clearly and it's difficult to breathe. I just want to scream! Driving in the car or walking at the mall it just stops me in my tracks . . . I'm paralyzed."

—Cancer patient

Anxiety disorders are among the most common of all psychiatric mood disorders. Cancer survival has improved greatly in the past 20 years increasing the prevalence and trajectory of fear and anxiety associated with the cancer diagnosis and recurrence. Mitchell, Ferguson, Gill, Paul, and Symonds' (2013) systematic review and mega-analysis suggests that anxiety rather than depression is a more prevalent problem to be addressed in long-term cancer survivors. Anxiety is common in patients with cancer and psychologically associated with a reduced quality of life, poor adherence to treatment and self-care, impaired physical, social, and family functioning, worse symptoms, and diminished will to live (Mitchell et al., 2011).

Clinical manifestation of general anxiety includes subjective and objective manifestations that include a pattern of worrying or anxiety that results in increased autonomic activity persisting for a period of at least 6 months (see Table 2.8). The behavior exhibited usually falls into one of four categories: acting out, somatization, immobilization or paralysis, and use of energy to seek other solutions.

The DSM-V identifies panic disorders as conditions in which an individual experiences intense fear or discomfort in which four or more of the following symptoms are developed abruptly and reach a peak within 10 minutes. Cancer patients suffering with anxiety exhibit varying symptoms. These include palpitations, pounding heart, or accelerated heart rate, sweating, trembling or shaking, sensations of shortness of breath or smothering, feelings of choking, chest pain or discomfort. Symptoms may also include nausea or abdominal distress, feeling dizzy, unsteady, lightheadedness, or faint, derealization (feeling of unreality) or depersonalization (being detached from oneself), fear of losing control or going crazy, fear of dying, paresthesias (numbness or tingling sensations), chills or hot flashes (American Psychological Association [APA], 2013).

Cancer survivors experience varying degrees of distress throughout the cancer continuum. Distress can range from feelings of vulnerability to disabling psychosocial symptoms. Stressors associated with the cancer experience shatter the individual's sense of normalcy, challenge functional ability, and alter patterns of everyday life that can create an overwhelming sense of threat for their life, lack of control, intense fear, and dread. Posttraumatic stress is theorized to result from the struggle to reconcile the shock of a traumatic event with core beliefs about oneself and the world. Cancer patients struggle to maintain a sense of normalcy and self often redefining those ideals along the cancer trajectory. The symptoms associated with posttraumatic stress disorder (PTSD) do not follow the usual stress resolution course of dissipating over time. Some cancer survivors are DSM-V classified with trauma and stress-related disorders that include PTSD and ASD. ASD and PTSD share several symptoms with the differences being the timeframe in which symptoms develop. ASD develops within 1 month of the traumatic event and lasts from 2 days to 3 weeks whereas PTSD the symptoms

Table 2.8 • **Clinical Manifestations of Anxiety**

Subjective	Objective
Increased tension	Facial tension
Apprehension and worry	Quivering voice
Pain and persistent increased helplessness	Insomnia
Uncertainty	Poor eye contact
Fear	Glancing about
Regret	Increased wariness
Overexcitement	Increased perspiration
Expressing concern regarding changes in life events	Sympathetic stimulation: tachycardia, superficial vasoconstriction, pupil dilation
Jitteriness	Restlessness
Shakiness	Trembling and hand tremors
Fear of unspecified consequences	Extraneous movements (foot shuffling, hand/arm movements)
Distress	Exaggerated startle response

are more enduring and have lasted for at least 1 month at the time of diagnosis. These debilitating stress disorders are the result of having experienced a catastrophic event and manifest initially by a sense of numbness, lack of emotional response, feelings of depersonalization or de-realization, confusion, and loss of memory of the original events. Extreme symptoms include increased sympathetic activation, such as sweating, trembling, shaking, chest pain, choking sensation, hypervigilance, and a pattern of reexperiencing the event through intrusive dreams, flashbacks, increased anxiety, rumination, insomnia, difficulty concentrating, and restlessness. ASD and PTSD individuals suffer diminished interest in relationships and external events. Their feeling of lack of control over distressing memories or dreams of the event with sudden sensations that the event is beginning again interferes with relationships, employment, and social interactions leading to loneliness and isolation (Rayner et al., 2010; Lethborg et al., 2000; Tedeschi & Calhoun, 2004).

Hildegard Peplau, a psychiatric nurse theorist, believed that anxiety is a normal part of the human experience and is necessary to change and develop better coping skills. Peplau proposed that there are four levels of anxiety: mild, moderate, severe, and panic, and those individuals have the capacity to learn from anxiety and adapt their behavior accordingly. Indeed if one believes that approach then the anxiety of illness has the potential to enrich, give meaning to and promote personal growth for the cancer survivor and family (Peplau, 1983). Tedeschi and Calhoun (2004) defined posttraumatic growth as the positive psychological change experienced as a result of the struggle with extreme life-altering events. Posttraumatic growth is represented by having met the challenge that represents something new and that the individual has benefited from the

Table 2.9 • Medications for the Treatment of Anxiety in the Medically Ill

Benzodiazepines	Cyclic Antidepressants
Diazepam (Valium and others)	Amitriptyline (Elavil and others)
Flurazepam (Dalmane and others)	Imipramine (Tofranil and others)
Halazepam (Paxipam)	Nortriptyline (Pamelor and others)
Chlordiazepoxide (Librium and others)	Protriptyline (Vivactil)
Alprazolam (Xanax)	Trazodone (Desyrel and others)
Triazolam (Halcion)	Desipramine (Norpramin and others)
Clorazepate (Tranxene)	Amoxapine (Asendin)
Prazepam (Centrax)	Maprotiline (Ludiomil)
Midazolam (Versed, IM, IV, and SC only)	Doxepin (Sinequan and others)
Quazepam (Doral)	Trimipramine (Surmontil)
Estazolam (ProSom)	
Clonazepam (Klonopin)	**Other Antidepressants**
Lorazepam (Ativan and others)	Fluoxetine (Prozac) an SSRI
Temazepam (Restorial and others)	Sertraline (Zoloft) an SSRI
Oxazepam (Serax amd others)	Paroxetine (Paxil) an SSRI
	Bupropion (Wellbutrin) dopamine reuptake blocker
	Nefazodone (Serzone) 5-HT2 receptor antagonist
Other Medications Selectively Used for Their Anxiolytic Effects	Venlafaxine (Effexor) serotonin/norepinephrine reuptake inhibitor
β-Adrenergic blocking agents such as propranolol	**Azapirones**
Monoamine oxidase inhibitors	Buspirone (Buspar)
Neuroleptics (antipsychotics) such as haloperidol	

From Valerand & Sanoski (2014).

experience. Perceived growth may help mitigate the negative events and losses associated with cancer and help preserve the belief that "the self" is both good and in control.

Anxiety, stress, and depression are common responses to cancer diagnosis that increase and decrease at transitional points along the disease trajectory of chronic and life-limiting illnesses. Nurses utilizing various counseling approaches singly or in conjunction with pharmacological agents promote supportive dialogs that validate the fluctuating emotions throughout cancer survival.

Pharmacologic interventions for anxiety include the use of antidepressant drugs as previously discussed and antianxiety pharmaceuticals (see Table 2.9).

Nurses as "frontline" healthcare providers are primary clinicians who assess, screen, and play an active role in the recognition and management of cancer survivor mood disorders. Early symptom recognition and diagnosis requires a multiprofessional psychological treatment approach that includes illness navigation, pharmacologic management, behavioral intervention programs, and psychotherapy that assist the cancer survivor and family throughout the cancer survivorship journey.

Living with cancer is living with symptoms associated with disease control and cure. Professional guidelines for practitioners promote adequate symptom management from cancer diagnosis through the uncertainty of illness treatment, cure, remission, recurrence, advanced disease, and/or terminal disease. Clinician's primary concern for patients and families is to provide comfort through symptom management, education, instruction, and interventions that diminish suffering and improve the quality of life for cancer survivors.

CASE STUDY **Part 1**

Directions: Discuss the biopsychosocial aspects of the following unfolding case study utilizing your knowledge of family dynamics, cancer symptom management, end of life, hospice/palliative care, and community health nursing. Include your ethical and advanced directives knowledge.

Gayle: Going Home

Gayle is a 58-year-old woman who was diagnosed with stage IV ovarian cancer 2 years ago. Primary treatment included pelvic exoneration surgery, insertion of chest Infusaport for chemotherapy infusion, and a Greenfield filter. Gayle received 6 months of intravenous chemotherapy. She was admitted to the hospital 3 days ago with a bowel obstruction, dehydration, and failure-to-thrive (this is the third admission for these same symptoms in the past month). After discussing possible further treatment with her physician (i.e., more chemotherapy, potential inclusion into a clinical trial, possible bone marrow transplant), Gayle and her husband, Tom, have decided to not continue further treatment and let "nature take its course." Gayle states, "I have lost 70 pounds in the last 10 months and I am now at 74 pounds. My body, mind, and spirit tell me I have had enough. I am at peace with this decision, please help me be comfortable."

As the RN caring for Gayle in the hospital, you have contacted the home hospice service about Gayle's wishes to go home. Your goal is to make the transition as easy as possible and alleviate persistent symptoms of abdominal pain, fatigue, anorexia, nausea, and constipation. The hospice nurse comes to the hospital to visit Gayle and Tom before she is discharged from the hospital. Tom confides to the hospice nurse that he is nervous and anxious to get his wife home. "I don't know what to expect once I get her home." "Do I have enough pain medicine for her and what if I run out?" "Will I be able to keep her comfortable?" "How will I know if she is actively dying?" "I am scared."

• Discussion Questions **Part 1**

1. What equipment, medications, and strategies would you discuss with Tom to assist with Gayle's symptoms?
2. As the hospice nurse, describe what you would assess once you arrived to Gayle and Tom's home for the first time?
3. Identify pharmacologic management of Gayle's pain, nausea, anorexia, malabsorption, and fatigue.
4. Discuss the dynamics of Gayle's psychological distress and strategies to promote well-being.

CASE STUDY **Part 2**

Three weeks after going home, Gayle becomes unconscious. The hospice nurse comes to make an assessment and to speak with Tom. Both agree that Gayle appears to be comfortable, though her breathing is quite labored. The hospice nurse recommends some morphine for this. Tom is afraid to give this to her, as he states, "I don't want to give her too many drugs or I will kill her. " You reassure him that he would not be giving her too much and that the goal of care is to keep his wife comfortable. You commend him on the excellent job he has done in honoring his wife's wishes of "just keep me comfortable." Five hours later, Gayle died.

• Discussion Questions **Part 2**

1. How would you address the statement "I don't want to give her too many drugs or I will kill her."
2. Describe the potential for using evidence-based practice in this situation.
3. What future research studies could be developed in similar situations?

References

Aaronson, L. S., Teel, C. S., Cassmeyer, V., Neuberger, G. B., Pallikkathayil, L., Pierce J., ... Wingate A. (1999). Defining and measuring fatigue. *Image—The Journal of Nursing Scholarship, 31*(1), 45–50.

American Cancer Society. (2014). Retrieved June 10, 2014 from http://www.cancer.org/

American Psychological Association (APA). (2013). *Diagnostic and statistical manual of mental disorders* (5th ed.). Washington, DC: American Psychological Association.

Anderson, J. G., & Gill Taylor, A. (2012). Use of complementary therapies for cancer symptom management: Results of the 2007 National Health Interview Survey. *Journal of Alternative and Complementary Medicine, 18*(3), 235–241. doi:10.1089/acm.2011.0022

Beck, A. T., Epstein, N., Grown, G., & Steer, R. A. (1988). An inventory for measuring clinical anxiety: Psychometric properties. *Journal of Consulting and Clinical Psychology, 56*(6), 893–897. doi:10.1037/0022-006X.56.6.893

Beck, A. T., Steer, R. A., & Brown, G. K. (2006). Beck Depression Inventory®—II (BDI®–II). Retrieved August 25, 2006 from http://harcourtassessment.com

Berger, A. M. (2009). Update on the state of the science: Sleep-wake disturbances in adult patients with cancer. *Oncology Nursing Forum, 36*(4), E165–E177.

Berger, A. M., NCCN Clinical Practice Guidelines in Oncology (NCCN Guidelines®) for Cancer Related Fatigue V.1. (2014). © 2014 National Comprehensive Cancer Network, Inc. Retrieved October 1, 2014 from NCCN.org.

Bisaga, W., Dorazil, M., Dobrogowski, J., & Wordliczek, J. (2010). A comparison of the usefulness of selected neuropathic pain scales in patient with chronic pain syndromes: A short communication. *Advances in Palliative Care, 9*(4), 117–121.

Boyle, D. A. (2006). Survivorship. *Clinical Journal of Oncology Nursing, 10*(3). 407–422.

Brant, J. M., & Wickham, R. S. (Eds.). (2004). *Statement on the scope and standards of oncology nursing practice.* Pittsburgh, PA: Oncology Nursing Society.

Crump-Woodward, S. (2011). Cognitive-behavior therapy for insomnia in patients with cancer. *Clinical Journal of Oncology Nursing, 15*(4), E42–E52. doi:10.1188/11

Davidson, J. R., Feldman-Stewart, D., Brennenstuhl, S., & Ram, S. (2007). How to provide insomnia interventions to people with cancer: Insights from patients. *Psycho-oncology, 16*(11), 1028–1038. doi:10.1002/pon.1183

Davidson, J. R., MacLean, A. W., Brundage, M. D., & Schulze, K. (2002). Sleep disturbance in cancer patients. *Social Science Medicine, 54,* 1309–1321.

Davies, A. (2011). The management of breakthrough cancer pain. *British Journal of Nursing, 20*(13), 803–807.

Davis, J., Ahlberg, F. M., Berk, M., Ashley, D. M., & Khasraw, M. (2013). Emerging pharmacotherapy for cancer patients with cognitive dysfunction. *BMC Neurology, 13,* 153–162. doi:101186/1471-2377-13-153

Deimling, G. T., Kahana, B., Bowman, K. F., & Schaefer, M. L. (2002). Cancer survivorship and psychological distress in later life. *Psycho-Oncology, 11*(6), 479–494.

Denlinger, C. S., Ligibel, J.A., Demark-Wahnefried, W., Dizon, D., Goldman, M., Jones, L.,... NCCN Clinical Practice Guidelines in Oncology (NCCN Guidelines®) for Survivorship V.2. (2014). © 2014 National Comprehensive Cancer Network, Inc. Retrieved October 1, 2014 from NCCN.org

DeSantis, C. E., Lin, C. C., Mariotto, A. B., Siegel, R. L., Stein, K. D., & Kramer, J. L.,...Jemal, A. (2014). Cancer treatment and survivorship statistics, 2014. *CA Cancer Journal for Clinicians, 64*(4), 252–271. Published online June 1, 2014. doi:10.3322/caac.21235

Dugan, W., McDonald, M. V., Passik, S. D., Rosenfeld, B. D., Theobald, D., & Edgerton, S. (1998). Use of the Zung self rating depression scale in cancer patients: Feasibility as a screening tool. *Psycho-Oncology, 7*(6), 483–493. doi:10.1002/(SICI)1099-1611(199811/12)

Dulko, D., Pace C. C., Dittius, K. L., Spraque, B. L., Pollack, L. A., Hawkins, N. A., & Geller, B. M. (2013). Barriers and facilitators to implementing cancer survivorship care plans. *Oncology Nursing Forum, 40*(6), 575–580. doi:101188/13

Ettinger, D.S., et al., NCCN Clinical Practice Guidelines in Oncology (NCCN Guidelines®) for Antiemesis V.2. 2014. © 2014 National Comprehensive Cancer Network, Inc. Retrieved October 1, 2014 from NCCN.org.

Ferrell, B. R., & Coyle, N. (2006). *Textbook of palliative care* (2 nd ed). New York: Oxford University Press.

Fleishman, S. (2012). *Manual of cancer treatment recovery what the practitioner needs to know and do.* New York: Demos Medical.

Flynn, K. E., Shelby, R. A., Mitchell, S. A., Fawzy, M. R., Hardy, N. C., Husain, A. M.,...Weinfurt, K.P. (2010). Sleep-wake functioning along the cancer continuum: Focus group results from the Patient- Reported Outcomes Measurement Information System (PROMIS®). *Psycho-Oncology, 19*(10), 1086–1093. doi:10.1002/pon.1664

Foley, E., Baillie, A., Huxter, M., Price, M., & Sinclair, E. (2010). Mindfulness-based cognitive therapy for individuals whose lives have been affected by cancer: A randomized controlled trial. *Journal of Consulting and Clinical Psychology, 78*, 72–79. doi:10.1037/a0017566

Feldt, K. S. (2000). The checklist of nonverbal pain indicators (CNPI). *Pain Management Nursing, 1*, 13–21.

Feldt, K. S., Ryden, M. B., & Miles, S. (1998). Treatment of pain in cognitively impaired compared with cognitively intact elder patients with hip fracture. *Journal of American Geriatric Society, 46*, 1079–1985.

Healthcare Technology Systems. (2006). Hamilton Anxiety Scale (HAMA)—IVR version. Retrieved August 25, 2006 from http://www.healthtechsys.com/ivr/assess/ivrhama.html

Herr, K., Bjoro, K., & Decker, S. (2006) Tools for assessment in pain in non-verbal older adults with dementia: A state of the art science review. *Journal of Pain Symptom Management, 31*(2), 170–192.

Herr, K., Spratt, K.F., Garand, L., & Li, L. (2007). Evaluation of the Iowa pain thermometer and other selected pain intensity scales in younger and older adult cohorts using controlled clinical pain: A preliminary study. *Pain Medicine, 8*(7), 585–600.

Hurley, A. C., Volicer, B. J., Hanrahan, P. A., Houde, S., & Volicer, L. (1992). Assessment of discomfort in advanced Alzheimer patients. *Restorative Nursing Health, 15*,369–377.

Institute of Medicine (IOM). (2008). *Cancer care for the whole patient.* Washington, DC: The National Academies Press.

Institute of Medicine (IOM). (2013). *Delivering high-quality cancer care: Charting a new course for a system in crisis.* Retrieved June 12, 2014 from www.iom.edu/reports/2013/

Jung-Eun, E. K., Dodd, M. J., Aouizerat, B. E., Jahan, T., & Miaskowski, C. (2009). A review of the prevalence and impact of multiple symptoms in oncology patients. *Journal of Pain and Symptom Management, 37*(4) 715–736.

Kuchinski, S. M., Reading, M., & Lash, A. A. (2009). Treatment-related fatigue and exercise in patients with cancer: A systematic review. *Medsurg Nursing, 18*(3) 174–180.

Kwekkeboom, K., Cherwin, C., Lee, J., & Wanta, B. (2010). Mind-body treatments for the pain-fatigue-sleep disturbance symptom cluster in persons with cancer. *Journal of Pain Symptom and Management. 39*(1), 126–138. doi:10.1016/j.jpainsymman.2009.05.022

Langford, D. J., Lee, K., & Miaskowski, C. (2012). Sleep disturbance interventions in oncology patients and family caregivers: A comprehensive review and meta-analysis. *Sleep Medicine Review, 16*, 397–414. doi:10.1016/j.smrv.2011.07.002

Larouche, S., & Edgar, L. (2004). The measure of distress: A practical thermometer for outpatient screening. *Oncology Exchange, 3*(3), 34–39. Retrieved July 5, 2005 from http://www.oncolo gyex.com/gif/archive/2004/vol3_no3/continuing_care.pdf

Lasheen, W., Walsh, D., Mahmoud, F., Davis, M. P., Rivera, N., & Khoshknabi, D. L. (2010). Methylphenidate side effects in advanced cancer; a retrospective analysis. *American Journal of Hospital Palliative Care, 27*(1), 16–23. doi:10.1177/1049909109345145

Lee, K. A., Hicks, G., & Nino-Murcia, G. (1991). Validity and reliability of a scale to assess fatigue. *Psychiatry Research, 36*, 291–298.

Lethborg, C. E., Kissane, D., Bursn, W. I., & Snyder, R. (2000). "Cast Adrift": The experience of completing treatment among women with early stage breast cancer. *Journal of Psychosocial Oncology, 18*, 73–90. doi:10.1300/J077v18n04

Lippincott. (2014). *Manual of nursing practice* (9th ed.). Phildelphia, PA: Wolters Kluwer/Lippincott Williams & Wilkins. Chapter 57.

Lou, Y., Yates, P., McCarthy, A., & Wang, H. (2013). Fatigue self-management: A survey of Chinese cancer patients undergoing chemotherapy. *Journal of Clinical Nursing, 22*(7/8), 1053–1065. doi:10.1111/jocn.12174

Lowe, B., Kroenke, K., Herzog, W., & Grafe, K. (2004). Measuring depression outcome with a brief self-report instrument: Sensitivity to change of the Patient Health Questionnaire PHQ-9. *Journal of affective disorders, 81*(1), 61–66. doi:10.1016/S0165-0327(03)00198-8

Madden, J. (2006). The problem of distress in patients with cancer: More effective assessment. *Clinical Journal of Oncology Nursing, 10*(5), 615–619.

McCorkle, R., & Young, K. (1978). Development of a symptom distress scale. *Cancer Nursing, 1*, 373–378.

Miller, K., Merry, B.A., & Miller, J. (2008). Seasons of survivorship revisited. *Cancer Journal, 14*(6), 369–374. doi:10.1097/PPO.0b013e31818edf60

Mitchell A. J., Chan, M., Bhatti, H., Halton, M., Grassi, L., Johansen, C., & Meader, N. (2011). Prevalence of depression, anxiety, and adjustment disorder in oncological, haematological, and palliative-care settings: A meta-analysis of 94 interview based studies. *Lancet Oncology, 12*(2), 160–174. doi:10.1016/S1470-2045(11)70002-X

Mitchell, A. J., Ferguson, D. W., Gill, J., Paul, J., & Symonds, P. (2013). Depression and anxiety in long term cancer survivors compared with spouses and health controls: A systematic review and meta-analysis. *The Lancet Oncology, 14*, 721–732. Retrieved from http://dx.doi.org/10.1016/S1470-2045(13)70244-4

Mock, V., Frangakis, C., Davidson, N. E., Ropka, M. E., Pickett, M., Poniatowski, B., ... McCorkle, R. (2005). Exercise manages fatigue during breast cancer treatment: A randomized controlled trial. *Psychooncology, 14*(6), 464–477.

Moyer, A., Goldenberg, M., & Hall, M. A. (2012). Mediators of change in psychosocial interventions for cancer patients: A systematic review. *Behavioral Medicine, 38*(3), 90–114. doi:10.1080/08964289.2012.695412

Mullan, F. (1983). *Vital signs: A young doctor's struggle with cancer.* Boston, MA: Farrar, Straus and Giroux.

Mullan F. (1985). Seasons of survival: Reflections of a physician with cancer. *New England Journal of Medicine, 313*, 270–273.

Mustian, K. M., Morrow, G. R., Carroll, J. K., Figueroa-Moseley, C. D., Jean-Pierre, P., & Williams, G. C. (2007). Integrative nonpharmacologic behavioral interventions for the management of cancer related fatigue. *Oncologist, 12*(Suppl 1), 52–67.

Comprehensive Care Network® (2014). NCCN® Clinical Practice Guidelines in Oncology. Retrieved from http://www.nccn.org/professionals/physician_gls

Nettina, S. M. (2014). *Lippincott manual of nursing practice* (10th ed.). Philadelphia, PA: Wolters Kluwer Health/Lippincott Williams & Wilkins.

Oniszczenko, W., & Laskowska, A. (2014). Emotional reactivity, coping style and cancer trauma symptoms. *Arch Medical Science, 10*(1), 110–116. doi:10.5114/aoms.2013.33069

Pasacreta, J., Minarik, P., & Nield-Anderson, L. (2006). Anxiety and depression. In B. R. Ferrell, & N. Coyle. (Eds.), *Textbook of palliative nursing* (2nd ed., pp. 375–400). New York: Oxford University Press.

Peplau, H. (1983). *Living and learning (Lecture).* Hartford, CT: Institute of Living. October 28.

Piper, B. F., Lindsey, A. M., Dodd, M. J., Kerketich, S., Paul, S. M., & Weller, S. (1989). The development of an instrument to measure the subjective dimension of fatigue. In S.G. Funk, E.M. Tornquist, M.T. Champagne, L.A. Copp, & R. Wiese (Eds.), *Key aspects of comfort* (pp. 199–208). New York: Springer.

Priest, H. M. (2006). Helping student nurses to identify and respond to the psychological needs of physically ill patients: Implications for curriculum design. *Nurse Education Today, 26*(5), 423–429.

Rayner, L., Lee, W., Price, A., Monroe, B., Sykes, N., Hansford, P., ... Hotopf M. (2010).The clinical epidemiology of depression in palliative care and the predictive value of somatic symptoms: Cross-sectional survey with four-week follow-up. *Palliative Medicine, 25*, 229–241.

Rhoten, D. (1982). Fatigue and postsurgical patient. In C. M. Norris (Ed.), *Concept clarification in nursing* (277–300). Rockville, MD: Aspen.

Shaw, C., & Taylor, L. (2012). Treatment-related diarrhea in patients with cancer. *Clinical Journal of Oncology Nursing, 16*(4), 413–417.

Snaith, R. (2003). The Hospital Anxiety and Depression Scale. *Health and Quality of Life Outcomes, 1*,29. Retrieved August 25, 2006 from http://www.hqlo.com/content/1/1/29

Snow, A. L., Weber, J. B., O'Malley, K. J., Cody, M., Beck, C., Bruera, E., ... Kunik, M.C. (2004). NOPAIN: A nursing assistant administered pain assessment instrument for use in dementia. *Dementia Geriatric Cognitive Disorder, 17*, 240–246.

Swann, J. (2010). Pain: Causes, effects and assessments. *Nursing and Residential Care, 12*(5), 212–215.

Swarm, R. A., et al., NCCN Clinical Practice Guidelines in Oncology (NCCN Guidelines®) for Adult Cancer Pain V.2. 2014. © 2014 National Comprehensive Cancer Network, Inc. Retrieved October 1, 2014 from NCCN.org

Tack, B. (1991). *Dimensions and correlated of fatigue in older adults with rheumatoid arthritis.* Unpublished doctoral dissertation. San Francisco, CA: University of California.

Tedeschi, R. G., & Calhoun, L. G. (2004). Posttraumatic growth: Conceptual foundations and empirical evidence. *Psychology Inquiry, 15*, 1–8.

Torta, R. G., & Ieraci, V. (2013). Pharmacological management of depression in patients with cancer: Practical considerations. *Drugs, 73*, 1131–1145. doi:10.1007/s40265-013-0090-7

Tyson, S. F., & Brown, P. (2014). How to measure pain in neurological conditions? A systematic review of psychometric properties and clinical utility of measurement tools. *Clinical Rehabilitation, 28*(7), 669–686. doi:01177/0269215513514231

Vallerand, A., & Sanoski, C. A., (2014). *Davis drug guide for nurses* (14th ed.). Philadelphia, PA: F.A. Davis Co.

Vena, C., Parker, K. P., Allen, R., Bliwise, D. L., Jain, S., & Kimble, L. (2006). Sleep-wake disturbances and quality of life in patients with advanced lung cancer. *Oncology Nursing Forum, 33*, 761–769. doi:10.1188/06.ONF.761-769

CHAPTER 3

PSYCHOLOGICAL DISTRESS

"From the moment I was told I had cancer, I have had this feeling of pervasive uneasiness. No matter what I do, I cannot shake the feeling. I see the world as black and white, no longer in color. I worry about being able to work and provide for my family as well as having insurance to pay for my health bills. I learned quickly who my friends were, and from whom I could ask for a favor. I worry that I am asking too much of my wife and my son. I worry about the cancer coming back. I always feel as if a sword is hanging over my head. I am convinced God has abandoned me."

—A cancer survivor

Key Terms

activities of daily living • family relationships • medical treatments • personal concerns • psychological distress • social support • spirituality

Upon completing this chapter, you will be able to do the following:

1. Define psychological distress.
2. Discuss the importance of screening for psychological distress.
3. Describe the influencing factors of psychological distress
4. Describe the use of the Distress Thermometer for psychological distress.
5. Discuss the role of nursing in addressing psychological distress.

Introduction

At the time of diagnosis, the patient with cancer marshals his/her inner strength to deal with the journey that lies ahead. A barrage of additional diagnostic procedures, decisions regarding treatments and their side effects, and the specter of a life-threatening illness, all challenge an individual diagnosed with cancer to maintain a routine that brings some order to the chaos that they are dealing with. Depending on the prescribed treatment(s), the individual may be able to maintain a routine that resembles life before diagnosis. The new routine may resemble what was before, but for many patients, a diagnosis of cancer shifts the sand beneath their feet and life does not feel routine or "normal." Historically, and in a practical sense, much of the emphasis of cancer care focused on the physical side effects of cancer treatments, which is the more immediate issue. One side effect that has not received sufficient attention is the impact of cancer on the individual's psyche and in fact, the care of the psychological side effects has lagged behind the care directly related to the disease (Institute of Medicine [IOM], 2008).

The lag in psychological care may be attributable to medicine's primary focus of "diagnosis, cure, and cost." Institutions have compounded the problem of psychological care by limiting the number of experts with mental healthcare background on healthcare teams (Pasacreta, Kenefick, & McCorkle, 2008). The limited number may be due to the salaries of these experts and, perhaps, their underutilization due to lack of appropriate referrals. In addition, patients perceive the stigma associated with the words "psychological," "psychiatric," and "emotional" as barriers to discussing their distress with healthcare providers and frequently do not discuss the full extent of the experience (Holland, 2014). Furthermore, the urging by physicians to fight and be positive concerning the cancer has been shown to be viewed by patients with cancer as a barrier to expressing their level of distress (Byrne, Ellershaw, Holcombe, & Salmon, 2002) as is the perception by patients not to reveal their distress to their physicians (Sellick & Edwardson, 2007). In addition, physicians may perceive psychological distress solely as a normal consequence of a diagnosis of cancer and not perceive the importance of providing referrals for appropriate psychological care (Greer, 2008).

For many patients, just the diagnosis of cancer alone generates a feeling of uncertainty (Kornblith, 1998) and part of the issue of cancer survivorship, which lasts from the moment of diagnosis until death (National Cancer Institute, 2010), is the uncertainty of sustaining remission and fear of recurrence. The feeling of uncertainty may exist despite aggressive and improved treatments (Zebrack, 2000) and persist beyond the treatment period (Henselmans, et al., 2010). The uncertainty associated with the diagnosis of cancer may give rise to psychological distress (Lubkin & Larsen, 2013), emphasizing the importance of understanding and discussing what psychological distress is, and what nurses and other healthcare providers can do to assist patients who report that they are experiencing it.

As survivorship becomes a reality for an increasing number of patients diagnosed with cancer, the need for interventions focused on the subjective experience of the survivors has become increasingly more important. Concerned about the lack of appropriate psychological care, the IOM (2008) has recommended the provision of funds to educate healthcare practitioners about the need for addressing the psychological care of cancer patients.

The National Comprehensive Cancer Network (NCCN) has recognized the presence and detrimental effects of psychological distress and has developed guidelines to assist healthcare practitioners in understanding, diagnosing, and treating patients experiencing this phenomenon (2014). Since 1999, NCCN has made available clinical guidelines for the management of psychological distress. These guidelines outline standards of care, provide a screening tool for assessment of psychological distress, and clinical pathways for treatment (Holland, 2014). The NCCN Clinical Practice Guidelines In

Oncology (NCCN Guidelines) for Distress Management are updated annually, ensuring that the latest information and treatment options are available to healthcare practitioners in the field of oncology.

In response to the IOM, The American College of Surgeons' Commission on Cancer has established two standards for accreditation addressing psychological care of cancer patients (2012). Standard 3.2 requires that psychological distress screening be conducted by a mental health professional whose expertise is in the psychosocial needs of cancer patients. Included in the standard is an outline indicating the requirements for timing, the method and tool to be used, assessment and referral process, as well as the necessary documentation. The standard does not specify which tool be used to screen psychological distress but does specify that it must be a standardized tool. Standard 3.3 outlines the requirements for survivorship care plans which includes documentation indicating assessment and implementation.

What Is Psychological Distress?

Psychological distress is a multifaceted, complex concept defined as a "multifactorial unpleasant emotional experience of a psychological (cognitive, behavioral, emotional), social, and/or spiritual nature that may interfere with the ability to cope effectively with cancer, its physical symptoms, and its treatment" (Holland, 2014). Psychological distress is also a "reaction to internal and external demands characterized by a heterogeneous set of psychological symptoms" (Antoine, Antoine, & Nandrino, 2008, p. 1175). Psychological distress exists on a continuum with anxiety and depression at the extreme end of clinical manifestations with sadness at the other end (Holland, 2014).

Psychological distress may occur at any point during the cancer experience, from the emergence of a clinical manifestation that inititiates the entry to healthcare system until death (Holland, 2014). Among all patients with cancer, psychological distress has been reported to be experienced by 35.1% (Zabora, Brintzenhofeszoc, Curbow, Hooker, & Piantadosi, 2001). The highest prevalence is among patients with lung cancer with reported ranges from 43.4% (Zabora et al., 2001) to 51% (Steinberg, et al., 2009), but high rates have also been reported among patients with advanced and recurring cancer of all sites (Arden-Close, Gidron, & Moss-Morris, 2008) and patients awaiting bone marrow transplants (Trask, et al., 2002). In addition, when comparing women and men, women are more likely to report that they are experiencing psychological distress as well as at higher levels (Enns, et al., 2013; Kantor, 2013).

The severity of psychological distress may fluctuate depending on where the patient is in terms of the cancer experience and whether the patient is dealing with the first diagnosis or recurrence (Zebrack, 2000). Psychological distress has also been reported to be higher in individuals approaching death (Gao, Bennett, Stark, Murray, & Higginson, 2010). This is consistent with Lazarus' (1999) view that the more catastrophic the individual perceives the cancer, the greater the psychological disturbances the individual is likely to experience.

Consequences of Psychological Distress

The need to understand, recognize, and screen for the presence of psychological distress is made clearer by its consequences. Psychological distress has been associated with a decrease in quality of life (Pasacreta et al., 2008; Thekkumpurath, Venkateswaran, Kumar, & Bennett, 2008). Psychological distress has also been associated with a decrease in cognition as well as a decrease in motivation which may then lead to decreased adherence to treatment regimens (Chen, et al., 2009; Jacobsen, et al., 2005; Madden, 2006;Ransom, Jacobsen, & Booth-Jones, 2006) and decreased survival rates (Hamer, Chida, & Molloy, 2009).

In addition, the higher the level of psychological distress, the lower the patient's perception of potential of survival (Hamer et al., 2009) and sense of control (Baker, Marcellus, Zabora, Polland, & Jodrey, 1997). Psychological distress has been associated with increased physical symptoms such as fatigue and pain (Bultz & Holland, 2006), side effects of radiation (Chen, et al., 2009), the side effects of chemotherapy (Trask, et al., 2002), and other general symptoms (Gibson, Lichtenthal, Berg, & Breitbart, 2006). Psychological distress has also been associated with difficulty coping (IOM, 2008), inability to sleep, decreased energy and motivation (Chen, et al., 2009), and financial worries (Bultz & Holland, 2006).

The NCCN (Holland, 2014) refers to psychological distress as "distress" because patients may feel a stigma when the words "psychological," "psychiatric," or "emotional" are included. In this textbook, the word "psychological" is used in conjunction with the word "distress" in order to differentiate the concept from spiritual distress (Kristeller, Zumbrun, & Schilling, 1999), moral distress (Hanna, 2004), and symptom distress (McCorkle & Young, 1978).

Measuring Psychological Distress

In the past, more than 40 scales have been used to measure psychological distress and the majority of these instruments focus on anxiety and depression (Vodermaier, Lindin, & Siu, 2009). The concept of psychological distress is broader than the clinical manifestations of anxiety and depression. Therefore, those scales are not effective tools in describing the patients' experiences with psychological distress. In addition, the large number of instruments utilized to measure psychological distress led to a lack of a uniform approach to identify patients experiencing the phenomenon and adequately measuring the degree of psychological distress among patients with cancer.

Two of these earlier instruments frequently used for assessment of psychological distress in patients with cancer are the Brief symptom inventory (BSI) and the Hospital anxiety and depression scale (HADS), originally developed for psychiatric patients (Thomas, Mohan, Thomas, & Pandey, 2002). The HADS scale has two subscales, anxiety and depression, and focuses on symptomatology related to these two disorders (Thekkumpurath et al., 2008) such as worrying, being fearful, and feeling tense. The BSI tool addresses nine symptom dimensions contained within three global scales and nine subscales that not only include anxiety and depression but also obsession-compulsion and hostility. Both instruments have high cut-offs focusing on those patients with high levels of anxiety and depression, therefore eliminating patients who are at lower levels or who are experiencing clinical manifestations other than anxiety and depression.

Given the context of a life-threatening illness, anxiety and depression is predictable for patients with a diagnosis of cancer (Ryan, et al., 2005), and most patients marshal their coping methods and demonstrate resilience (Wool & Mor, 2005). Wool and Mor (2005) stated that the depression noted in patients with cancer may be related to specific cancers in which there is a delay in seeking a diagnosis, hence the disease being more wide spread. Coordinators at bone marrow transplant centers perceived psychological distress as "synonymous" with anxiety while patients perceived psychological distress as synonymous with depression (Trask, et al., 2002). This study also revealed that the coordinators underestimated the number of patients who were experiencing psychological distress.

The focus on the manifestations of anxiety and depression may originate from healthcare providers perceiving these reactions as the priority as well as the ease of administration of the most frequently used tools for assessment of psychological distress, which, as stated previously, focus on anxiety and depression. The emergence of studies looking at the concept of demoralization as experienced by these patients reflects the growing understanding of the differences regarding anxiety and depression in this patient population (Cherny, 2010).

Recognizing the need for an easy-to-administer screening tool, the NCCN developed the distress thermometer (DT) and Problem List to screen for psychological distress. Available since the Fall of 1999, the DT is a self-administered visual analog scale and asks patients to rate their degree of psychological distress on a scale of 0 to 10, with 0 indicating no distress and 10 indicating extreme distress (Fig. 3.1). The tool also provides patients the opportunity to identify the source of their distress but these responses are not part of the computed score. The score of 4 or more on the DT as a cut-off for moderate to severe psychological distress, was established by a study that compared the

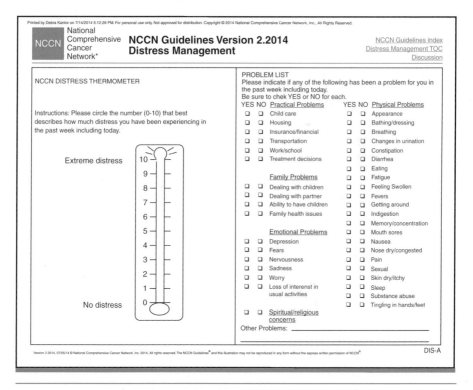

Figure 3.1 • NCCN guidelines version 2.2014: Distress management. (Holland, J. C. (2014). NCCN Clinical Practice Guidelines in Oncology (NCCN Guidelines) Distress Management Version 2. © 2014 National Comprehensive Cancer Network, Inc. Retrieved from NCCN.org.)

DT with the BSI and HADS (Jacobsen, et al., 2005). The NCCN Guidelines for Distress Management V.2.2014 suggest referrals for patients reporting a distress level of 4 or higher (Holland, 2014). Since patients are able to identify sources of their psychological distress, the healthcare practitioner is cued in to what issues are contributing to the patient's subjective report.

As stated previously, the NCCN (Holland, 2014) has developed clinical practice guidelines for (psychological) distress management. The guidelines were created by expert panel members, comprising various members of the healthcare team, including nurses. The guidelines emphasize the need for a collaborative approach for early and appropriate identification of (psychological) distress and utilization of available resources to care for oncology patients. Within the distress management guidelines, nursing's role is identified at the assessment level, leaving interventions to social workers and pastoral members. However, nursing has a wide range of independent nursing interventions, including therapeutic communication and offering of self in assisting these patients.

Factors Influencing Psychological Distress

Psychosocial factors influencing psychological distress directly relate to the experience of patients diagnosed with cancer. These factors include medical treatments, personal concerns, family relationships, social support, spirituality, activities of daily living, and uncertainty. To fully understand the concept of psychological distress, a discussion of these factors is necessary.

Cancer has become a chronic disease due to the advancement of cancer treatments (IOM, 2008) and these treatments have inherent consequences including expected side effects, untoward side effects, and risks. Each patient must make decisions regarding treatment options that include specialists for each approach. Medical treatments often result in temporary or permanent disfigurement and/or functioning of body systems which may contribute to psychological distress (IOM, 2008). Medical treatments can lead to changes in role performance and interactions between the patients, their families, and friends. In addition, patients may have other co-morbidities such as cardiac, respiratory, or renal disease at the time of their cancer diagnosis, which may directly affect treatment options and overall prognosis

Patients diagnosed with cancer must contend with immediate, long-term, and late effects of the treatments. For example, patients undergoing surgical resection of a cancerous tumor must recover from the surgical procedure itself. The recovery period includes the direct effects of anesthesia; pain; decreased self-care ability; and, depending on the type of surgery, alteration in body image and disfigurement. In addition, the recovery period depends on factors such as age, type of cancer, and the extent of the surgery. General long-term and late effects of surgery include paresthesia, pain, loss of range of motion, and lymphedema.

Initial chemotherapy protocols for specific cancers such as breast, colon, and prostate cancer, have finite treatment lengths frequently lasting months. Metastatic disease treatments are often ongoing and last as long as the patient survives and/or the side effects are tolerable. A wide range of side effects of chemotherapy exists. Some side effects are immediate such as nausea and vomiting, anemia, hair loss, and weight loss. Other side effects are categorized as long term and late effects, such as fatigue, hair loss, weight gain, changes in sexual function, and neuropathy. An additional side effect of chemotherapy and/or radiation is the emergence of secondary cancers because of the carcinogenic effects of these treatments.

Personal concerns are the specific concerns related to the diagnosis of cancer. These include fear of recurrence and self-perception of body image. Others are financial worries, side effects of treatments, and sustaining the day-to-day routines and role expectations.

A primary issue for patients diagnosed with cancer is the fear of recurrence described by some as the "sword of Damocles." The more advanced the cancer at the time of diagnosis the greater the fear of recurrence (Kornblith, 1998) and the greater the level of psychological distress (Levin & Kissane, 2006). In addition, patients who have experienced recurrence have greater levels of psychological distress than patients who remain cancer free (Burgess et al., 2005).

Patients diagnosed with cancer face changes in their health status and the impact of cancer on various areas of their lives. These areas include changes in body functions and personal appearance from the side effects of treatments. In addition, there may be a financial impact along with the ability to continue to work, family and social relationships, side effects such as fatigue and pain, and the ability to conduct and carry out normal activities of daily living.

A diagnosis of cancer frequently causes patients to assess their personal values and beliefs and re-order their priorities. A qualitative study of 59 women with breast cancer (Arman, Rehnsfeldt, Carlsson, & Hamrin, 2001) revealed that the participants had developed an increased positive outlook on life and that life gave them a "deeper value" (p.196). Another study (Rinaldis, Pakenham, & Lynch, 2010) of 1,757 participants diagnosed with colorectal cancer, of which 59.9% were men, revealed an increase in interpersonal growth in areas of "increased awareness, appreciation, and quality of relationships with others; and acceptance" (p. 270).

The literature also reports that a diagnosis of cancer "erodes self-concept and confidence" (Emmanuel, Ferris, von Gunten, & Van Roenn, 2011) and leads to the emergence of "problems associated with personal and relationship issues [which] are commonly manifested in the form of psychological distress" (Sellick & Edwardson, 2007, p. 535). In addition, studies have indicated that patients diagnosed with cancer report a loss of control and mastery, leading to greater difficulty in psychological adjustment (Thompson & Collins, 1995). One qualitative study of 16 participants (Taylor, Richardson, & Cowley, 2010) treated for colorectal cancer revealed that participants sought to achieve a sense of control over their bodies but were not always successful. Another recent study of 133 women with breast cancer revealed a direct relationship between sense of control and the ability to adapt (Henselmans et al., 2010).

A consequence of the disease process and/or medical treatments is the inability to participate in self-care activities and "age-appropriate physical and cognitive activities" (IOM, 2008) at the levels prior to diagnosis. Body alterations and the presence and level of pain and fatigue may limit or cause fluctuations in an individual's ability to participate in self-care activities and may result in the need for assistance.

The ability to participate in activities of daily living and the inherent functional limitations due to treatments and/or disease progression has been studied in the literature. In one study, when compared to other individuals with the same age, gender, and level of education, adults with a history of cancer were more apt to request assistance with activities of daily living (Yancik & Ries, 2000). Another study revealed that cancer survivors without a history of other chronic illnesses when compared with individuals without a diagnosis of cancer or other chronic illnesses, reported a higher degree of difficulty in participating in activities of daily living (Grov, Fossa, & Dahl, 2010). A more recent study revealed among hospitalized elderly diagnosed with cancer, 38% were found to have difficulty participating in activities of daily living (Hamaker et al., 2011). Regarding older patients diagnosed with cancer, assessment of their ability to participate in activities of living has been encouraged because of the impact on their quality of life (Given & Given, 2010) and the limited resources and support that may exist.

A diagnosis of cancer permanently alters the lives of the patient and family members. The initial period of treatment may "set the tone for future spousal interactions" (Badr & Taylor, 2008, p. 616). Strong interpersonal relationships between the patient and spouse and other family members correlate negatively to psychological distress (Hagedoorn, Sanderman, Bolks, Tuinstra, & Coyne, 2008). Families with poor cohesiveness have been associated with poor psychosocial outcomes for all family members (Kissane, Bloch, McKenzie, McDowall, & Nitzan, 1998). Therefore, patient and family needs is an area that must be identified and included in the plan of care (Sellick & Edwardson, 2007).

Lewis (2010) discussed "stuck points" in terms of the family and adjustment to a cancer diagnosis. One stuck point is spouses not having the necessary skills to communicate with their spouse, and vice versa, thereby resulting in increased discordance in the marriage. Another is the effect of the patient and spouse's depression on other family members. A third is the effect of the marital tension on children, especially those still living in the home. A fourth is the coping methods utilized by the family members in an attempt to deal with the diagnosis of cancer.

The problems that arise between the patient diagnosed with cancer and the individual's relationships with others, are "commonly manifested" as psychological distress (Sellick & Edwardson, 2007). The impact of the cancer and cancer treatments result in "considerable emotional and social burden" on patients and families, which in turn is measurable in terms of clinical manifestations of psychological distress (Sellick & Edwardson, 2007). Studies have shown a direct relationship between unsupportive behavior from spouses and higher psychological distress (Druley & Townsend, 1998; Koopman, Hermanson, Diamond, Angell, & Spiegel, 1998).

The fish bowl–like existence of a cancer patient and family members uncovers the means in which a family communicates especially in high stress situations and illnesses such as cancer can alter family relationships. Family members of cancer survivors have reported reactions to the diagnosis that are greater than the survivors themselves, which may have a direct impact on family relationships (Bowman, Rose, & Deimling, 2006). In fact adjustments related to the caregiver role by the spouse establishes a change in the relationship between the patient with cancer and the spouse (Arrington, 2005).

A diagnosis of cancer can threaten the economic well-being of the family and may result in a change in which partner is the primary wage earner. In addition, there may be unexpected role changes for the cancer patient's spouse in regards to household chores as well as caregiver (Syse, Tretli, & Kravdal, 2009). A large population-based study of 1.1 million participants with 17, 250 cancer survivors revealed that female patients with cancer did not affect their spouses' salaries; however, male cancer patients adversely affected their wives' earnings (Syse, et al., 2009).

Other issues include the importance of close personal relationships to patients in the terminal stages of cancer and that the presence of family members and strong interpersonal relationships are "reasons for living" (Prince-Paul, 2008, p. 367). Patients diagnosed with cancer may feel the need to "protect" family members and friends and healthcare providers and not disclose their distress (Byrne et al., 2002). The primary caretaker of patients diagnosed with cancer due to cigarette smoking or other lifestyle choices may display anger toward the patient, which may result in inadequate or inconsistent care and support. In addition, the anger may also arise from lack of lifestyle changes after diagnosis.

Social support assists individuals in dealing with changes in health status and is derived from family, friends, and the community, which provide socio-economical, informational, and/or instrumental support. Social support may have a positive influence on the feeling of control over a health issue and may reduce "negative factors that cause social strain" (Sjölander & Berterö, 2008, p. 182). Success in establishing a new normal following a diagnosis of cancer has been associated with informal support networks (Wool & Mor, 2005). The presence of social support has been associated with improved adjustment to uncertainty in patients with breast cancer (Sammarco, 2001).

A diagnosis of cancer has specific needs brought on by the uniqueness of facing a life-threatening illness, which may require more long-term support from a wide range of sources. Social support was found to assist in the reappraisal of uncertainty associated with a life-threatening illness such as HIV/AIDS (Brashers, Neidig, & Goldsmith, 2004). Breast cancer patients with higher level of psychological distress required more social support than those with lower levels (Lepore, Glaser, & Roberts, 2008); patients with low social support have higher levels of psychological distress (Levin & Kissane, 2006; Thomas , Pandey, Ramdas, & Nair, 2002); and perceived social support reduced psychological distress in patients with advanced cancer (Zabalegui, 1997).

An established social support system contributes to the successful mediation of emotions by most patients upon learning of a diagnosis of cancer (Wool & Mor, 2005). This finding is consistent with studies of patients with other diagnoses. For example, a study of patients with coronary artery disease revealed a possible connection between social support and adherence to the medical regimen, improved dietary intake, and reduction of exposure to inherent stressors (Peterson, et al., 2010). A study of patients with HIV/AIDS confirmed the importance of outreach programs in improving retention of patients in treatment protocols through the provision of education, assistance with access and insurance, and referrals to formal support groups (Rajabiun, et al., 2007). A study of male patients with diabetes mellitus suggested a positive relationship between health benefits and reciprocal peer support (Helsler, Vijan, Makki, & Plette, 2010).

Spirituality is a personal experience and a standard definition for spirituality is elusive due to the subjectivity of the concept (Cawley, 1997). Coyle (2002) argued that spirituality is "defined within transcendence, value guidance, or religiosity" (p. 594) and that spirituality provides "meaning and purpose" for individuals. Transcendence is the belief of being connected to God or to higher being. Value guidance arises from one's beliefs and values and may lead to a sense of empowerment. Religiosity is connected to the practices and beliefs learned from being a member of an organized religion (Coyle, 2002). Together, these dimensions of spirituality may provide benefits when an illness occurs (Coyle, 2002). Spirituality "motivates, enables, empowers, and provides hope" (Coyle, 2002, p. 592). In differentiating spirituality from religion, spirituality is something that occurs at a personal level while religion occurs at the community or social level (Crane, 2009).

Due to the personal nature of spirituality, assessment of spiritual well-being may be difficult. However, omission of a spiritual assessment prevents a clear understanding because the actual impact of the cancer diagnosis may not be accurate. Both the IOM and the NCCN identified the need for the assessment of spiritual and religious concerns. The IOM identified spiritual and existential issues as part of the emotional health problems faced by patients diagnosed with cancer (2008). The clinical practice guidelines for distress management developed by the NCCN (Holland, 2014) include the spiritual dimension in its definition of distress. Within the NCCN Guidelines for Distress Management V.2.2014, oncology team members are expected to initiate referrals to pastoral services for treatment for spiritual and religious concerns. Specific areas for the clergy to address include both spiritual and religious concerns and the clergy may make additional referrals for social work or mental health services (Holland, 2014). Patients are given an opportunity to identify that they have spiritual/religious concerns in the problem list that accompanies the DT (Holland, 2014).

Numerous studies have been conducted regarding spirituality and a diagnosis of cancer. One study revealed that African-Americans have a strong belief in the relationship between spirituality and coping and surviving cancer (Schulz, et al., 2008). Another reported that older, more educated patients with long-term advanced cancer frequently report high levels of spiritual well-being with lower levels of anxiety and depressed mood (Blank & Bellizzi, 2008; Rose, et al., 2009). In addition, patients diagnosed with cancer have reported an increase in spirituality and spiritual practices (Becker-Schutte, 2003). Assessment of spiritual needs is not always conducted but certainly should be considered (see Chapter 18: "Role of the Clergy").

Healthcare providers through their role as professional providers of care, are able to reduce levels of uncertainty through their expertise in their discipline and the image and confidence that they project (Mishel & Clayton, 2008). The more trust and confidence the patient has in the healthcare provider, the more valuable the healthcare provider is in reducing the level of uncertainty (Mishel, 1988) and therefore the degree of psychological distress.

The ability to establish rapport, and therefore establish trust and confidence, is contingent on the communication skills of the healthcare provider (IOM, 2008) and extends beyond merely providing information concerning the illness or treatment options. The IOM has identified communication skills as an essential component not only in being valuable as a clinician but also in being a "supportive partner," which the IOM refers to as a characteristic of high-quality health care and healthcare professionals (2003). The IOM's recognition of the importance of communication and establishing rapport is consistent with Watson's Caring Science. Listed among the carative factors of Caring Science is the need to be "sensitive to one's self and to others" and "the development of a helping–trusting relationship" (Watson, 2005). Research has shown that caring interactions by nurses positively influence the emotional–spiritual, physical, and social well-being of patients (Swanson, 1999). Therefore, caring interactions, including the offering of self, establishing rapport, assessing and addressing patient concerns, and providing health education may directly impact the psychological distress of patients with cancer.

In a study of patients with HIV, the ability of the healthcare provider and patient to form a partnership in developing the plan of care was "important for patient uncertainty management" (Brashers, Hsieh, Neidig, & Reynolds, 2006, p. 224). A study of patients with inoperable lung cancer revealed the importance that these participants placed on being able to trust the professionals involved in their care in terms of information and care as well as support (Dale & Johnston, 2011). The influence that a nurse may have on reducing psychological distress was revealed in a study that examined the role of the oncology nurse navigator in psychological distress management. Psychological distress scores, as measured by the DT, were lower for patients of age 65 and younger who were seen by the oncology nurse navigator (Swanson & Koch, 2010).

Nursing Implications

Studies have shown that nurses, believing they lack the necessary skills to assess psychological factors, do not routinely screen for psychological distress (Fulcher & Gosselin-Acomb, 2007), cite discomfort regarding discussing "patient concerns" (Robbins, 2007), and demonstrate a "lack of awareness" (Fulcher & Gosselin-Acomb, 2007). In addition, lack of time and insufficient experience with screening tools has also been cited (Chen & Raingruber, 2014). Interpersonal skills, of which communication is a part, provide the opportunity not only to extract necessary information from the patient regarding their illness, but also to establish trust and rapport and engage in conversations geared toward the subjective experience of the illness. Since patients may be reluctant to express their feelings about their disease, nurses need to take the time to inquire and determine what assistance would benefit the patient.

Nurses are in the unique position through their contact with patients in various cancer treatment areas, to develop therapeutic relationships, assess patients, identify psychological distress, and make appropriate referrals. In order to provide holistic care, individualized plans of care and appropriate referrals are dependent on the appropriate assessment of psychological distress experienced by these patients. The ability to provide holistic care is dependent on an understanding of the physiological and psychological needs of the patient. Nurses should be made aware of resources such as the NCCN and the resources that they have to assist healthcare professionals who care for oncology patients. To view the most recent and complete version of the NCCN Guidelines, go online to NCCN.org. Referrals for patients with lower levels of psychological distress may include support groups, nutritionists, or clergy, and recognition of the need for a financial planner and earlier interventions may decrease the number of patients experiencing high levels of psychological distress.

Summary

Psychological distress is a multifaceted, complex concept defined as a "multifactorial unpleasant emotional experience of a psychological (cognitive, behavioral, emotional), social, and/or spiritual nature that may interfere with the ability to cope effectively with cancer, its physical symptoms, and its treatment" (Holland, 2014). While nurses are not the only ones who can assess for psychological distress, their understanding of the concept, what influences may exist, and the means to screen for it, will all contribute to improving the care that patients dealing with cancer receive. Ultimately, through their caring demeanor, communication skills, and advocacy role, nurses are frequently the positive influence in the patient's perception of their experience. The influencing factors of psychological distress are dynamic and fluctuate depending where the patient with cancer is in terms of the disease trajectory. An understanding of the psychosocial needs of these patients and including those needs in plans of care is essential in providing holistic care.

CASE STUDY

MJ, a 60-year-old male, has been diagnosed with Stage IV lung cancer following a 40-year history of cigarette smoking. Treatment has not yet begun, the patient is considering his options. His wife nor his three adult children smoke. All three children are married and live within a 30-minute drive. His wife is an elementary school teacher and works fulltime. The patient was asked to complete the DT by the nurse. He circled the number 8 on the scale and on the accompanying problem list, checked dealing with partner, worry, appearance, tingling in hands and feet, and spiritual/religious concerns.

1. What additional psychosocial assessments are necessary?
2. What interventions should the nurse consider?
3. What referrals would benefit this patient?
4. What psychosocial issues are the priorities for this patient?

References

American College of Surgeons. (2012). *Commission on cancer*. Retrieved August 11, 2014, from American College of Surgeons: https://www.facs.org/~/media/files/quality%20programs/cancer/coc/programstandards2012.ashx

Antoine, P., Antoine, C., & Nandrino, J. L. (2008). Development and validation of the cognitive inventory of subjective distress. *International Journal of Geriatric Psychiatry, 23*, 1175–1181.

Arden-Close, E., Gidron, Y., & Moss-Morris, R. (2008). Psychological distress and its correlates in ovarian cancer. *Psycho-Oncology, 17*, 1061–1072.

Arman, M., Rehnsfeldt, A., Carlsson, M., & Hamrin, E. (2001). Indications of change in life perspective among women with breast cancer admitted to complementary care. *European Journal of Cancer Care, (10)*, 192–200.

Arrington, M. I. (2005). "She's right behind me all the way": An analysis of prostate cancer narratives and changes in family relationships. *The Journal of Family Communication, 5*(2), 141–162.

Badr, H., & Taylor, C. L. (2008). Effects of relationship maintenance on psychological distress and dyadic adjustment among couples coping with lung cancer. *Health Psychology, 27*(5), 616–627.

Baker, F., Marcellus, D., Zabora, J., Polland, A., & Jodrey, D. (1997). Psychological distress among adult patients being evaluated for bone marrow transplantation. *Psychosomatics, 38*(1), 10–19.

Becker-Schutte, A. M. (2003). Exploring the experience of spirituality in midwestern American women with breast cancer. Retrieved from ProQuest Dissertations & Theses (288105040).

Blank, T. O., & Bellizzi, K. M. (2008). A gerontological perspective on cancer and aging: Multiple trajectories, multiple influences and differential outcomes. *Cancer, 112*, 2569–2576.

Bowman, K. F., Rose, J. H., & Deimling, G. T. (2006). Appraisal of the cancer experience by family members and survivors in long-term survivorship. *Psychooncology, 15*(9), 834–845.

Brashers, D. E., Hsieh, E., Neidig, J. L., & Reynolds, N. R. (2006). Managing uncertainty about illness: Health care providers as credible authorities. In R. M. Dailey, & B. A. LePoire

(Eds.), *Applied interpersonal communication matters: Family, health, and community relations* (pp. 219–240). New York, NY: Peter Lang Publishing.

Brashers, D. E., Neidig, J. L., & Goldsmith, D. J. (2004). Social support and the management of uncertainty for people living with HIV or AIDS. *Health Communication, 16*, 305–331.

Bultz, B. D., & Holland, J. C. (2006). Emotional distress in patients with cancer: The sixth vital sign. *Community Oncology, 3*(5), 311–314.

Burgess, C., Cornelius, V., Love, S., Graham, J., Richards, M., & Ramirez, A. (2005). *Depression and anxiety in women with early breast cancer: Five year observational study.* Retrieved June 6, 2010, from BMJ Online First: http://www.ncbi.nlm.nih.gov/pmc/articles/PMC555631/pdf/bmj33000702.pdf. doi:10.1136/bmj.38343.670868.D3

Byrne, A., Ellershaw, J., Holcombe, C., & Salmon, P. (2002). Patients' experience of cancer: Evidence of the role of 'fighting' in collusive clinical communication. *Patient Education and Counseling, 48*(1), 15–21.

Cawley, N. (1997). Towards defining spirituality: An exploration of the concept of spirituality. *International Journal of Palliative Nursing, 1*, 31–36.

Chen, A. M., Jennelle, R. L., Grady, V., Tovar, A., Bowen, K., Simonin, P., … Vijayakumar, S. (2009). Prospective study of psychological distress among patients undergoing radiotherapy for head and neck cancer. *International Journal Radiation Oncology, 73*(1), 187–193.

Chen, C., & Raingruber, B. (2014). Educational needs of inpatient oncology nurses in providing psychosocial care. *Clinical Journal of Oncology Nursing, 18*(1), E1–E5. doi: 10.1188/14.CJON.

Cherny, N. (2010). *Taxonomy of distress: Including spiritual suffering and demoralization.* Retrieved from Supportive Oncology: www.SupportiveOncology.net/journal/articles/0801013.pdf

Coyle, J. (2002). Spirituality and health: Towards a framework for exploring the relationship between spirituality and health. *Journal of Advanced Nursing, 37*(6), 589–597.

Crane, J. N. (2009). Religion and cancer: Examining the possible connections. *Journal of Psychosocial Oncology, 27*, 469–486. doi: 10.1080/07347330903182010

Dale, M. J., & Johnston, B. (2011). An exploration of the concerns of patients with inoperable lung cancer. *International Journal of Palliative Nursing, 17*(6), 285–290.

Druley, J. A., & Townsend, A. L. (1998). Self- esteem as a mediator between spousal support and depressive symptoms: A comparison of healthy individuals and individuals coping with arthritis. *Health Psychology, 17*, 255–261.

Emmanuel, L., Ferris, F. D., von Gunten, C. F., & Van Roenn, J. H. (2011). *EPEC-O palliative care educational materials.* Retrieved 2011, from National Cancer Institute: http://www.cancer.gov/cancertopics/cancerlibrary/epeco/selfstudy/module-4

Enns, A., Waller, A., Groff, S. L., Bultz, B. D., Fung, T., & Carlson, L. E. (2013). Risk factors for continuous distress over a 12-month period in newly diagnosed cancer patients. *Journal of Psychological Distress, 31*(5), 489–506. doi: 10.1018/07347332.2013.822052

Fulcher, C. D., & Gosselin-Acomb, T. K. (2007). Distress assessment: Practice change through guideline implementation. *Clinical Journal of Oncology Nursing, 11*(6), 817–821.

Gao, W., Bennett, M. I., Stark, D., Murray, S., & Higginson, I. J. (2010). Psychological distress in cancer from survivorship to end of life care: Prevalence, associated factors and clinical implications. *European Journal of Cancer, 46*, 2036–2044. doi: 10.1016/j.ejca.2010.03.033

Gibson, C. A., Lichtenthal, W., Berg, A., & Breitbart, W. (2006). Psychologic issues in palliative care. *Anesthesiology clinics of North America, 24*, 61–80.

Given, B. A., & Given, C. W. (2010). The older patient. In J. C. Holland, W. S. Breitbart, P. B. Jacobsen, M. S. Lederberg, M. J. Loscalzo, & R. McCorkle (Eds.), *Psycho-oncology* (2nd ed., pp. 491–496). Oxford: Oxford University Press.

Greer, S. (2008). CBT for emotional distress of people with cancer: Some personal observations. *Psycho-Oncology, 17*, 170–173. doi: 10.1002/pon.1205

Grov, E. K., Fossa, S. D., & Dahl, A. A. (2010). Activity of daily living problems in older cancer survivors: A population-based control study. *Health and social care in the community, 18*(4), 396–406.

Hagedoorn, M., Sanderman, R., Bolks, H. N., Tuinstra, J., & Coyne, J. C. (2008). Distress in couples coping with cancer: A meta-analysis and critical review of role and gender effects. *Psychological Bulletin, 134*(1), 1–30.

Hamaker, M. E., Buurman, B. M., van Munster, B. C., Kuper, I., Smorenburg, C. H., & de Rooij, S. E. (2011). The value of a comprehensive geriatric assessment for patient care in acutely hospitalized older patients with cancer. *The Oncologist, 16*(10), 1403–1412.

Hamer, M., Chida, Y., & Molloy, G. J. (2009). Psychological distress and cancer mortality. *Journal of Psychosomatic Research, 66*, 255–258.

Hanna, D. (2004). Moral distress: The state of the science. *Research & Theory for Nursing Practice, 18*(1), 73–93.

Helsler, M., Vijan, S., Makki, F., & Plette, J. D. (2010). Diabetes support with reciprocal peer support versus nurse care management. *Annals of Internal Medicine, 153*(8), 507–515.

Henselmans, I., Sanderman, R., Helgeson, V. S., de Vries, J., Smink, A., & Ranchor, A. V. (2010). Personal control over the cure of breast cancer: Adaptiveness, underlying beliefs and correlates. *Psycho-Oncology, 19*(5), 525–534.

Holland, J. C. (2014). NCCN Clinical Practice Guidelines in Oncology (NCCN Guidelines®) Distress Management Version 2. © 2014 National Comprehensive Cancer Network, Inc. Retrieved from NCCN.org. Accessed October 1, 2014.

Institute of Medicine. (2008). In N. E. Adler, & A. E. K. Page, (Eds.), *Cancer care for the whole patient*. Washington, DC: The National Academies Press.

IOM. (2003). In A. Greiner, & E. Knebel (Eds.), *Health professions education: A bridge to quality*. Washington, DC: The National Academies Press.

Jacobsen, P. B., Donovan, K. A., Trask, P. C., Fleishman, S. B., Zabora, J., Baker, F., & Holland, J. G. (2005). Screening for psychologic distress in ambulatory cancer patients. *Cancer, 103*(7), 1494–1502.

Kantor, D. (2013). Factors influencing psychological distress in patients with cancer. Retrieved from Pro Quest (1431183258).

Kissane, D., Bloch, S., McKenzie, M., McDowall, C., & Nitzan, R. (1998). Family grief therapy: A preliminary account of a new model to promote healthy family functioning during palliative care and bereavement. *Psycho-oncology, 7*, 14–25.

Koopman, C., Hermanson, K., Diamond, S., Angell, K., & Spiegel, D. (1998). Social support, life stress, pain, and emotional adjustment to advanced breast cancer. *Psycho-Oncology, 7*(2), 101–111.

Kornblith, A. B. (1998). Psychosocial adaptation of cancer survivors. In J. C. Holland (Ed.), *Psycho-oncology* (pp. 223–238). New York, NY: Oxford University Press.

Kristeller, J. L., Zumbrun, C. S., & Schilling, R. F. (1999). 'I would if I could': How oncologists and oncology nurses address spiritual distress in cancer patients. *Psycho-Oncology, 8*, 451–458.

Lazarus, R. (1999). *Stress and emotion*. New York, NY: Springer Publishing Company.

Lepore, S., Glaser, D. B., & Roberts, K. J. (2008). On the positive relation between received social support and negative affect: A test of the triage and self-esteem threat models in women with breast cancer. *Psycho-Oncology, 17*. 1210–1215. doi: 10.1002/pon.1347

Levin, T., & Kissane, D. W. (2006). Psychooncology—the state of its development in 2006. *European Journal of Psychiatry, 20*(3), 183–197.

Lewis, F. M. (2010). The family's "stuck points" in adjusting to cancer. In J. C. Holland, W. S. Breitbart, P. B. Jacobsen, M. S. Lederberg, M. J. Loscalzo, & R. McCorkle (Eds.), *Psycho-oncology* (2nd ed., pp. 511–515). New York, NY: Oxford University Press.

Lubkin, I. M., & Larsen, P. D. (2013). *Chronic illness: Impact and intervention* (8th ed.). Burlington, MA: Jones and Bartlett Learning.

Madden, J. (2006). The problem of distress in patients with cancer: More effective assessment. *Clinical Journal of Oncology Nursing, 10*(5), 615–619.

McCorkle, R., & Young, K. (1978). Development of a symptom distress scale. *Cancer Nursing, 1*(5), 373–378.

Mishel, M. H. (1988). Uncertainty in illness. *Image: Journal of Nursing Scholarship, 20*(4), 225–232.

Mishel, M. H., & Clayton, M. F. (2008). Theories of uncertainty. In M. J. Smith, & P. R. Liehr (Eds.), *Middle range theory for nursing* (2nd ed., pp. 55–84). New York, NY: Springer.

Pasacreta, J. V., Kenefick, A. L., & McCorkle, R. (2008). Managing distress in oncology patients. *Cancer Nursing, 31*(6), 485–490.

Peterson, J. C., Alegrante, J. P., Pirraglia, P. A., Robbins, L., Lane, K. P., Boschert, K. A., & Charlson, M. E. (2010). Living with heart disease after angioplasty: A qualitative study of patients who have been successful or unsuccessful in multiple behavior change. *Heart & Lung: The Journal of Acute and Chronic Care, 39*(2), 105–115.

Prince-Paul, M. (2008). Understanding the meaning of social well-being at the end of life. *Oncology Nursing Forum, 35*(3), 365–371.

Rajabiun, S., Mallinson, R. K., McCoy, K., Coleman S., Drainoni, M. L., Rebholz, C., & Holbert, T. (2007). "Getting me back on track": The role of outreach interventions and retaining of people living with HIV/AIDS in medical care. *AIDS Patient Care STDs, 21*, s20–s29.

Ransom, S., Jacobsen, P. B., & Booth-Jones, M. (2006). Validation of the distress thermometer with bone marrow transplant patients. *Psycho-Oncology, 15*, 604–612.

Rinaldis, M., Pakenham, K. I., & Lynch, B. M. (2010). Relationships between quality of life and finding benefits in a diagnosis of colorectal cancer. *British Journal of Psychology, 101*, 259–275. doi: 10.1248/000712609×448676

Robbins, M. A. (2007). Barriers to using the National Comprehensive Cancer Network (NCCN) distress management tool: Does it cause more stress? *Oncology Nursing Forum, 34*(2), 503.

Rose, J. H., Kypriotakis, G., Bowman, K. F., Einstadter, D., O'Toole, E. E., Mechekano, R., & Dawson, N. (2009). Patterns of adaptation in patients living long term with advanced cancer. *Cancer, 115*(18Suppl), 4298–4310.

Ryan, H., Schofield, P., Cockburn, P., Butow, P., Tattersall, M., Turner, J., … Bowman, D. (2005). How to recognize and manage psychological distress in cancer patients. *European Journal of Cancer Care, 14*, 7–15.

Sammarco, S. (2001). Perceived social support, uncertainty, and quality of life of younger breast cancer survivors. *Cancer Nursing, 24*, 212–219.

Schulz, E., Holt, C. L., Caplan, L., Blake, V., Southward, P., Buckner, A., & Lawrence, H. (2008). Role of spirituality and in cancer coping African Americans: A qualitative examination. *Journal of Cancer Survivorship: Research and Practice, 2*(2), 104–115.

Sellick, S. M., & Edwardson, A. D. (2007). Screening for new cancer patients for psychological distress using the hospital anxiety and depression scale. *Psycho-Oncology, 16*, 534–542. doi: 10.1002/pon.1085

Sjölander, C., & Berterö, C. (2008). The significance of social support and social networks among newly diagnosed lung cancer patients in Sweden. *Nursing and Health Sciences, 10*, 182–187.

Steinberg, T., Roseman, M., Kasymjanova, G., Dobson, S., Lajeunesse, L., Dajczman, E., … Small, D. (2009). Prevalence of emotional distress in newly diagnosed lung cancer patients. *Support Cancer Care, 17*, 1493–1497. doi: 10.1007/s00520–009–0614–6

Swanson, J., & Koch, L. (2010). The role of the oncology nurse navigator in distress management of adult inpatients with cancer: A retrospective study. *Oncology Nursing Forum, 37*(1), 69–76.

Swanson, K. (1999). What is known about caring in nursing research: A literary meta-analysis. In A. S. Hinshaw (Ed.), *Handbook of clinical nursing research* (pp. 31–60). Thousand Oaks, CA: Sage Publications, Inc.

Syse, A., Tretli, S., & Kravdal, O. (2009). The impact of cancer on spouses' labor earnings. *Cancer, 115*(18), 4350–4361. doi: 10.1002/cncr.24582

Taylor, C., Richardson, A., & Cowley, S. (2010). Restoring embodied control following surgical treatment for colorectal cancer: A longitudinal study. *International Journal of Nursing Studies, 47*(8), 946–956. doi: 10.1016/j.ijnurstu.2009.12.008

Thekkumpurath, P., Venkateswaran, C., Kumar, M., & Bennett, M. I. (2008). Screening for psychological distress in palliative care: A systematic review. *Journal of Pain and Symptom Management, 36*(5), 520–528.

Thomas, B. C., Pandey, M., Ramdas, K., & Nair, M. K. (2002). Psychological distress in cancer patients: Hypothesis of a distress model. *European Journal of Cancer Prevention, 11*, 179–185.

Thomas, B., Mohan, V. N., Thomas, I., & Pandey, M. (2002). Development of a distress inventory for cancer: Preliminary results. *Journal of Postgraduate Medicine, 48*, 16–20.

Thompson, S., & Collins, M. (1995). Applications of perceived control to cancer: An overview of theory and measurement. *Journal of Psychosocial Oncology, 13*, 1–21.

Trask, P., Paterson, A., Riba, M., Brines, B., Griffith, K., Weich, J., … Ferrara, J. (2002). Assessment of psychological distress in prospective bone marrow transplant patients. *Bone Marrow Transplantation, 29*, 917–925.

Vodermaier, A., Lindin, W., & Siu, C. (2009). Screening for emotional distress in cancer patients: A systematic review of assessment instruments. *Journal of the National Cancer Institute, 101*(21), 1464–1488.

Watson, J. (2005). *Caring science as sacred science.* Philadelphia, PA: F. A. Davis Company.

Wool, M. S., & Mor, V. (2005). A multidimensional model for understanding cancer pain. *Cancer Investigation, 23*, 727–734. doi: 10.108/07357900500360032

Yancik, R., & Ries, L. A. (2000). Aging and cancer in America. *Hematology/Oncology Clinics in North America, 14*(1), 17–23.

Zabalegui, A. (1997). *Perceived social support, coping, and psychological distress in advanced cancer patients (Doctoral dissertation).* Retrieved from Dissertations & Theses Full Text (AAT 9737488)

Zabora, J., Brintzenhofeszoc, K., Curbow, B., Hooker, C., & Piantadosi, S. (2001). The prevalence of psychological distress by cancer site. *Psycho-Oncology, 10*, 19–28.

Zebrack, B. (2000). Cancer survivors and quality of life: A critical review of the literature. *Oncology Nursing Forum, 27*(9), 1395–1401.

PSYCHOSOCIAL ISSUES OF CANCER SURVIVORSHIP

CHAPTER 4

FAMILY RELATIONSHIPS, SOCIAL SUPPORT, FEAR OF RECURRENCE, AND FINANCES

"There are days where things seem normal to me but at other times I feel as if things will never be the same. My husband was supportive during my treatment but now at times seems distant. We depleted our savings because I could not work for six months. I feel as if I lost valuable time with my daughter, time that I can never get back."

—A cancer survivor

Key Terms

Damocles syndrome • recurrence anxiety • secondary survivors

Upon completing this chapter, you will be able to do the following:

1. Identify psychosocial issues in patients with cancer.
2. Discuss how family relationships can be impacted with a diagnosis of cancer.
3. Discuss the role of social support.
4. Discuss the fear of recurrence in patients with cancer.
5. Discuss the role of nursing in addressing psychological issues of cancer survivorship.

Family Relationships

Overview

The stress that cancer creates affects family members as well as the diagnosed individual. Considered "secondary survivors," families have unique issues and provocations as they cope with life after cancer (Boyle et al., 2000; Mellon, 2002). Family members must adapt to the changes brought on by cancer such as role changes, economic shifts, ongoing care needs, lingering effects of the illness for the survivor, and learning to live with potential uncertainty about the future. They express concerns that are similar to those of the cancer survivor. For example, family members may experience frustration, feel isolated, and feel worn down by the competing demands of work and routine family care in conjunction with accommodating the survivors' needs. Frequently, families receive medical information secondhand and worry in isolation about the future. They may have feelings of guilt and question themselves. They may wonder if they should have recognized the symptoms earlier, been more forceful regarding seeking out the healthcare practitioner, and may blame themselves for being preoccupied and not recognizing the weight loss. After the survivor completes treatment, family members frequently have an expectation that the individual will return to "normal," return to previous activities and roles, and put the cancer experience behind them (Hara & Blum, 2009; Oktay, Bellin, Scarvalone, Appling, & Helzlsouer, 2011). In addition, family members may expect the survivor to feel relieved that the treatment is over. However, resumption of life as it was before the cancer diagnosis is not consistent with the experience of the overwhelming majority of cancer survivors (Murphy, Morris, & Lange, 1997).

Effect on Family Members

The ability of a family to cope with the stress of a member dealing with a diagnosis of cancer is influenced by several factors. These include persistent symptoms of distress, anxiety, depression, uncertainty, hopelessness, concurrent stressors, and role problems. Furthermore, a family's ability to adapt is influenced by the developmental phase of the family. An example of these differences is a young family with small children trying to balance the needs of the children with work demands versus an older couple who are retired (Jensen & Given, 1993). Coping by family members is also influenced by previous life experiences, personality, feelings, quality of the relationships among family members, family belief systems, cultural and racial characteristics, and finances (Lauria, Clark, & Hermann, 2001).

As part of the healthcare team, collaboration with an oncology social worker is essential since they will be able to assess the coping strategies of the family, recognize the presence of dysfunctional coping mechanisms, and tailor interventions for the families accordingly. When providing support for the family, the oncology social worker will view the family as a unit, communicate with them as an entity, and help them communicate with one another (Lauria, et al., 2001). Interventions conducted by oncology social workers to promote coping with family caregivers alone or in combination with the survivors have been shown to result in less depression, lower mood disturbance, greater confidant support, greater marital satisfaction, less emotional discomfort, higher sexual satisfaction, greater use of adaptive coping, and more positive growth (Alfano & Rowland, 2006; Bultz, Speca, Brasher, Geggie, & Page, 2000; Hara & Blum, 2009; Manne, Babb, Pinover, Horowitz, & Ebbert, 2004; Pasacreta, Barg, Nuamah, & McCorkle, 2000; Toseland, Blanchard, & McCallion, 1996).

Effect on Spousal/Partner Relationship

As in many chronic illnesses, treatment of cancer and its aftereffects place an enormous burden on the physical and emotional responses of a couple (Galbraith, Fink, & Wilkins, 2011). Difficulties with communication and intimacy are common and if not addressed, they can have negative effects on a couple's physiological, psychosocial, and relational health.

Many cancer survivors question their partner's relational commitment. Some partners of cancer survivors may experience uncertainty about continuing the marriage, while for others, the illness may serve to strengthen the partnership bonds. Couples in the childbearing years may have questions regarding the ability to have children in the future or may wonder about the hereditary nature of the cancer and ultimately question the desire to have biological children. They may also be concerned about the effect of the cancer on the childrearing process.

Partners of prostate cancer survivors have their own unique experiences as they live through the survivorship process and often experience more distress than the patient themselves (Galbraith, Hays, & Tanner, 2012). Partners of prostate cancer survivors with sexual dysfunction report less communication and increased relational distress (Badr & Taylor, 2009). Men describe frustrations with their relationship and their ability to cope effectively with emotions and concerns expressed by their partner (Couper et al., 2009).

Increased support and better communication can help couples develop strategies to improve their ability to cope with the disruptions in their relationship (Sanders, Pedro, O'Carroll-Bantum, & Galbraith, 2006). Research suggests that the way survivors and partners help each other cope with the stressors related to the cancer, handle changes in relationship priorities, and try to maintain a sense of normalcy in the relationship, impacts the quality of the relationship.

Communication

Communication is important to the quality of life of cancer survivors, their partners, and their family members. Family members frequently differ in their communication styles. Many men have difficulty expressing feelings; women might have the need to talk. If a family member's way of communicating conflicts with the survivor, the survivor and family member will experience greater stress in times of crisis. Communication styles will either enhance or compromise intimacy, depending on the specific communication strategies they use (Manne, Badr, Zaider, Nelson, & Kissane, 2010). Couples who have been able to maintain communication related to sexuality and intimacy report a higher quality of life (Galbraith et al., 2011). The Relationship Intimacy Model of Cancer Adaptation (Manne & Badr, 2008) proposes that the relationship communication style influences a family member's or couple's psychological adaptation by its effects on relational intimacy. According to this model, there are two types of communication: relationship-enhancing and relationship-compromising. Relationship-enhancing communication improves relationship closeness and includes mutual discussion and feelings regarding cancer-related concerns. This type of communication creates a perception that both parties are expressing feelings, discussing concerns and solutions for how to manage the issues, and both parties feel understood. Relationship-compromising behaviors such as holding back concerns, actively avoiding cancer-related discussions, and placing pressure or demands to discuss concerns while the other partner withdraws can reduce relationship closeness. This type of communication behavior has been associated with greater relationship, marital, and psychological distress.

Interventions

According to the Institute of Medicine [IOM] (2005), caregivers and family members often require, but do not receive, the respite, healthcare, psychosocial, and financial assistance they need in meeting the many needs of cancer survivors in their lives. Research indicates that family members, like survivors, may exhibit emotional adjustment problems after treatment ends (Ell, Nishimoto, Mantell, & Hamovitch, 1988; Hagedoorn, Bunk, Kuijer, Wobbies, & Sandermen, 2000). The exact length of time family members' distress continues after cancer treatment has ended is not known; however, 45% of caregivers reported experiencing mild fatigue, 25% moderate fatigue, and 28% severe fatigue related to the caregiving role (Jensen & Given, 1993).

Seeking outside professional help can provide support to the family members as well as the survivor, and provide the courage to discuss concerns and to listen and validate feelings. A study conducted by Woods and Earp (1978) described an association between breast cancer survivors' need to communicate their concerns regarding fear of recurrence and the families' desires to avoid this conversation. This phenomenon, termed "conversational isolation," amplifies how breast cancer survivors triggered emotional distress in their families by disclosing their fears about cancer recurrence and the possibility of premature death (Woods & Earp, 1978). Families responded by avoiding these conversations, which ultimately left the survivors feeling isolated and without significant support.

For the psychological and physical well-being of the couple, it is essential that both members be included in any intervention design (Galbraith et al., 2011). Couples who are seeking to reduce psychological distress may benefit from counseling that enhances relationship closeness by learning how to facilitate constructive discussions about concerns, reduce the use of mutual avoidance, and facilitate greater responsiveness. Learning the use of "I" messages, active listening skills, and role playing may facilitate improved communication for family members, couples, and survivors (Stanley, 2003). Cancer survivors with sexual performance issues such as patients with prostate cancer have identified important issues when planning interventions. These include intracouple communication, information needs about intimacy, and how to manage treatment-related sexual challenges. Survivors and their spouses have reported increased self-efficacy, increased coping skills, and better communication with each other when a family-based intervention designed to improve their coping skills was offered (Harden et al., 2009).

Social Support

Overview

Most people are not equipped on their own to cope with a serious illness or how to solve the emotional and practical problems it creates (Murphy et al., 1997). To address these challenges at the beginning of a cancer diagnosis, during treatment, and especially during survivorship, where one may still be grappling with the long-term consequences of this devastating disease, the support of other people, family, friends, colleagues, religious groups, and helping professionals is paramount. Social support takes many forms. Assistance can be someone offering assistance with transportation to a medical appointment or from members of a support group who share similar experiences and feelings. Cancer is a life crisis that nobody would willingly seek out; still, many people discover that the experience presents an opportunity to rediscover the importance of life, connections to other people and society as a whole (Murphy et al. 1997).

Why Is Social Support Important?

Most cancer survivors experience an increase in distress at the completion of active treatment (IOM, 2005). Conclusion of treatment is a time when predictable routines end, leaving survivors with a sense of loss and uncertainty. Faced with the unknown future, cancer survivors perceive themselves as having limited social support or not needing support at all. However, taking active steps in creating a support network can instill a sense of empowerment and lead to positive healing for many cancer survivors.

Individuals in a cancer survivor's support network can help recognize signs of declining mood, encourage the survivor to stay connected to others, and seek appropriate help if needed. A cancer survivor that feels understood and cared for is more likely to try to stay healthy by eating well and exercising. The support of others can also prevent destructive habits such as smoking and alcohol use (Murphy et al., 1997).

Types of Social Support

Informal Support

Informal support for the cancer survivor may come in the form of family, friends, neighbors, colleagues, and coworkers, or other individuals the survivor may turn to for support and comfort. Survivors should be encouraged to ask for what they need and those offering support should be clear as to what they can offer. However, an informal support network is not without some limitations. The changes that have occurred in family life and countless concerns for the survivor may result in the spouse or partner feeling overwhelmed. The most important part of the informal support are often the spouse or partner; however, research shows that one in four people with cancer have problems communicating with their partners (Murphy et al., 1997). The majority of those reporting such problems are women, who often state that they want to talk openly about their fears and anxieties but that their husbands tend to discount such feelings (Murphy et al., 1997).

Types of Formal Support

Examples of formal support are groups, mental health professionals, social workers, religious institutions, and advocacy organizations. Formal support should not be a substitute for informal support, but should complement a cancer survivor's informal support network. Living through cancer can be a lonely experience, even for those who are surrounded by family and friends. Oftentimes a person in a survivor's life may not know how to be helpful. Some may withdraw themselves from the survivor due to one's overwhelming feelings regarding the survivor's illness. The cancer survivor themselves may be reluctant to share what they are experiencing for fear of becoming a burden. Cancer survivors benefit from guidance that will help better understand their cancer journey; participating in a group can normalize their fear and anxiety. Helping professionals or group members can alleviate this sense of isolation and ostracism.

Formal support is often given in a group setting which offers support from others living the path of cancer survivorship. Self help and support groups are forums to share knowledge and strategies that can promote effective coping. The stories and struggles of survival exchanged in a group setting help the participants recognize the reality and validity of their deepest feelings.

Group counseling can be an effective intervention for cancer survivors and their families. The ability to meet others in similar circumstances, to share methods of coping, and to develop new relationships at a time of perceived isolation are all factors that can promote healthy survivorship (Lauria, et al., 2001). Group experiences can broaden a cancer survivor's social network by the development of new friendships that are built on mutual concern and sharing as well as increasing their knowledge of resources and techniques in navigating the complex healthcare system.

Oncology social workers can connect the survivor to appropriate agencies that can offer information on employment, insurance, or other relevant issues. In addition, the oncology social worker can provide counseling for both the cancer survivor and his or her family members that can address their fears, concerns, and any practical problems that may arise.

Professionally Facilitated Support Groups

A professionally facilitated support group is a structured group designed to address the concerns of cancer survivors. These groups are facilitated by a professional (social worker or nurse) trained in the issues related to cancer survivors. Trained professionals in group work have the experience to manage group members that monopolize conversations or deal with members who are upset that a group is not providing support.

Some of these groups charge a fee, but many are subsidized by healthcare facilities. Sessions can have a planned topic of discussion, a scheduled presenter, or simply be an open forum for the purpose of discussion being formulated by issues of the participants.

Self-Help Groups

Self-help groups, also referred to as peer support networks, differ from support groups in that they do not involve facilitation by a professional and may concentrate on more practical, how to issues. These groups are usually free of charge, held in homes, community centers or religious facilities, and facilitated by the members themselves. Self-help groups not only focus on feelings but offer problem-solving strategies on survivorship. Groups can be organized by stage of disease, diagnosis, age, or other common factors such as treatment modality (Lauria et al., 2001).

Which group the cancer survivor will choose depends solely on their needs and interests, and/or what is available in the community. Ideally, a group size should be no larger than ten members. The discussion of private issues may be easier for the survivor if the support group is limited to their own sex, type of cancer, or a specific number of participants. Selection may also be based on scheduling frequency. A group might meet weekly, twice a month, or run for a specified length of time (6 to 12 sessions). Some groups are open-ended and accept new members for as long as the group functions. Other groups are closed to new members after the first meeting. Both open-ended and time-limited groups may provide education through speakers or educational DVDs. Oncology social workers often encourage the cancer survivor to participate in more than one group as each group has something different to offer. For those with physical limitations or time restraints, possibly in the case of a caregiver, telephone and internet support groups are becoming more popular. A well-facilitated group puts no pressure on a member to "open up" or share their feelings. The most important task for the leader in any support group is to provide a safe atmosphere in which members feel free to participate without fear, judgment, or ridicule (Lauria et al., 2001).

Supportive Psychotherapy

The purpose of support psychotherapy is to facilitate coping rather than personality change. Psychotherapy can be delivered in a group setting, individually, or with family members. Oncology social workers who are Clinical Social Workers, as designated by the state in which they practice, are skilled in recognizing the fundamental issues related to cancer and survivorship and will explore approaches to resolving these issues. Private sessions offer the chance to express thoughts and feelings that do not emerge in other formal or informal settings. Those in individual therapy have the full attention of the professional for the length of the session. The confidentiality and objectivity in therapy can be valuable. The frequency of visits may vary from very few to extending over months, or even years. Joint sessions with couples or family members present can provide an opportunity for airing concerns in an aired structured way. In addition, mental health professionals can evaluate anxiety and changes in mood and make appropriate referrals if psychopharmacology is advised. Most health insurance plans and Medicare/Medicaid cover mental health; however, there can be a limit in the number of sessions allowed.

Religious and Spiritual Support

Many cancer survivors seek the support of their faith or religious organization to provide solace and strength while adjusting to life after cancer treatment. Spirituality and religiousness may decrease anxiety, pain, and hostility; encourage cooperation; improve interpersonal relationships; increase satisfaction with life; and decrease depression (Miller, 2005). In addition to offering spiritual guidance, the religious community can offer support with practical issues like transportation, meals, and assistance with daily household tasks.

Finances

Overview

"You completely deplete your savings, investment funds, and IRAs. You drain that out. A lot of people are living off their credit cards. You don't have the money, but you need groceries, you need to pay your bills, so you end up putting it all on your credit card" (Newfield, 2008).

"You move suddenly from a middle-income home to a lower-income home because your medical expenses are growing. Insurance only covers 80% of the medical costs, so you are left with the 20% co-pay. The physician is now prescribing you designer drugs, and you are being reimbursed with your prescription coverage. These medicines can cost up to $10000 a month in the case of leukemia, or for solid tumors it can easily reach to $70000 a month" (Newfield, 2008).

These are just two stories from cancer survivors discussing the financial impact of cancer. Cancer is not just physically disruptive; it is economically disruptive to the comfort level of each person in the home (Newfield, 2008). The issue of finances is a crucial part of a cancer survivor's experience. The survivor may face loss of or limited employment, restricted health plans, high out-of-pocket expenses for prescription drugs, and expenses related to co-insurance and co-payments. Employment, insurance, and economic issues may pose an overwhelming burden to the survivor and their family.

Employment

Employment provides not only financial support but also a sense of identity and self-worth. The majority of cancer survivors, who have worked before their diagnosis, return to work following their treatment. Retaining one's employment status has obvious financial benefits and is often necessary for health insurance coverage, self-esteem, and social support. For many, surviving cancer may prompt retirement from an undesirable occupation. Many employed survivors work in excess of 40 hours per week, and some report various degrees of disability that interfere with job performance. According to the analysis of the 2000 National Health Interview Survey (NHIS), cancer survivors were found to have poorer outcomes across all employment-related burden measures relative to matched control subjects (Yabroff, Lawrence, Clauser, Davis, & Brown, 2004). Cancer survivors are more likely to be unable to work because of health problems, and typically have more days lost from work. Needing to work fewer hours, taking on lighter job responsibilities, or requiring more frequent breaks are a few examples of adaptations required (Bloom et al., 1993; Joly et al., 1996). As many as one in five individuals who work at the time of diagnosis have cancer-related limitations in ability to work 1 to 5 years later. Half of those with limitations are unable to work at all (Short, Vasey, & Tunceli, 2005b). It is important that the cancer survivor, if age appropriate, return to productive work in some capacity, learn a new skill, launch a new career, or go back to school. The office of vocational rehabilitation (OVR) has state agencies that assist those whose ability to work has been affected by illness and possibly re-train a survivor for another field of employment.

Discrimination

All survivors are at risk of experiencing subtle discrimination. Concern over employment discrimination is significant. Cancer survivors have reported problems in the workplace that include dismissal, failure to hire, demotion, denial of promotion, undesirable transfer, denial of benefits, and hostility (Fesco, 2001; Hoffman, 2004b).

Cancer survivors have the same rights as does anyone else to employment befitting their skills, training, and experience; they should never have to accept a position they never would have considered before their illness, and hiring, promotion, and treatment in the workplace should depend entirely on ability and qualifications (Murphy et al., 1997).

In reality, however, cancer survivors face many employment and workplace discrimination issues for which outside assistance is necessary. Due to their fear of revealing they had cancer on an employment application, cancer survivors may feel locked into positions they would like to leave due to their fear they will not be hired into a new setting or position. Others continue to work in positions that are unfulfilling or physically too demanding. In addition, the survivor may continue to work past planned early retirement due to financial need.

Federal laws enacted in the 1990s which include the American Disabilities Act (ADA), Family Medical Leave Act (FMLA), and the Employee Retirement and Income Security

Act (ERISA) have offered cancer survivors some protection from discriminatory practices such as firing or denial of benefits because of cancer (IOM, 2005). Common accommodations offered by employers are reduced and flexible schedules. However, some survivors have not been fully protected from job loss and access to accommodations.

The ADA of 1990 prohibits employers from discriminating against qualified individual with disabilities in the job application process, hiring, firing, advancement, compensation, and job training. A qualified employee with a disability is an individual who with or without reasonable accommodations can perform the essential functions of one's job. The FMLA of 1993 requires employers who employ 50 or more to provide certain benefits for serious medical illnesses:

- Provide 12 weeks of unpaid leave
- Provide health insurance during leave period
- Restore employees to the same or equivalent position
- Allow leave time to care for a spouse, child, or parent who has a serious health condition
- Allow leave because a serious health condition renders the employee "unable to perform" the functions of the position.

The ERISA prohibits an employer from discriminating against an employee in collecting benefits under an employee benefit plan. Employee benefits are defined as health insurance benefits, disability, or unemployment benefits.

Employer's Perspective

From an employer's perspective, cancer represents a potential health and productivity burden. There are concerns about absenteeism from work, disability program use, worker's compensation programs costs, turnover, family medical leave, and on-the-job productivity losses. According to Pyenson and Zenner (2002), cancer accounts for about 10% of an employer's or insurer's annual medical claim costs, 10% of short-term disability claim costs, and 10% of long-term disability costs. Employers, supervisors, and coworkers may assume that cancer survivors are not able to perform job responsibilities as well as they did before, and perceive them as a poor risk for promotion. Survivors themselves may have misconceptions about their ability to resume their employment following treatment. Limitations in performing physical tasks such as lifting heavy loads, or mental tasks requiring concentrating for long periods of time, analyzing data, and learning new things may interfere with a cancer survivor's work performance.

Some prejudices still exist in the workplace with employers reacting to the diagnosis of cancer as an unspecified danger or unpleasant reminder of their own mortality. Some employers may be afraid of the lower production or financial losses because of the survivor's diminished capability or time taken off for treatment.

Financial Assistance

There are many replacement sources for cancer survivors who have had extended time away from employment or who are disabled and can no longer work.

- Short- and long-term disability: provides financial assistance through employers to individuals who have exhausted their sick and annual leave at work. These benefits are not offered by all employers.

- Federal Social Security Administration Programs:
  - Supplemental Security Income (SSI) has a guaranteed minimum level of income for needy aged, blind, or disabled individuals. To be considered disabled, an individual must have a medically determinable physical or mental impairment that is expected to last at least 12 months. SSI is means tested and does not require prior participation in the labor force (IOM, 2005).
  - Social Security Disability Insurance (SSDI) is an insurance program that provides payments to persons with disabilities based on their history of social security covered earnings. To be eligible, an individual must be unable to work for 12 months or be in terminal stages of an illness (IOM, 2005).

Health Insurance Issues

Cancer is one of the five most costly medical conditions in the United States and many survivors' feel the financial squeeze of treating their disease and are among those who are most likely to have difficulties navigating the U.S. health insurance system (Schwartz, Claxton, Martin, & Schmidt, 2009; Soni, 2007). They may face significant barriers to coverage, access to individual health insurance may be denied in certain states due to a cancer history, or face surcharged premiums for coverage. Despite having private insurance or public insurance, some cancer survivors may still face high healthcare costs. Some cancer survivors may find that their insurance caps their benefits or will not pay for treatments recommended by their doctor, thus leaving them effectively uninsured for much of the cost of their cancer treatment with inadequate financial resources to pay for all of the care and services they need. A 2006 poll conducted by USA Today, the Kaiser Family Foundation, and the Harvard School of Public Health found that 5% of insured cancer patients reported delaying their treatment or deciding not to get care because of costs (USA Today, 2006).

Patients and survivors who lose their jobs, decide to change jobs, or otherwise lose their group insurance can be denied coverage in the individual market because of a cancer diagnosis and can ultimately be left uninsured. Eleven percent of adult cancer survivors under the age of 65 are uninsured and for these people the cost of cancer is financially devastating (USA Today, 2006).

Out-of-network doctors may be difficult to avoid for survivors, whose insurers have a limited provider network. Patients who seek care out-of-network often have to pay higher cost sharing for these doctors and are frequently billed for the balance of the physician's total charges after the insurance company reimburses the physician (Schwartz et al., 2009). For cancer survivors with employer-sponsored coverage, changing employers may lead to a change in health plans and insurance networks. Such a change could lead to a new network of doctors and a new set of benefits. Cancer patients may be reluctant to take the chance that their physicians would be out-of-network if they switched insurers, since that can lead to significant increases in costs.

Public Insurance

Medicare is a federally funded health insurance program for those of 65 years of age and older regardless of income. Individuals under 65 that are disabled and who are receiving SSDI, because they are no longer able to work as a result of an illness, can be eligible to enroll in Medicare 2 years after SSDI payments begin. Medicare consists of four parts:

Part A is hospital coverage.

Part B covers physician visits.

Parts C provides Medicare-managed care plans.

Part D is prescription drug coverage.

Medicaid is a state-funded social service program that provides health insurance to children and needy families and individuals who meet income requirements. In 2014, to receive Medicaid, the income requirement for a family of four was $23,850.

Assistance

Cancer patients who are not healthy enough to work or lose their job are in jeopardy of losing their health insurance. The Consolidated Omnibus Budget Reconciliation Act of 1985 (COBRA) was designed to help people maintain their health coverage after leaving a job (Schwartz et al., 2009). COBRA allows people to temporarily continue the health insurance they had through their employer by paying the full cost of the insurance themselves. However, COBRA is expensive and the coverage usually lasts for 18 months, so many individuals instead seek coverage on the individual market or now through the Affordable Care Act (ACA). The ACA is designed to provide the uninsured access to health care through either a State or Federally run Marketplace. Through online access consumers can shop for health insurance across multiple carriers, apply for financial assistance, and purchase coverage. Consumers can choose among four different levels of health coverage, and premiums are based on percentage of income ranging from 2% to 9.5%.

Health Insurance policies, managed care plans, and government assistance vary widely in their coverage of cancer treatments, prescriptions, and restorative procedures. The Lance Armstrong Foundation, Cancer Care, and the Patient Advocate Foundation all provide information to assist cancer survivors with some of these issues.

Fear of Recurrence

Overview

Although relieved to be ending cancer treatment, cancer survivors report being unprepared to manage the concern of cancer's adverse late effects that may arise after treatment ends or the possibility of recurrence (Alfano & Rowland, 2006). Fear of recurrence of cancer is experienced by 5% to 89% of cancer survivors, across disease sites (Kornblith et al., 1998; Ronson & Body, 2002). With little guidance or information to guide through this adaptation, survivors and families face this experience feeling illequipped to master this new challenge (Carroll-Johnson, Gorman, & Bush, 2006). Referred to as the "Damocles syndrome," it is a nagging and disabling fear that cancer will reappear at some point. Blended with the relief of no longer having to endure the rigors and hardship of treatment is the apprehension of not knowing what to expect and dreading that recurrence is what awaits (Koocher & O'Malley, 1981).

Although it diminishes over time, the degree of worry about recurrence may fluctuate and be triggered by a variety of sources including doctor visits, unexplained symptoms, reports of cancer in the media, death of fellow survivors, and learned reminders of the experience (e.g., smell of alcohol, sight of the cancer center) (Gil et al., 2004; Mast, 2002).

When no longer in active treatment, the survivor can feel abandoned by the healthcare team with whom they were so closely involved. Survivors rated losing the support and reassurance of hospital staff the most common fear around treatment completion, in terms of intensity and frequency (Jefford et al., 2008). The treatment gives them something to work toward and gives them a sense of control. The sense of control is replaced with worry and fear. Follow-up appointments may trigger feelings of ambivalence and anxiety prior to the appointment, followed by a sense of relief when nothing abnormal is found. Advising the survivor that the fear of recurrence is normal and that in the beginning it will be at the forefront of the person's mind but with time the person will adjust to thinking about it less and less, can be helpful to the emotional health of the survivor.

Emotional Responses

Many disease-free cancer survivors experience some degree of anxiety over the possibility of a cancer recurrence. Anxiety levels may be as high as when the survivor was diagnosed and received treatment which may result in disruptive behaviors such as frequent self-examination for signs and symptoms of a recurrence, anxiety around follow-up doctor visits, worry about the future, preoccupation with health, inability to plan for the future, and despair.

Recurrence anxiety is worry focused on the possibility that the cancer will return. It is pervasive and, at times, overwhelming dread experienced by survivors as well as families (Dow, 1992; Welch-McCaffrey, Hoffman, Leigh, Loescher, & Meyskens, 1989). Anxiety is the coping response that all survivors can expect to experience. Recurrence anxiety can be described as "walking through life with a dark cloud hanging over your head, never knowing if or when the cancer will recur" or "sitting on a powder keg waiting for it to go off" (Schmale et al., 1983). The pattern of recurrence anxiety is erratic with the exception of the immediate period following treatment where concerns are the most intense (Cella & Tross, 1986; Fobair & Mages, 1981). The anxiety of recurrence can become a preoccupation and cancer survivors are extremely vulnerable for up to 1 year after treatment. Those with low tolerance for ambiguity or with preexisting anxiety disorders or other emotional problems are likely to be the most vulnerable and suffer ongoing distress following the ending of cancer treatment (Lauria et al., 2001).

Recurrence anxiety can produce two distinct behaviors. Hypochondria may evolve as the survivor proposes that a somatic change or new symptom concludes the cancer has returned. Avoidance behaviors may occur in terms of visits to the physician in order to avoid being told that the cancer has returned. Episodic worry, incited by symptom suspicion, return doctor visits, or exposure to fellow cancer survivors with progressive cancer can evoke chronic anxiety in cancer survivors (Powel & McFadden, 1995).

Recurrence anxiety may also be observed in families, prompting "hovering behaviors" and persistent scrutiny of the cancer survivors' physical status (Carroll-Johnson et al., 2006). This may solicit conflict within the family or couple as the survivor attempts to dismiss the presence of cancer while the family will focus on its possible return. Within time, recurrence anxiety diminishes, with periodic episodes resurfacing around physician visits and the presence of somatic complaints.

Feeling one's future may be cut short is a central element in the fear of cancer recurrence. It is also a defining symptom used to diagnose posttraumatic stress disorder (PTSD) in cancer survivors (Andrykowski, Lykins, & Floyd, 2008). The possibility that cancer survivors might experience PTSD as a result of trauma associated with their cancer experiences has been a recent focus of study (Kangas, Henry, & Bryant, 2002). Up to 32% of cancer survivors are estimated to experience PTSD due to the trauma associated with their cancer experience following completion of cancer treatment (Kangas et al., 2002). Cancer survivors may experience "flash backs," a survivor-specific emotional response similar to PTSD (Amir & Ramati, 2002; Carter, 1993; Kwekkeboom & Seng, 2002; Yehuda, 2002). However, a clear diagnosis of PTSD can be difficult as the defining symptoms of PTSD, including memory, concentration difficulties, cognitive avoidance, hyper vigilance, and sleep disruption, could be direct effects of cancer disease or treatment.

Interventions

Few studies have reported on interventions to address fear of recurrence specifically; however, interventions that effectively reduce stress and improve a sense of well-being might result in decreased worry about disease recurrence. Survivors of cancer suggest that for many people thinking of the disease as a long term, chronic condition can help in coping with the fear of recurrence (Murphy et al., 1997). The type of intervention provided by oncology social workers will depend on the preference of the patient. Intervention options include forums to minimize uncertainty, dispel misconceptions, and enhance coping skills as well as techniques such as cognitive reframing, promoting survivor and healthcare professional communication, teaching coping skills, relaxation exercises, and calming self-talk (Mishel et al., 2005). Counseling can address the emotional components of coping with survivorship, and assist in strengthening personal coping mechanisms for long-term survival.

Educational and psychotherapeutic approaches explore what precipitates the survivor's anxiety. Identifying irrational thoughts and behavioral psychotherapeutic approaches may be of benefit for survivors who have excessive body checking of signs and symptoms of recurrence (Lee-Jones, Humphries, Dixon, & Hatcher, 1997).

This could include techniques to assist survivors to manage panic attacks following a somatic sensation that may precipitate a fear of recurrence. Several therapeutic treatment modalities encourage the expression of feelings and identify irrational thoughts. In many cases, brief screening tools can be used to identify individuals with symptoms of distress so that clinical assessment by the primary oncology team and referral to psychosocial providers can take place (Trask, 2004). For example, the Distress Thermometer is a visual analogue scale that the National Comprehensive Cancer Network (NCNN) guidelines suggest for the screening of psychological distress (NCNN, 1999).

CASE STUDY

At 38 years old, Janice was diagnosed with Stage IIIC ovarian cancer and underwent successful surgery followed by six cycles of chemotherapy. She achieved a complete remission but struggled with feelings of anxiety and panic of fear of recurrence.

Janice is married with a 4-year-old daughter. She would like to have other children but is concerned about the effects of chemotherapy on her fertility.

Janice's husband supported Janice emotionally during her treatment and took over the most of the caregiving for their 4-year-old daughter. Since her remission, Janice has found that her husband is expecting their life to return to normal. Presently, Janice has found herself to be overwhelmed and fatigued with her home responsibilities.

Janice was employed as an accountant full time, but her employer has since reduced her hours to part time and is giving new assignments to other employees. Janice holds her health insurance for the family and is concerned about losing her health insurance benefits if she is terminated by her employer. In addition, Janice has been receiving medical bills and has been informed that her health insurance is not covering all of her medical expenses. At a recent follow-up visit with her physician, Janice is very tearful as she expresses her difficulty in coping with life as a cancer survivor.

• Critical Thinking **Questions**

1. What issues do you surmise may have occurred during Janice's treatment period regarding her relationship with her family and her family finances?
2. What role does social support have during treatment and posttreatment for cancer?
3. How would you categorize Janice's fear of recurrence? How would you address her concerns?
4. What are the employment rights of individuals with cancer?
5. What options are available for individuals with cancer who lose their health insurance?
6. What can a couple do to enhance their relationship following cancer treatment?
7. What role does nursing have in assisting patients with cancer in terms of addressing psychosocial issues?

References

Alfano, C. M., & Rowland, J. J. (2006). Recovery issues in cancer survivorship: A new challenge for supportive care. *The Cancer Journal. 12*(5), 432–443.

Amir, M., & Ramati, A. (2002). Post-traumatic symptoms, emotional distress and quality of life in long term-survivors of breast cancer: A preliminary research. *Journal of Anxiety Disorders. 16*, 195–206.

Andrykowski, M. A., Lykens, E., & Floyd, A. (2008). Psychological health in cancer survivors. *Seminars in Oncology Nursing. 24*(3), 193–201.

Badr, H., & Taylor, C. (2009). Sexual dysfunction and spousal communication in couples coping with prostate cancer. *Psychosocial Oncology. 2*, 23–35.

Bloom, J. R., Fobair, P., Gritz, E., Wellisch, D., Spiegel, D., Varghese, A. & Hoppe, R. (1993). Psychosocial outcomes of cancer: Comparative analysis of Hodgkin's disease and testicular cancer. *Journal of Clinical Oncology. 11*, 979–988.

Boyle, D. A., Blodgett, L., Gnesdiloff, S., White, J., Bamford, A. M., Sheridan, M. & Beveridge, R. (2000). Caregiver quality of life after autologous bone marrow transplantation. *Cancer Nursing. 23*, 193–205.

Bultz, B. D., Speca, M., Brasher, P. M., Geggie, P. H. & Page, S. A. (2000). A randomized controlled trail of a brief psycho educational support group for partner of early stage breast cancer patients. *Psycho Oncology. 9*(4), 303–313.

Carroll-Johnson, R. M., Gorman, L. M. & Bush, M. J. (2006). *Psychosocial nursing care along the cancer continuum* (2nd ed.). Pittsburgh, PA: Oncology Nursing Society.

Carter, B. (1993). Long term survivors of breast cancer: A qualitative descriptive study. *Cancer Nursing. 16*, 354–361.

Cella, D. F., & Tross, S. (1986). Psychological adjustment to survival from Hodgkin's disease. *Journal of Consulting and Clinical Psychology 54*, 616–622.

Couper, J., Block, S., Love, A., Duchesne, G., Macvean, M., & Kissane, D. (2009). Coping patterns and psychosocial distress in female partners of prostate cancer patients. *Psychosomatics. 50*(4), 375–382.

Dow, H. (1992). On the nature and meaning of locally recurrent breast cancer. *Quality of Life-A Nursing Challenge. 1*, 27–34.

Ell, K., Nishimoto, R., Mantell, J. & Hamovitch, M. (1988). Longitudinal analysis of psychological adaptation among family members of patients with cancer. *Journal of Psychosomatic Research, 32*(4–5), 429–438.

Fesco, S. L. (2001). Workplace experiences of individuals who are HIV+ and individuals with cancer. *Rehabilitation Counseling Bulletin, 45*(1), 2–11.

Fobair, P., & Mages, N. L. (1981). *Psychological morbidity among cancer patient survivors. Living and Dying with Cancer.* New York: Elsevier.

Galbraith, M.E., Fink, R., & Wilkins, G.G. (2011). Couples surviving prostate cancer: Challenges in their lives and relationships. *Seminars in Oncology Nursing. 27*(4), 300–308.

Galbraith, M.E., Hays, L., & Tanner, T. (2012). What men say about surviving prostate cancer: Complexities represented in a decade of comments. *Clinical Journal of Oncology Nursing. 16*(1),65–72.

Gil, K. M., Mishel, M. H., Beleya, M., Germino, B., Germino, L. S. Porter, L. … Stewart, J. (2004). Triggers of uncertainty about recurrence and long term treatment side effects in older African Americans and Caucasian breast cancer survivors. *Oncology Nursing Forum. 31*(3), 633–639.

Hagedoorn, M., Bunk, B. P., Kuijer, R. G., Wobbies, T., & Sandermen, R. (2000). Couples dealing cancer: Role and gender differences regarding psychological distress and quality of life. *Psycho Oncology. 9*(3), 232–242.

Hara, R., & Blum, D. (2009). Social well-being and cancer survivorship. *Oncology. 23*(2), 40–50.

Harden, J., Falahee, M., Bickes, J., Schafenacker, A., Walker, J., Mood, D., & Northouse, L. (2009). Factors associated with prostate cancer patients' and their spouses' satisfaction with a family-based intervention. *Cancer Nursing. 3*, 271–280.

Hoffman, B. (2004). *Working it out: Your employment rights. A cancer survivor's almanac: Charting your journey* (3rd ed.). Hoboken, NJ: John Wiley & Sons.

Institute of Medicine. (2005). *From cancer survivor: Lost in transition.* Washington, DC: The National Academies Press.

Jefford, M., Karahalios, E., Pollard, A., Baravelli, C., Carey, M., Franklin, J., … Schofield, P. (2008). Survivorship issues following treatment completion-results from focus groups with Australian cancer survivors and health professionals. *Journal of Cancer Survivorship. 2*(1), 20–31.

Jensen, S., & Given, B. (1993). Fatigue affecting family caregivers of cancer patients. *Supportive Care Center. 1*(6), 321–325.

Joly, F., Henty-Amar, M., Arveux, P., Reman, O., Tanguy, A., Peny, A.M., … Leporrier, M. (1996). Late psychosocial sequelae in Hodgkin's disease survivors: A French population based case control study. *Journal of Clinical Oncology. 14*(9), 2444–2453.

Kangas, M., Henry, J.L., & Bryant, R. A. (2002). Posttraumatic stress disorder following cancer: A conceptual and empirical review. *Clinical Psychology Review. 22*, 499–524.

Koocher, G. P., & O'Malley, J. E. (1981). *The damocles syndrome: Psychosocial consequences of surviving childhood cancer.* New York, NY: McGraw Hill.

Kornblith, A. B., Herndon, J. E., Zuckerman, E., Cella, D. F., Cherin, E., Wolchok, S., ... Holland, J. C. (1998). Comparison of psychosocial adaption of advanced stage Hodgkin's disease and acute leukemia survivors. Cancer and Leukemia Group B. *Annals of Oncology. 9*(3), 297–306.

Kwekkeboom, K. L., & Seng, J. S. (2002). Recognizing and responding to post traumatic stress disorder in people with cancer. *Oncology Nursing Forum. 29*, 643–650.

Lauria, M. M., Clark, E. & Hermann, J. F. (2001). *Social work in oncology: Supporting survivors, families, and caregivers.* Atlanta, GA: American Cancer Society.

Lee-Jones, C., Humphries, G., Dixon, R., & Hatcher, M. B. (1997). Fear of cancer recurrence: A literature review and proposed cognitive formulation to explain exacerbation of recurrence fears. *Psycho Oncology. 6*, 95–105.

Manne, S., Babb, J., Pinover, W., Horowitz, E., & Ebbert, J. (2004). Psycho educational group interventions for wives of men with prostate cancer. *Psycho Oncology. 13*(1)37–46.

Manne, S. & Badr, H. (2008). Intimacy and relationship processes in couples' psychosocial adaption to cancer. *Cancer. 112*(11), 2541–2555.

Manne, S., Badr, H., Zaider, T., Nelson, C., & Kissane, D. (2010). Cancer-related communication, relationship intimacy, and psychological distress among couples coping with localized prostate cancer. *Journal of Cancer Survivorship. 4*, 74–85.

Mast, M. E. (2002). Survivors of breast cancer: Illness uncertainly, positive reappraisal and emotional distress in later life. *Psycho Oncology. 11*(6), 479–494.

Mellon, S. (2002). Comparisons between cancer survivors and family members on meaning of illness and family quality of life. *Oncology Nursing Forum. 29*, 1117–1125.

Miller, B. (2005). Spiritual journey during and after cancer treatment. *Gynecologic Oncology. 99*, S129–S130.

Mishel, M. H., Germino, B. B., Gil, K. M., Belyea, M., Laney, I. C., Stewart, J., ... Clayton, M. (2005). Benefits from an uncertainty management intervention for African American and Caucasian older long term breast cancer survivors. *Psychooncology. 14*(11), 962–978.

Murphy, G. P., Morris, L. B., & Lange, D. (1997). *Informed decisions: The complete book of cancer diagnosis, treatment and recovery.* New York, NY: Penguin Books.

NCNN (National Comprehensive Cancer Network). (1999). NCCN practice guidelines for the management of psychological distress. *Oncology. 13*(5A), 113–147.

Newfield, N. A. (2008). Dealing with cancer debt. *Social Work Today. 8*(3)

Oktay, J. S., Bellin, M. H., Scarvalone, S., Appling, S., & Helzlsouer, K. J. (2011). Managing the impact of post-treatments fatigue on the family: Breast cancer survivors share their experiences. *Families, Systems & Health. 29*(2), 127–137.

Pasacreta, J. V., Barg, F., Nuamah, I., & McCorkle, R. (2000). Participant characteristics before and months after attendance at a family caregiver cancer education program. *Cancer Nursing. 23*(4), 295–303.

Powel L., & McFadden M. E. (1995). Repercussions of cancer treatment: Long term physiological and psychological sequelae. *Quality of Life-A Nursing Challenge. 4*(2):33–39.

Pyenson, B., & Zenner, P. A. (2002). The Cost of Cancer to the Worksite. New York, NY: Milliman.

Ronson, A., & Body, J. J. (2002). Psychosocial rehabilitation of cancer patients after curative therapy. *Supportive Care in Cancer. 10*(4), 281–291.

Sanders, S., Pedro, L.W., O'Carroll-Bantum, E., & Galbraith, M. E. (2006). Couples' surviving prostate cancer: Long-term intimacy needs and concerns following treatment. *Clinical Journal of Oncology Nursing. 10*(4), 503–508.

Schmale, A. H., Morrow, G. R., Schmitt, M.H., Adler, L.M., Enelow, A., Murawski, B.J., & Gates, C. (1983). Well-being of cancer survivors. *Psychosomatic Medicine. 45*, 163–169.

Schwartz, K., Claxton, G., Martin, K., & Schmidt, C; American Cancer Society. (2009). Spending time to survive: Cancer patients confront holes in the health insurance system. Retrieved

April 30, 2014 from http://www.cancer.org/acs/groups/content/@corporatecommunications/documents/document/acsq-017518.pdf

Short, P. F., Vasey, J. J., & Tunceli, K. (2005). Employment pathways in a large cohort of adult cancer survivors. *Cancer. 103*(6), 1292–1301.

Soni, A. (2007). *The five most costly conditions, 2000 and 2004: Estimates for the U.S. civilian non institutionalized population.* Rockville, MD: Medical Expenditure Panel Survey, Agency for Healthcare Research and Quality.

Stanley, S. M. (2003). Strengthening marriages in a skeptical culture: Issues and opportunities. *Journal of Psychology and Theology. 31*, 224–230.

Toseland, R.W., Blanchard, C.G., & McCallion, P. (1996). A problem solving intervention with spouses of cancer patients. *Journal of Psychosocial Oncology. 14*, 1–21.

Trask, P. C. (2004). Assessment of depression in cancer patients. *Journal National Cancer Institute Monographs. 32*, 80–92.

USA Today. (2006). The Kaiser Family Foundation, The Harvard School of Public Health. National survey of households affected by cancer, August 1–September 14, (#7591).

Welch-McCaffrey, D., Hoffman, B., Leigh, S. A., Loescher, L. J., & Meyskens, L. (1989). Surviving adult cancers. Part 2: Psychosocial implications. *Annals of Internal Medicine. 111*, 517–524.

Woods, N. F., & Earp, J. L. (1978). Women with cured breast cancer: A study of mastectomy patients in North Carolina. *Nursing Research. 27*, 279–285.

Yabroff, K. R., Lawrence, W. F., Clauser, S., Davis, W. W., & Brown, M. L. (2004). Burden of illness in cancer survivors: Findings from a population-based national sample. *Journal National Cancer Institute. 96*(17), 1322–1330.

Yehuda, R. (2002). Post-traumatic stress disorder. *New England Journal of Medicine. 346*, 108–114.

CHAPTER **5**

SPIRITUALITY

"My belief in God has helped me through this ordeal. I truly believe that with God's help I will overcome this."

—A cancer survivor

Key Terms

religious/religiousness • spirituality • theistic/nontheistic worldview

Upon completing this chapter, you will be able to do the following:

1. Differentiate religion and spirituality.
2. Discuss religion and spirituality and their role in the care of cancer survivors.
3. Describe the relationship between religion and spirituality and a sense of psychological well-being in the patient with cancer.

Introduction

Since the 1980s, religion and spirituality (R/S) have been studied in an attempt to understand how individuals cope with chronic or severe illnesses, including cancer. The literature supports a significant link between R/S and psychological well-being (Fisher, 2011; Schreiber & Brockopp, 2012; Thomas, Burton, Griffin, & Fitzpatrick, 2010), psychological distress (Ellison & Lee, 2010; Rawdin, Evans, & Rabow, 2013; Schreiber, 2011; Schreiber & Brockopp, 2012), and quality of life (Edmondson, Park, Blank, Fenster, & Mills, 2008; Kristeller, Sheets, Johnson, & Frank, 2011; Whitford & Olver, 2012). The relationship between R/S and experience of side effects (Anandarajah & Hight, 2001; Büssing, Fischer, Ostermann, & Matthiessen, 2008; Wonghongkul, Dechaprom, Phumivichuvate, & Losawatkul, 2006) and survival (King et al., 2013; Van Ness, Kasl, & Jones, 2003) is much less clear. The vast majority of studies regarding R/S and health and cancer are cross-sectional and qualitative. The work has advanced in recent years to include more quasi-experimental studies and a few true randomized control trials (Rosmarin, Wachholtz, & Ai, 2011). Why is this so? How can we move forward with R/S research which would enable us to provide quality, evidence-based care? This chapter will discuss definitions, related and/or overlapping concepts, theoretical frameworks, ways of measuring R/S, evidence-based interventions, resources, and future directions for understanding R/S and its role in the care of cancer survivors.

Conceptual Definitions

When discussing issues of R/S, there are four main conceptual definitions to consider—spirituality, religion, religions, and theistic/nontheistic worldview. Although it may seem that there is not much of a difference between these four concepts, there is. Failure to consider the definition of a concept being discussed or studied may result in confusion, misinterpretation of results due to unclear variables, and collection of information that is not particularly useful within the clinical interaction between survivors and healthcare professionals. A concept analysis on spirituality, religion, and religions identified similarities and clear differences (Lazenby, 2010). The terms "religion" and "spirituality" are considered to be very similar and overlapping, where the individual experiences and reacts to life in the context of a belief in God/Higher Power/Energy characterized by a sense of the transcendent. "Religions," on the other hand, is the concept of the objectification of beliefs into particular attitudes, behaviors, and rituals associated with a named object of belief.

Religion. An analysis of the conceptualization and definition of religion and spirituality from 2000 was the first paper to try to identify commonalities and differences between the two concepts (Hill et al., 2000). The definition of religion is as follows:

> The feelings, thoughts, experiences, and behaviors that arise from a search for the sacred. The term "search" refers to attempts to identify, articulate, maintain, or transform. The term "sacred" refers to a divine being, divine object, Ultimate Reality, or Ultimate Truth as perceived by the individual. (p. 66)

The conclusion was that this core definition was the sole criterion for spirituality and was the core criteria for religion in addition to two other criteria related to the means and methods of the search for the sacred. Other definitions of religion include "…is defined as religious practice, religious coping, perception of God, and religious support (Hill et al., 2000, p. 83)."

Spirituality. A consensus statement from a conference designed to examine spirituality in palliative care, in which there was an agreement on what directions to go in the future, was published in 2009 (Puchalski et al., 2009). The definition of spirituality is as follows:

> Spirituality is the aspect of humanity that refers to the way individuals seek and express meaning and purpose and the way they experience their connectedness to the moment, to self, to others, to nature, and to the significant or sacred. (p. 887)

This definition is very close to the definition of Hill et al. in 2000 referred to in the religion section. Along with the conceptual definition, there are many recommendations from the Consensus Conference on how to move the science around R/S forward.

Religions/Religiousness. The terms religions and religiousness are essentially the same. Both terms convey the sense of specified beliefs, attitudes, and behaviors associated with particular creeds or belief systems. People with similar views of God, divine being, Ultimate Reality/Truth, or the transcendent will often also share beliefs of how the world works, attitudes toward the source of meaning in their lives, and behaviors arising from those beliefs that help to reinforce them (Audi, 2008; Park, Edmondson, Hale-Smith, & Blank, 2009; Stark, Hamberg, & Miller, 2005).

Individuals who associate themselves with organized or "churched" religions follow a common creed or doctrine. Stark et al. (2005) defined "unchurched" religions as those without formal congregations that can vary, from having a specific creed to very individualized beliefs, but that influence and direct behaviors and the search for ultimate meaning in life. Any group that identifies itself with a name ending in "ism" can be considered a group with inherently religious beliefs and practices. Merriam-Webster dictionary defines *-ism* as "a distinctive doctrine, cause, or theory" (Merriman-Webster, 2007). When individuals rally around a doctrine, cause, or theory, behaviors associated with commonly accepted religious behaviors arise: guidelines for living, "good" and "bad" behaviors, devotion to the principles of the *ism,* and the desire to influence or convert others to their beliefs.

Theistic/Nontheistic Worldview (TNW). Religious, spiritual, or existential questions are frequently raised by patients and survivors after a diagnosis of cancer (Albaugh, 2003; Baker, 2003; Fabricatore, Handal, Rubio, & Gilner, 2004; Koenig, 2004). An individual's religious—spiritual—existential worldview is the primary driving force directing most people's behaviors.

Each person's ultimate concern is the search for transcendent meaning or striving to answer fundamental questions: Why am I here? Or, what is my purpose in life? (Archer, Collier, & Porpora, 2004; Frankl, 1978; Reker & Chamberlain, 2000). The search for meaning and the pursuit of "the ultimate" are universal themes within one's TNW (Baldacchino & Draper, 2001; Chan, Ng, Ho, & Chow, 2006; Emmons, 2000; Weber, Pargament, Kunik, Lomax, & Stanley, 2012).

Worldviews are comprehensive views or philosophies of how human life interacts with the world or environment (Carvalho, 2006; McSherry & Cash, 2004). Vidal (2008) identifies six fundamental questions: (1) What is? (ontology-model of being); (2) Where does it all come from? (explanation-model of the past); (3) Where are we going? (prediction-model of the future); (4) What is good and what is evil? (axiology-theory of values); (5) How should we act? (praxeology-theory of action); and (6) What is true and what is false? (epistemology-theory of knowing). Other works discussing worldviews present variations on these fundamental questions (Sire, 2004; Vidal, 2012). Worldviews influence personal choices and require or mandate specific behaviors (Buck, Baldwin, & Schwartz, 2005; Kagee & Dixon, 2000). One's worldview is expressed through actions and behaviors that are congruent with underlying beliefs (Koltko-Rivera, 2004). Answers to these questions and common behaviors based on shared responses may be theistic or nontheistic in nature.

Related Concepts

There are many concepts that overlap with the concepts of R/S. These include, but are not limited to: (1) meaning and purpose in life; (2) hope; (3) connectedness; (4) love; and (5) forgiveness (Henoch & Danielson, 2009; Whitford & Olver, 2012). Underlying much of the variation difficulty in teasing out what part of each of these concepts is independent from R/S is definitional inconsistency and a multiplicity of measures used to evaluate R/S. Other concepts may not overlap with R/S but are strongly related, such as: (1) anxiety; (2) depression; (3) demoralization; (4) psychological well-being; and (5) quality of life (Henoch & Danielson, 2009; Sansone & Sansone, 2010; Sawatzky, Ratner, & Chiu, 2005; Schreiber & Brockopp, 2012; Whitford & Olver, 2012).

Meaning and Purpose in Life. Although there are measures of meaning and purpose independent of R/S (Reker, 1992; Reker, 2005; Reker & Chamberlain, 2000), one frequently used measure of spirituality, the FACIT-SP (Functional Assessment of Chronic Illness-Spiritual), has three subscales—Meaning, Peace, and Faith (Bredle, Salsman, Debb, Arnold, & Cella, 2011). Meaning and purpose are inherent in currently accepted definitions of spirituality.

Hope. R/S is closely associated with hope. Hope is often interchanged with optimism (Wills, 2007). What does one hope for, or is optimistic about? The object of hope may be in practical everyday issues such as minimal symptoms or side effects of disease and its treatment. It may also be for cure, strength, or a particular outcome in the future (Carifio & Rhodes, 2002; Stanton, Danoff-Burg, & Huggins, 2002). What is the source of hope? For many, their source of hope is the focus of their theistic/nontheistic worldview: God, eternal life, karma, reincarnation, or leaving a legacy (Audi, 2008; Wills, 2007). Demonstrating this interconnectedness is a study by Rawdin and colleagues (2013), where high levels of hope were associated with increased spiritual well-being scores and decreased pain intensity, pain interference with functioning, anxiety, and depression. When depression and spiritual well-being were controlled, for the relationship between hope and pain was not supported, leading to the conclusion that when someone has lost hope, the healthcare professional should "…look beyond pain measures and explore psychological adjustment and spiritual concerns." (p. 171)

Connectedness. Connectedness is a sense of relationship to God or a Higher Power or to others (Coyle, 2002; Pesut, 2008; Villagomeza, 2005). Facing a significant illness, such as cancer, is difficult. When someone feels alone and disconnected, the challenges of the illness may be overwhelming. Studies (Chan et al., 2006; Lin & Bauer-Wu, 2003; Pesut, 2008; Villagomeza, 2005) and measures (de Jager Meezenbroek et al., 2012) have consistently included a sense of connectedness as a component of R/S. Connecting with others, a Higher Power, or God, imparts a sense of support and belonging which increases one's inner strength (Villagomeza, 2005).

Love. Love is a universal human need (Maslow, 1943). According to Maslow's theory of human motivation, love and belonging comes after basic physiologic and safety needs and need to be met before esteem and self-actualization issues can be addressed. Love is identified as a need and component of the spiritual (Lane, 2005; Taylor, 2003; Wright, 2002). Love, belonging, and connectedness are interrelated and overlap with the spiritual well-being (Frankl, 2000; Pargament, 2007), usually in the context of discussing what is sacred and vital to well-being in life.

Forgiveness. Many people dealing with life-threatening issues have a need for forgiveness from God, others, or themselves (Pargament, Koenig, & Perez, 2000; Puchalski et al., 2009; Romero et al., 2006). A sense of a need for forgiveness is based on an individual sense of failure to adhere to a moral standard based on one's theistic/nontheistic worldview. Forgiveness is only needed when relational issues and conflicts arise; conflicts can be bi-directional and open or often are one-sided and internalized. Lack of forgiveness is a major stressor in palliative care settings (Friedman et al., 2010; Romero et al., 2006) and in survivorship (Johnstone et al., 2012; Worthington, Lin, & Ho, 2012). Spirituality and religion are sources of moral authority and avenues for finding forgiveness and peace.

Psychological Distress. Concepts commonly used as proxies for psychological distress—anxiety and depression—have consistently strong associations with measures of R/S (Johnson et al., 2011; King et al., 2013; Rawdin et al., 2013; Schreiber, 2011; Schreiber & Brockopp, 2012). In general, as R/S measures increase, anxiety and depression decrease (Schreiber & Brockopp, 2012). Reports of increased anxiety and depression have been noted when individuals use "turning to religion" as a key coping mechanism (Gall, Kristjansson, Charbonneau, & Florack, 2009; Schreiber & Brockopp, 2012). This association, at first glance, may seem to be unexpected; however, if someone has not been relying on their R/S resources for support they may "turn to religion" for support when they experience anxiety and depression. If the event causing the distress is not resolved in the way they expected by turning to religion, one's anxiety and depression may increase as they perceive that religion did not solve their problems.

Anxiety and depression are treated with medications, psychotherapy, or both (Liu et al., 2008; Mueller, Plevak, & Rummans, 2001; Sheard & Maguire, 1999). Antidepressants do not work for everyone and may be a source of major drug interactions (Lal et al., 2012). Often a survivor does not clearly present as anxious or depressed, yet is experiencing distress. A lesser known, or discussed, diagnosis may be demoralization and apathy. Demoralization is considered a dysphoric state where the individual experiences existential distress feeling a sense of despondency, despair, or futility (Sansone & Sansone, 2010; Vehling et al., 2011; Vehling & Mehnert, 2013). There are differences between grief—an emotional response, usually time limited, anhedonic depression—where there is an absence of pleasure in all areas of life, and demoralization—where a range of emotions can be expressed in areas where the person is not demoralized (Wellen, 2010). This description of demoralization may be true for many cancer survivors. They can enjoy their child's graduation, wedding, or another event in the moment, but be despondent and despairing about their own future. Recent research has begun to include measures of demoralization when assessing psychological distress in cancer patients (Vehling et al., 2011, Vehling et al., 2012; Vehling & Mehnert, 2013).

Psychological Well-Being/Quality of Life. Like psychological distress, psychological well-being and quality of life are strongly associated with R/S factors. Survivors who view God as loving or engaged with the world and with themselves report higher levels of well-being and quality of life (Fisher, 2011; Schreiber, 2011; Stroope, Draper, & Whitehead, 2013; Whitford & Olver, 2012). Survivors who utilize active coping or positive religious coping also report higher levels of well-being and quality of life (Gall, 2004; Gall, Guirguis-Younger, Charbonneau, & Florack, 2009). One issue in data interpretation is that many of the studies linking quality of life to spiritual well-being is the use of the FACIT-Sp. Some of the questions in the spiritual portion of the measure are asking about spiritual well-being and the other four subscales are physical, emotional, functional, and social well-being, which may amplify the associations (Bredle et al., 2011; Monod et al., 2011). Considerations for future work will need to focus on which specific pieces or measures of R/S measure a construct separate from well-being or any other related concepts discussed in this section.

Theoretical Frameworks

There are many theoretical frameworks describing the role and measurement of R/S factors. A sampling of frameworks based on three main foci—behaviors, attitudes, and theistic/nontheistic worldviews—will be discussed. Frameworks that clearly present each view, or are the most commonly used will be highlighted.

Behaviors. Spiritual Intelligence as a framework was brought forward by Robert Emmons (2000). Spiritual intelligence is the ability for people to solve problems and attain goals utilizing a set of spiritual capacities and abilities (Fig. 5.1). Five core components are listed related to transcendence, heightened consciousness, sanctification of experiences, use of spiritual resources, and virtuousness.

The Spiritual Framework of Coping was developed by Gall and colleagues as an adaptation of the Transactional Model of Coping (Fig. 5.2; Gall et al., 2005). This framework incorporates spirituality into the appraisal process, spiritual coping behaviors, spiritual connections, and person factors leading to meaning making which impacts well-being. The framework was reviewed by clergy representing a variety of faiths—Muslim, Christian, Jewish, Secular Humanism, and Hinduism—who found that the Spiritual Framework of Coping fit each of their faith traditions.

Attitudes. The most significant framework associated with the individual's coping and attitude toward R/S was developed by Pargament (2007). He believes that spirituality is the core function of religion as people search for the sacred (Fig. 5.3; Pargament, 2013). Religious coping mechanisms are used to conserve spiritual resources or to deal with spiritual struggles: successful coping results in transformation and unsuccessful coping results in spiritual disengagement which culminates in either growth or decline.

Theistic/Nontheistic Worldviews. Frameworks based on behaviors, coping, or attitudes have produced improved understanding of how outward manifestations of R/S relate to the individual and the world. Some scientists are asking not how do beliefs manifest themselves in behaviors, coping, and attitudes, but what does one's fundamental belief about how God, Higher Power, Ultimate Source interacts with individuals and the world have to do with the role of R/S and health (Ironson et al., 2011; Josephson & Peteet, 2007; Schreiber & Edward, 2014). Whether one believes about the existence of God or not and how God interacts with the individual and world or not is the basis for

Core Components of Spiritual Intelligence

1. The capacity to transcend the physical and material.

2. The ability to experience heightened states of consciousness.

3. The ability to sanctify everyday experience.

4. The ability to utilize spiritual resources to solve problems.

5. The capacity to be virtuous.

Figure 5.1 • Core components of spiritual intelligence. (Emmons, R. A. (2000). Is spirituality an intelligence? Motivation, cognition, and the psychology of ultimate concern. *International Journal for the Psychology of Religion. 10*(1), 3. Reprinted by permission of Taylor & Francis Ltd, http://www.tandf.co.uk/journals.)

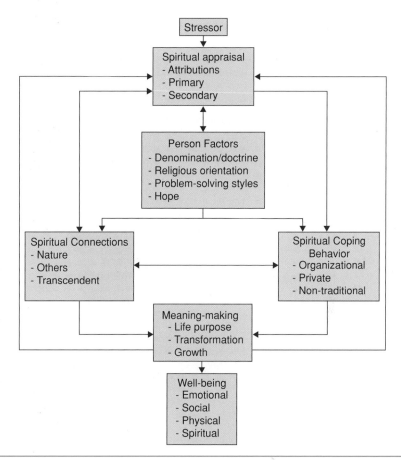

Figure 5.2 • The Spiritual Framework of Coping (an adaptation/applicationof the transactional model). (From Gall, T. L., Charbonneau, C., Clarke, N. H., Grant, K., Joseph, A., & Shouldice, L. (2005). Understanding the nature and role of spirituality in relation to coping and health: a conceptual framework. *Canadian Psychology. 46*(2), pp. 88–104. Copyright 2005, Canadian Psychological Association. Permission granted for use of material.)

answering key life questions such as, what is right/wrong? Is there good/evil? Is there life after death? What kind of life after death?

The Relational Model of Image of God in Cancer Survivorship was developed from a mixed methods approach with early breast cancer survivors (Fig. 5.4; Schreiber & Edward, 2014). Women who believed in a highly engaged (HE) God reported higher psychological well-being and lower psychological distress than women who believed in a lesser engaged (LE) God (Schreiber, 2011). Based on this finding, qualitative descriptive data was analyzed for two groups: those viewing God as HE and those viewing God as LE. Comparing where they were after treatment to where they were before their diagnosis, women with an HE view reported strengthening their relationship with God, personal growth, improved relations with others, and a transformed life. Women with an LE view reported personal growth based on their own activities and personal endeavors and a focus on making life good for them.

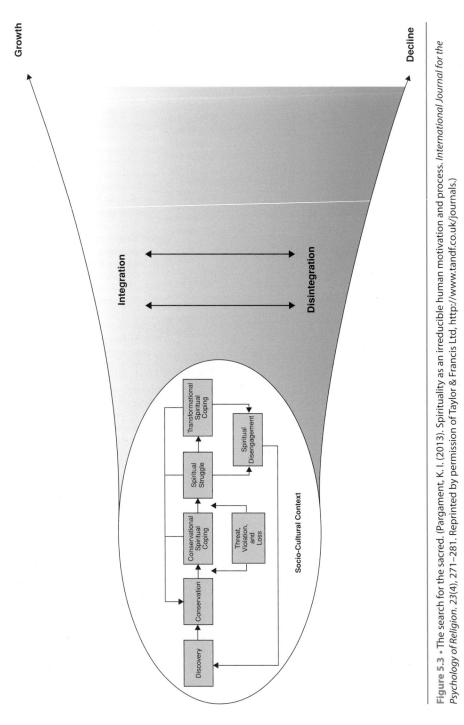

Figure 5.3 • The search for the sacred. (Pargament, K. I. (2013). Spirituality as an irreducible human motivation and process. *International Journal for the Psychology of Religion. 23*(4), 271–281. Reprinted by permission of Taylor & Francis Ltd, http://www.tandf.co.uk/journals.)

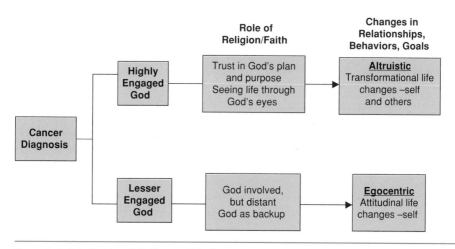

Figure 5.4 • Relational model of image of God in cancer survivorship. (With kind permission from Springer Science+Business Media. Schreiber, J. A., & Edward, J. (2014). Image of god, religion, spirituality and life changes in breast cancer survivors: a qualitative approach. *Journal of Religion and Health, Advanced Online Publication. 54*(2), 612–622.)

Spirituality Across the Cancer Experience

R/S impacts all aspects of the cancer experience from screening through end-of-life. A clear picture of the true role of R/S in the cancer experience is quite difficult to paint; there are more than 120 measures of R/S and multiple measures of related concepts resulting in an infinite number of combinations—all of which are purported to measure the same thing (de Jager Meezenbroek et al., 2012; Hall, Meador, & Koenig, 2008; Schreiber & Brockopp, 2012).

An individual's R/S beliefs, or theistic/nontheistic worldviews, are associated with their willingness to participate in cancer screening and treatment decisions (El Turabi, Abel, Roland, & Lyratzopoulos, 2013; Gall, Kristjansson, et al., 2009; Johnson, Elbert-Avila, & Tulsky, 2005; Mohamed, Skeel Williams, Tamburrino, Wryobeck, & Carter, 2005; True et al., 2005; Underwood & Powell, 2006). If operating from a fatalistic view, a survivor may choose to delay seeking help or ignore early symptoms believing that what happens, happens and that there is no way to change events or outcomes in life. Others may believe that although they have been diagnosed with cancer, through their efforts alone, their efforts in conjunction with God/Higher Power/Ultimate Source, or God/Higher Power/Ultimate Source acting alone, the outcome of their diagnosis is not set in stone. A sense of fatalism or a sense of hope and action often results in vastly different choices about whether to be screened, the urgency of seeking treatment, need for information, and participation in treatment decisions (Kub et al., 2003). Understanding the worldview that underlies the survivor's responses and decisions is vital to understanding why certain decisions are made, and to inform the delivery of education (Josephson & Peteet, 2007).

Studies regarding R/S and worldviews are most prevalent in populations of cancer survivors, conducted from the initial treatment period through the end-of-life. R/S plays a strong role in survivors' coping processes, psychological well-being, fear of recurrence, and ability to face death and dying well first, whether measured with general coping scales or specific religious coping scales. R/S factors, such as seeking God's help and preserving R/S beliefs (positive religious coping), are generally associated with improved psychosocial outcomes such as increased sense of well-being, decreased anxiety and depression, less death anxiety, lower fear of recurrence, and improved quality of life (Burton et al., 2012; Schreiber, 2011; Schreiber & Brockopp, 2012; Thune-Boyle, Stygall, Keshtgar, & Newman, 2006; van Laarhoven, Schilderman, Vissers, Verhagen, & Prins, 2010). However, some studies have found an increase in anxiety and depression with some aspects of R/S, particularly with survivors who "turn to God/religion" once diagnosed, those who see God/Higher Power/Ultimate Source as primarily good/positive, or those who are experiencing spiritual struggles (negative religious coping) (Büssing et al., 2008; Gall, Kristjansson, et al., 2009; Tarakeshwar et al., 2006). One possible explanation for a decrease in psychological well-being may be that the survivor is turning to God or expecting God to cure them, take away the cancer, or save them from cancer.

Second, R/S has been studied extensively related to psychological well-being and distress with the vast majority of studies, mostly cross-sectional, generally supporting a positive relationship between R/S and psychological well-being and an inverse relationship with distress (Laubmeier, Zakowski, & Bair, 2004; Manning-Walsh, 2005; Schreiber & Brockopp, 2012). Regardless of a survivor's theistic/nontheistic worldview whether atheistic, secular humanistic, deistic, or theistic, its positive or negative impact on psychological well-being and distress is most significantly affected by their sense of coherence/certainty or struggle with their stated worldview or belief system. The more certain a survivor is about the truth of their worldview, the more likely they are to report better psychological well-being and less distress (Ellison & Lee, 2010; Schreiber, 2011; Weber et al., 2012; Zwingmann, Wirtz, Müller, Körber, & Murken, 2006). Survivors who report an existential crisis or struggle with their worldview in the presence of their diagnosis, treatment, and survival also report more distress and less psychological well-being (Ellison & Lee, 2010; Hills, Paice, Cameron, & Shott, 2005; Mako, Galek, & Poppito, 2006; Schreiber, 2011; Zwingmann et al., 2006).

Third, a recent survey of survivors reported that fear of recurrence/living with uncertainty were among the top concerns (Ness et al., 2013). Fear or concern of recurrence in relation to R/S has not been studied much; however, a couple of studies found decreased fear of recurrence in survivors who reported a higher level of religiosity or higher level of God's engagement (Hamrick & Diefenbach, 2006; Schreiber, 2011). A view of God/Higher Power/Ultimate Truth who is actively involved with the survivors' life appears to be distinct and survivors with this view do report significant differences from survivors with other theistic/nontheistic worldviews.

Fourth, how a survivor approaches or feels about death and end-of-life has also been linked with R/S views. Although many studies have examined R/S and dying, the majority have been cross-sectional or qualitative. Data from these types of studies provide a lot of information regarding R/S and end-of-life; however, they are snapshots of many at the time of the survey or videos of the individual experiences of a few. Longitudinal studies and those designed to specifically compare people with varying theistic/nontheistic worldviews are not common. A recent longitudinal study with three time points ($n = 170$) compared the person's strength of belief to their levels of anxiety, depression, and use of psychotropic drugs and concluded that there were no differences between groups (King et al., 2013). Some issues to consider in interpreting these findings include the fact that at time 2, 33 participants (19%) were lost to follow-up and at time 3, 57 participants (33.5%) were lost to follow-up; data was imputed and according to the authors did not significantly change the results (King et al., 2013). Also, the comparator was the strength of belief, not what the participants believed. Death awareness and the person's beliefs about God/Allah/Buddha among Christians, Muslims, Atheists, and Agnostics was examined (Vail, Arndt, & Abdollahi, 2012). When confronted with a death reminder, Christians and Muslims reported stronger belief in their worldview and less belief in other worldviews, Atheists did not report any difference, and Agnostics reported an increased belief in God, Allah, or Buddha (Vail et al., 2012). The authors concluded that whatever the person's theistic/nontheistic worldview was prior to the death reminder, it was increased or strengthened for Christians, Muslims, and Agnostics. Only Atheists reported no difference in the strength/importance of their worldview.

Across the cancer survivor continuum, R/S has been identified as a significant factor in the person's experience. Reactions to a cancer diagnosis, treatment, and issues of survivorship are influenced by the survivor's theistic/nontheistic worldview. What a survivor believes about the existence of God/Higher Power/Ultimate Truth or that there is nothing beyond humankind, forms the base for beliefs of how the world works. These beliefs, whether consciously acknowledged or not, are the lens by which each person looks out at the world and how they interpret events in the world (Koltko-Rivera, 2004).

R/S Assessment in Research

In the last two decades, researchers have attempted to develop measures of R/S that grasp essential conceptual components. In the process, some measures specifically focus on particular aspects, ethnic viewpoints, and faith traditions. Other measures, attempting to measure a concept of R/S that encompasses or transcends all belief systems, are quite broad in scope. As a result, there are well over 100 measures of religion and spirituality, with more being developed and tested each year (Hill & Hood, 1999). A number of systematic reviews have examined measures of R/S from different perspectives (Berry, Bass, Forawi, Neuman, & Abdallah, 2011; de Jager Meezenbroek et al., 2012; Monod et al., 2011; Selman, Harding, Gysels, Speck, & Higginson, 2011). Due to the large number of measures available, this section will review the three most commonly reviewed measures of R/S based on the measure's perspective: (1) spiritual well-being; (2) attitudinal/behavioral; and (3) theistic/non-theistic worldview.

Spiritual Well-Being. The two most commonly used measures are the Functional Assessment of Chronic Illness Therapy-Spiritual (FACIT-Sp) and the Spiritual Well-Being Scale (Bredle et al., 2011; Kapuscinski & Masters, 2010; Paloutzian & Ellison, 1982; Peterman, Fitchett, Brady, Hernandez, & Cella, 2002). The FACIT-Sp was designed to inclusively measure spirituality (Peterman et al., 2002). The FACIT-Sp is a specific, 12-item subscale added to the core measure—Functional Assess of Cancer Therapy-General (FACT-G), 27-items which measure four well-being domains: (1) physical; (2) functional; (3) social/family; and (4) emotional. The FACT-G provides a total quality of life score and subscales can be scored individually, with good internal consistency reliability scores, $\alpha = 0.72$ to 0.85 (Peterman et al., 2002). The FACIT-SP originally had two subscales: peace/meaning and faith (Peterman et al., 2002); however, further psychometric studies have supported a three-factor model: peace, meaning, and faith (Bredle et al., 2011; Canada, Murphy, Fitchett, Peterman, & Schover, 2008). The Spiritual Well-Being Scale is a 20-item measure of spiritual quality of life with two subscales, religious well-being and existential well-being. It is a self-report measure with initial internal consistency reliabilities of $\alpha = 0.87$ to 0.89 (Paloutzian & Ellison, 1982).

Attitudinal/Behavioral. There are three frequently used measures related to attitudinal and behavioral aspects of R/S: the RCOPE (Pargament et al., 2000), the Multidimensional Measure of Religiousness/Spirituality (MMRS) (Fetzer Institute National Institute on Aging Working Group, 1999), and the Daily Spiritual Experience Scale (DESS) (Underwood & Teresi, 2002). The RCOPE is a measure of religious coping mechanisms that currently has four versions: (1) RCOPE, 105 items: 21 subscales with 5 items per subscale; (2) RCOPE-Short Form, 63 items: 21 subscales with 3 items per subscale; (3) BriefRCOPE, 11 items: one overall question and two subscales, positive and negative coping, with 5 items per subscale; and (4) BriefRCOPE-Short Form, 7 items: one overall question and two subscales, positive and negative coping, with 3 items per subscale (Pargament et al., 2000). A more recent publication, reports on a 14-item measure with two subscales, positive and negative religious coping. Internal consistency reliability was reported based on pooled data from 30 studies across a variety of populations: positive religious coping median $\alpha = 0.92$ and negative religious coping median $\alpha = 0.81$ (Pargament, Feuille, & Burdzy, 2011).

The MMRS is a comprehensive general measure of R/S across 12 domains identified by the Fetzer Institute, National Institute on Aging Working Group (1999). The 12 domains include daily spiritual experiences, meaning, values, beliefs, forgiveness, private religious practices, religious/spiritual coping, religious support, religious/spiritual history, commitment, organizational religiousness, and religious preference. There are two versions: the long version with 88 items and the short version with 38 items with internal consistency reliabilities ranging from $\alpha = 0.54$ to 0.91 across disparate samples (Fetzer Institute National Institute on Aging Working Group, 1999; Monod et al., 2011).

The DSES is a 16-item measure designed to assess experiences of spirituality such as inner peace, joy, and awe (Fetzer Institute National Institute on Aging Working Group, 1999; Underwood & Teresi, 2002); what the person perceives as transcendent and their interaction with the transcendent in life. Questions are reflective of the person's feelings and desires related to the transcendent (i.e., "I feel...," "I am spiritually touched...," "I desire...") (Underwood & Teresi, 2002). Internal consistency reliability is strong with $\alpha = 0.94$ to 0.95 (Underwood & Teresi, 2002). The DSES is positively associated psychological variables and with social support (Underwood & Teresi, 2002).

Theistic/Nontheistic Worldviews. There are two measures of how people view God and God's interaction with the world that have been studied in health research: the Image of God Scale (IGS) (Bader & Froese, 2005; Schreiber, 2011) and the View of God Inventory (VOG) measure (Ironson et al., 2011). The IGS is a 14-item measure with two subscales: engagement (8 items) and judgment (6 items) (Bader & Froese, 2005). The two subscales can also be combined to identify four images of God: Benevolent, Authoritarian, Distant, and Critical (Bader & Froese, 2005). Internal consistency reliabilities are reported as $\alpha = 0.89$ to 0.91 for Engagement and $\alpha = 0.80$ to 0.85 (Bader & Froese, 2005; Schreiber, 2011). The VOG Inventory is a 12-item, measure with two subscales: Positive View of God (benevolent/loving/merciful/forgiving) and Negative View of God (harsh/judgmental/punishing) (Ironson et al., 2011). Internal consistency reliability was good: Positive View of God, $\alpha = 0.86$ and Negative View of God, $\alpha = 0.78$ (Ironson et al., 2011).

The concept of theistic/nontheistic worldviews as a measure of R/S is not totally new; however, older measures tended to be rather long and did not make significant inroads into health research. Over the past two decades, the number of R/S studies and measures has burgeoned. Due to this interest in R/S research there is a breadth of knowledge about the relationship of R/S to cancer survivorship issues, but there is limited depth of information on meaningful R/S interventions and activities that transcend belief systems or are appropriate based on different R/S beliefs. One reason may be that the majority of the studies related to R/S examine attitudes, behaviors, and well-being associated with a person's theistic/nontheistic worldview, not the worldview itself. Whether someone perceives God/Higher Power/Ultimate Truth to be in ultimate control, believes that there is collaboration between themselves and God/Higher Power/Ultimate Truth, or believes that their effort is all that matters, what the person thinks and how they behave in relation to cancer survivorship flows from their view of how the world works.

R/S Interventions

Intervention studies for R/S factors in improved psychological well-being and quality of life have been infrequent and findings from these studies have limited usage in general practice, but the science is young. A burst of new studies have been published in the last 2 years, making the studies referenced a representation, not an exhaustive list, of what is in the literature. Most intervention studies related to R/S and cancer survivors employ mindfulness, creative arts, prayer, or cognitive therapy/meaning making. Mindfulness studies have consistently reported improvements in psychological well-being, quality of life, stress, and pain (Ando et al., 2009; Bränström, Kvillemo, & Moskowitz, 2012; Garland, Thomas, & Howard; Lengacher et al., 2014; Moadel et al., 1999; Targ & Levine, 2002). Creative arts therapies have been used for many years; study results have supported positive effects on sense of psychological well-being, quality of life, and spirituality (Hodge, 2005; Lane, 2008; Puig, Lee, Goodwin, & Sherrard, 2006; Tuck, 2004; Wood, Molassiotis, & Payne, 2011). Intercessory or centering prayer has been linked to improved quality of life, psychological well-being, and physical symptoms; most interesting is that the intercessory prayer studies have been double- or triple-blinded so participants are not even aware that prayer is part of the study (Heiney et al., 2003; Johnson et al., 2009; Olver & Dutney, 2012; Palmer, Katerndahl, & Morgan-Kidd, 2004). The most frequently used intervention is cognitive therapy/meaning making, either individually or through group activities. Improved emotional, psychological, physical, and functional well-being have been reported after cognitive therapy/meaning making (Breitbart et al., 2012; Breitbart et al., 2010; Cole & Pargament, 1999; Lee, 2008; Miller, Chibnall, Videen, & Duckro, 2005).

The rapid increase in intervention studies since the mid-2000s is an exciting step forward in R/S research. Studies confirming methodologies such as mindfulness-based therapies and other cognitive therapies in diverse cancer survivor populations will solidify the effectiveness of these interventions, refine the interventions, and ultimately improve the implementation of evidence-based R/S interventions.

R/S Resources

R/S resources are available from nursing, social work, chaplaincy, and behavioral medicine sources. At this time, few of the resources will be as up-to-date as a literature search for R/S issues or interventions that are of interest to you. New data related to interventions and understanding R/S in cancer survivorship is increasing exponentially. With that caveat, there are some well-maintained and updated resources on the Internet. George Washington University hosts The George Washington Institute for Spirituality and Health (http:/smhs.gwu.edu/gwish). The Center for Spirituality, Theology, and Health is based in the Duke University Center for Aging and Human Development (www.spiritualityandhealth.duke.edu). The Institute for Studies of Religion is based in the Sociology Department at Baylor University, but has an interdisciplinary focus (www.baylorisr.org). The Oncology Nursing Society has many resources available by searching the term "Spiritual Care" on their website (www.ons.org). The American Cancer Society also has links to numerous resources by searching "spiritual" on their website (www.cancer.org). The National Cancer Institute has the Spirituality in Cancer Care report in two versions, health professional and patient, along with many other resources by searching "spiritual" (www.cancer.gov/cancertopics/pdq/supportivecare/spirituality/HealthProfessional; www.cancer.gov/cancertopics/pdq/supportivecare/spirituality/Patient).

CASE STUDY

Randy and Jean Cooper have been married for 8 years. They have four children: Ben, a healthy 6-year-old who is in first grade; Susie, their outgoing 5-year-old; and Caleb and Connor, very active 15-month-old twins. Jean worked as a secretary until the twins were born. At that time they decided they would be better off financially if Jean stayed home with the children, since the cost of daycare would be almost as much as Jean made in a year. Randy is an outside sales person with a busy territory that causes him to have dinner meetings at least one night a week. The family moved to a new town, 100 miles away, when Randy switched territories 4 months ago, so that he could be home more often since he was out of town one to two nights a week. Randy does not think his demanding boss will be very accommodating of any changes in his schedule or work plan.

Jean is a survivor of Stage II Hodgkin lymphoma below the diaphragm, having completed her treatment shortly before the move. Prior to moving, the Cooper's were very active in their hometown church they attended since before they married. Many long-term friends and family had helped with childcare, housework, and meals during treatment. Even after the move, family and friends made the trip to their new home to help for a few days at a time. Randy and Jean do not know how they would have been able to cope with everything if they had not had the help.

Since the move, they spent a few months finding a new church home where they have attended regularly for the last 5 months. They are friendly with a number of other parents they have met at church, but have not yet developed deep friendships. Now that Jean is a "survivor" and "back to normal," the visits from old family and friends have dropped off. Randy feels that Jean is "short-tempered" and "withdrawn from their relationship and from activities with the children." Jean comes to the oncology clinic for her 6-month follow-up visit and tells you that she feels abandoned by her family, friends, and God. She also states that she is depressed because "... everyone keeps congratulating me on being a 'survivor.'

They think that everything is back to 'normal' now and I should get on with my life. 'You have everything to live for…a great husband, children…' is what they keep saying. I know they're trying to be encouraging and I know that I am blessed. I've always believed that God is in control, but right now I feel a dread that the disease will come back, that I'm no longer the Jean that everyone used to know, I feel like I'm playing a part in all my relationships—including with Randy, and that no one understands—they are not Hodgkin survivors."

• Critical Thinking Questions

1. How would you initially respond to Jean's questions and concerns? (Give specific actions.)

2. What questions would you ask her related to her spiritual life? (Write the questions out.)

3. What actions or behaviors would you encourage her to pursue? Why?

4. What resources would you offer Jean? Would you make the referral or would you simply give the information to Jean?

References

Albaugh, J. A. (2003). Spirituality and life-threatening illness: A phenomenologic study. *Oncology Nursing Forum. 30*(4), 593–598. doi: 10.1188/03.ONF.593–598

Anandarajah, G., & Hight, E. (2001). Spirituality and medical practice: Using the HOPE questions as a practical tool for spiritual assessment. *American Family Physician. 63*(1), 81–89.

Ando, M., Morita, T., Akechi, T., Ito, S., Tanaka, M., Ifuku, Y., & Nakayama, T. (2009). The efficacy of mindfulness-based meditation therapy on anxiety, depression, and spirituality in Japanese patients with cancer. *Journal of Palliative Medicine. 12*(12), 1091–1094. doi: 10.1089/jpm.2009.0143

Archer, M. S., Collier, A., & Porpora, D. V. (2004). *Transcendence: Critical realism and God.* London: Routledge.

Audi, R. (2008). Belief, faith, and acceptance. *International Journal for Philosophy of Religion. 63*(1–3), 87–102. doi: 10.1007/s11153–007–9137–6

Bader, C., & Froese, P. (2005). Images of God: The effect of personal theologies on moral attitudes, political affiliations, and religious behavior. *Interdisciplinary Journal of Research on Religion. 1*(Article 11), 1–24. Retrieved from www.religjournal.com

Baker, D. C. (2003). Studies of the inner life: The impact of spirituality on quality of life. *Quality of Life Research. 12*(Suppl 1), 51–57.

Baldacchino, D., & Draper, P. (2001). Spiritual coping strategies: A review of the nursing research literature. *Journal of Advanced Nursing. 34*(6), 833–841.

Berry, D. M., Bass, C. P., Forawi, W., Neuman, M., & Abdallah, N. (2011). Measuring religiosity/spirituality in diverse religious groups: A consideration of methods. *Journal of Religion & Health. 50*(4), 841–851. doi: 10.1007/s10943–011–9457–9

Bränström, R., Kvillemo, P., & Moskowitz, J. T. (2012). A randomized study of the effects of mindfulness training on psychological well-being and symptoms of stress in patients treated for cancer at 6-month follow-up. *International Journal of Behavioral Medicine. 19*(4), 535–542. doi: 10.1007/s12529–011–9192–3

Bredle, J. M., Salsman, J. M., Debb, S. M., Arnold, B. J., & Cella, D. (2011). Spiritual well-being as a component of health-related quality of life: The Functional Assessment of Chronic Illness Therapy—Spiritual Well-Being Scale (FACIT-Sp). *Religions. 2*(1), 77–94. doi: 10.3390/rel2010077

Breitbart, W., Poppito, S., Rosenfeld, B., Vickers, A. J., Li, Y., Abbey, J., ... Cassileth, B. R. (2012). Pilot randomized controlled trial of individual meaning-centered psychotherapy for patients with advanced cancer. *Journal of Clinical Oncology. 30*(12), 1304–1309. doi: 10.1200/JCO.2011.36.2517

Breitbart, W., Rosenfeld, B., Gibson, C., Pessin, H., Poppito, S., Nelson, C., ... Olden, M. (2010). Meaning-centered group psychotherapy for patients with advanced cancer: A pilot randomized controlled trial. *Psycho-Oncology. 19*(1), 21–28. doi: 10.1002/pon.1556

Buck, T., Baldwin, C. M., & Schwartz, G. E. (2005). Influence of worldview on health care choices among persons with chronic pain. *Journal of Alternative & Complementary Medicine. 11*(3), 561–568. doi: 10.1089/acm.2005.11.561

Burton, A. M., Sautter, J. M., Tulsky, J. A., Lindquist, J. H., Hays, J. C., Olsen, M. K., ... Steinhauser, K. E. (2012). Burden and well-being among a diverse sample of cancer, congestive heart failure, and chronic obstructive pulmonary disease caregivers. *Journal of Pain & Symptom Management. 44*(3), 410–420. doi:10.1016/j.jpainsymman.2011.09.018

Büssing, A., Fischer, J., Ostermann, T., & Matthiessen, P. F. (2008). Reliance on God's help, depression and fatigue in female cancer patients. *International Journal for Psychiatry Medicine. 38*(3), 357–372.

Canada, A. L., Murphy, P. E., Fitchett, G., Peterman, A. H., & Schover, L. R. (2008). A 3-factor model for the FACIT-Sp. *Psycho-Oncology. 17*(9). 908–916. doi: 10.1002/pon.1307

Carifio, J., & Rhodes, L. (2002). Construct validities and the empirical relationships between optimism, hope, self-efficacy, and locus of control. *Work. 19*(2), 125–136.

Carvalho, J. J. (2006). Overview of the structure of a scientific worldview. *Zygon®. 41*(1), 113–124. doi:10.1111/j.1467–9744.2006.00729.x

Chan, C. L., Ng, S. M., Ho, R. T., & Chow, A. Y. (2006). East meets West: Applying Eastern spirituality in clinical practice. *Journal of Clinical Nursing. 15*(7), 822–832. doi: 10.1111/j.1365–2702.2006.01649.x

Cole, B., & Pargament, K. (1999). Re-creating your life: A spiritual/psychotherapeutic intervention for people diagnosed with cancer. *Psycho-Oncology. 8*(5), 395–407.

Coyle, J. (2002). Spirituality and health: Towards a framework for exploring the relationship between spirituality and health. *Journal of Advanced Nursing. 37*(6), 589–597.

de Jager Meezenbroek, E., Garssen, B., van den Berg, M., van Dierendonck, D., Visser, A., & Schaufeli, W. B. (2012). Measuring spirituality as a universal human experience: A review of spirituality questionnaires. *Journal of Religion & Health. 51*(2), 336–354. doi: 10.1007/s10943–010–9376–1

Edmondson, D., Park, C. L., Blank, T. O., Fenster, J. R., & Mills, M. A. (2008). Deconstructing spiritual wellbeing: Existential well-being and HRQOL in cancer survivors. *Psycho-Oncology. 17*(2), 161–169.

El Turabi, A., Abel, G., Roland, M., & Lyratzopoulos, G. (2013). Variation in reported experience of involvement in cancer treatment decision making: Evidence from the National Cancer Patient Experience Survey. *British Journal of Cancer. 109*, 780–787.

Ellison, C., & Lee, J. (2010). Spiritual struggles and psychological distress: Is there a dark side of religion? *Social Indicators Research. 98*(3), 501–517. doi: 10.1007/s11205–009–9553–3

Emmons, R. A. (2000). Is spirituality an intelligence? Motivation, cognition, and the psychology of ultimate concern. *International Journal for the Psychology of Religion. 10*(1), 3.

Fabricatore, A. N., Handal, P. J., Rubio, D. M., & Gilner, F. H. (2004). Stress, religion, and mental health: Religious coping in mediating and moderating roles. *The International Journal for the Psychology of Religion. 14*(2), 91–108.

Fetzer Institute National Institute on Aging Working Group. (1999). *Multidimensional measurement of religiousness, spirituality for use in health research.* Kalamazoo, MI: Fetzer Institute.

Fisher, J. (2011). The four domains model: Connecting spirituality, health and well-being. *Religions, 2*(1), 17–28.

Frankl, V. E. (1978). *The Unheard Cry for Meaning: Psychotherapy and Humanism.* New York, NY: Simon & Schuster.

Frankl, V. E. (2000). *Man's Search for Ultimate Meaning.* New York, NY: Basic Books.

Friedman, L. C., Barber, C. R., Chang, J., Tham, Y. L., Kalidas, M., Rimawi, M. F., ... Elledge, R. (2010). Self-blame, Self-forgiveness, and spirituality in breast cancer survivors in a public sector setting. *Journal of Cancer Education. 25*(3), 343–348. doi: 10.1007/s13187–010–0048–3

Gall, T. L. (2004). The role of religious coping in adjustment to prostate cancer. *Cancer Nursing. 27*(6), 454–461.

Gall, T. L., Charbonneau, C., Clarke, N. H., Grant, K., Joseph, A., & Shouldice, L. (2005). Understanding the nature and role of spirituality in relation to coping and health: A conceptual framework. *Canadian Psychology-Psychologie Canadienne. 46*(2), 88–104.

Gall, T. L., Guirguis-Younger, M., Charbonneau, C., & Florack, P. (2009). The trajectory of religious coping across time in response to the diagnosis of breast cancer. *Psycho-Oncology. 18*(11), 1165–1178.

Gall, T. L., Kristjansson, E., Charbonneau, C., & Florack, P. (2009). A longitudinal study on the role of spirituality in response to the diagnosis and treatment of breast cancer. *Journal of Behavioral Medicine. 32*(2), 174–186. doi: 10.1007/s10865–008–9182–3

Garland, E. L., Thomas, E., & Howard, M. O. (2014). Mindfulness-oriented recovery enhancement ameliorates the impact of pain on self-reported psychological and physical function among opioid-using chronic pain patients. Advance online publication. *Journal of Pain & Symptom Management.* doi: 10.1016/j.jpainsymman.2014.03.006

Hall, D. E., Meador, K. G., & Koenig, H. G. (2008). Measuring religiousness in health research: Review and critique. *Journal of Religion & Health. 47*(2), 134–163. doi: 10.1007/s10943–008–9165–2

Hamrick, N., & Diefenbach, M. A. (2006). Religion and spirituality among patients with localized prostate cancer. *Palliative & Supportive Care. 4*(04), 345–355. doi:10.1017/S1478951506060457

Heiney, S. P., McWayne, J., Walker, S., Bryant, L. H., Howell, C. D., & Bridges, L. (2003). Evaluation of a therapeutic group by telephone for women with breast cancer. *Journal of Psychosocial Oncology. 21*(3), 63–80.

Henoch, I., & Danielson, E. (2009). Existential concerns among patients with cancer and interventions to meet them: An integrative literature review. *Psycho-Oncology. 18*(3), 225–236. doi: 10.1002/pon.1424

Hill, P. C., & Hood, R. W. (1999). *Measures of religiosity.* Birmingham, AL: Religious Education Press.

Hill, P. C., Pargament, K. I., Hood, R. W., McCoullough, M. E., Swyers, J. P., Larson, D. B., & Zinnbauer, B. J. (2000). Conceptualizing religion and spirituality: Points of commonality, points of departure. *Journal for the Theory of Social Behaviour. 30*(1), 51–77.

Hills, J., Paice, J. A., Cameron, J. R., & Shott, S. (2005). Spirituality and distress in palliative care consultation. *Journal of Palliative Medicine. 8*(4), 782–788. doi:10.1089/jpm.2005.8.782

Hodge, D. R. (2005). Spiritual lifemaps: A client-centered pictorial instrument for spiritual assessment, planning, and intervention. *Social Work. 50*(1), 77–87.

Ironson, G., Stuetzle, R., Ironson, D., Balbin, E., Kremer, H., George, A., ... Fletcher, M. (2011). View of God as benevolent and forgiving or punishing and judgmental predicts HIV disease progression. *Journal of Behavioral Medicine. 34*(6), 414–425. doi: 10.1007/s10865–011–9314–z

Johnson, K., Tulsky, J., Hays, J., Arnold, R., Olsen, M., Lindquist, J., & Steinhauser, K. (2011). Which domains of spirituality are associated with anxiety and depression in patients with advanced illness? *Journal of General& Internal Medicine. 26*(7), 751–758. doi: 10.1007/s11606–011–1656–2

Johnson, K. S., Elbert-Avila, K. I., & Tulsky, J. A. (2005). The influence of spiritual beliefs and practices on the treatment preferences of African Americans: A review of the literature. *Journal of the American Geriatrics Society.* *53*(4), 711–719.

Johnson, M. E., Dose, A. M., Pipe, T. B., Petersen, W. O., Huschka, M., Gallenberg, M. M., … Frost, M. H. (2009). Centering prayer for women receiving chemotherapy for recurrent ovarian cancer: A pilot study. *Oncology Nursing Forum.* *36*(4), 421–428. doi: 10.1188/09.ONF. 421–428

Johnstone, B., Yoon, D., Cohen, D., Schopp, L., McCormack, G., Campbell, J., & Smith, M. (2012). Relationships among spirituality, religious practices, personality factors, and health for five different faith traditions. *Journal of Religion & Health.* *51*(4), 1017–1041. doi: 10.1007/s10943012–9615–8

Josephson, A. M., & Peteet, J. R. (2007). Talking with patients about spirituality and worldview: Practical interviewing techniques and strategies. *Psychiatric Clinics of North America.* *30*(2), 181–197. doi: 10.1016/j.psc.2007.01.005

Kagee, A., & Dixon, D. N. (2000). Worldview and health promoting behavior: A causal model. *Journal of Behavioral Medicine, 23*(2), 163–179.

Kapuscinski, A. N., & Masters, K. S. (2010). The current status of measures of spirituality: A critical review of scale development. *Psychology of Religion & Spirituality, 2*(4), 191–205. doi: 10.1037/a0020498

King, M., Llewellyn, H., Leurent, B., Owen, F., Leavey, G., Tookman, A., & Jones, L. (2013). Spiritual beliefs near the end of life: A prospective cohort study of people with cancer receiving palliative care. *Psycho-Oncology.* doi: 10.1002/pon.3313

Koenig, H. G. (2004). Religion, spirituality, and medicine: Research findings and implications for clinical practice. *Southern Medical Journal.* *97*(12), 1194–1200.

Koltko-Rivera, M. E. (2004). The psychology of worldviews. *Review of General Psychology.* *8*(1), 3–58. doi: 10.1037/1089–2680.8.1.3

Kristeller, J. L., Sheets, V., Johnson, T., & Frank, B. (2011). Understanding religious and spiritual influences on adjustment to cancer: Individual patterns and differences. *Journal of Behavioral Medicine.* *34*(6), 550–561. doi: 10.1007/s10865–011–9335–7

Kub, J. E., Nolan, M. T., Hughes, M. T., Terry, P. B., Sulmasy, D. P., Astrow, A., & Forman, J. H. (2003). Religious importance and practices of patients with a life-threatening illness: Implications for screening protocols. *Applied Nursing Research.* *16*(3), 196–200.

Lal, L., Zhuang, A., Hung, F., Feng, C., Arbuckle, R., & Fisch, M. (2012). Evaluation of drug interactions in patients treated with antidepressants at a tertiary care cancer center. *Supportive Care in Cancer.* *20*(5), 983–989. doi: 10.1007/s00520–011–1170–4

Lane, M. R. (2005). Spirit body healing–A hermeneutic, phenomenological study examining the lived experience of art and healing. *Cancer Nursing.* *28*(4), 285–291.

Lane, M. R. (2008). Spirit-body healing II: A nursing intervention model for spiritual/creative healing. *Cancer Nursing.* *31*(3), E24–E31.

Laubmeier, K. K., Zakowski, S. G., & Bair, J. P. (2004). The role of spirituality in the psychological adjustment to cancer: A test of the transactional model of stress and coping. *International Journal of Behavioral Medicine.* *11*(1), 48–55. doi: 10.1207/s15327558ijbm1101_6

Lazenby, J. M. (2010). On "spirituality," "religion," and "religions": A concept analysis. *Palliative & Supportive Care.* *8*(04), 469–476. doi:10.1017/S1478951510000374

Lee, V. (2008). The existential plight of cancer: Meaning making as a concrete approach to the intangible search for meaning. *Supportive Care in Cancer.* *16*(7), 779–785.

Lengacher, C., Shelton, M., Reich, R., Barta, M., Johnson-Mallard, V., Moscoso, M., … Kip, K. (2014). Mindfulness based stress reduction (MBSR(BC)) in breast cancer: Evaluating fear of recurrence (FOR) as a mediator of psychological and physical symptoms in a randomized control trial (RCT). *Journal of Behavioral Medicine.* *37*(2), 185–195. doi: 10.1007/s10865–012–9473–6

Lin, H. R., & Bauer-Wu, S. M. (2003). Psycho-spiritual well-being in patients with advanced cancer: An integrative review of the literature. *Journal of Advanced Nursing. 44*(1), 69–80.

Liu, C. J., Hsiung, P. C., Chang, K. J., Liu, Y. F., Wang, K. C., Hsiao, F. H., …Chan, C. L. (2008). A study on the efficacy of body-mind-spirit group therapy for patients with breast cancer. *Journal of Clinical Nursing. 17*(19), 2539–2549. doi: 10.1111/j.1365-2702.2008.02296.x

Mako, C., Galek, K., & Poppito, S. R. (2006). Spiritual pain among patients with advanced cancer in palliative care. *Journal of Palliative Medicine. 9*(5), 1106–1113. doi: 10.1089/jpm.2006.9.1106

Manning-Walsh, J. K. (2005). Psychospiritual well-being and symptom distress in women with breast cancer. *Oncology Nursing Forum. 31*(3), E56–E62.

Maslow, A. H. (1943). A theory of human motivation. *Psychological Review. 50*(4), 370–396.

McSherry, W., & Cash, K. (2004). The language of spirituality: An emerging taxonomy. *International Journal of Nursing Studies. 41*(2), 151–161.

Merriman-Webster. (2007). Merriman-Webster online dictionary. Retrieved from November 30, 2997 http://www.m-w.com/dictionary/ism

Miller, D. K., Chibnall, J. T., Videen, S. D., & Duckro, P. N. (2005). Supportive-affective group experience for persons with life-threatening illness: Reducing spiritual, psychological, and death-related distress in dying patients. *Journal of Palliative Medicine. 8*(2), 333–343.

Moadel, A., Morgan, C., Fatone, A., Grennan, J., Carter, J., Laruffa, G., …Dutcher, J. (1999). Seeking meaning and hope: Self-reported spiritual and existential needs among an ethnically-diverse cancer patient population. *Psycho-Oncology. 8*(5), 378–385.

Mohamed, I. E., Skeel Williams, K., Tamburrino, M., Wryobeck, J., & Carter, S. (2005). Understanding locally advanced breast cancer: What influences a woman's decision to delay treatment? *Preventive Medicine. 41*(2), 399–405. doi: 10.1016/j.ypmed.2004.12.012

Monod, S., Brennan, M., Rochat, E., Martin, E., Rochat, S., & Bula, C. J. (2011). Instruments measuring spirituality in clinical research: A systematic review. *Journal of General & Internal Medicine. 26*(11), 1345–1357. doi: 10.1007/s11606-011-1769-7

Mueller, P. S., Plevak, D. J., & Rummans, T. A. (2001). Religious involvement, spirituality, and medicine: Implications for clinical practice. *Mayo Clinic Proceedings. 76*(12), 1225–1235.

Ness, S., Kokal, J., Fee-Schroeder, K., Novotny, P., Satele, D., & Barton, D. (2013). Concerns across the survivorship trajectory: Results from a survey of cancer survivors. *Oncology Nursing Forum. 40*(1), 35–42. doi: 10.1188/13.ONF.35–42

Olver, I. N., & Dutney, A. (2012). A randomized, blinded study of the impact of intercessory prayer on spiritual well-being in patients with cancer. *Alternative Therapies in Health & Medicine. 18*(5), 18–27.

Palmer, R. F., Katerndahl, D., & Morgan-Kidd, J. (2004). A randomized trial of the effects of remote intercessory prayer: Interactions with personal beliefs on problem-specific outcomes and functional status. *Journal of Alternative & Complementary Medicine. 10*(3), 438–448. doi: 10.1089/1075553041323803

Paloutzian, R. F., & Ellison, C. W. (1982). Loneliness, spiritual well-being, and quality of life. In L. A. Peplau & D. Perlman (Eds.), *Loneliness: A sourcebook of current theory, Research & Therapy.* New York, NY: Wiley.

Pargament, K., Feuille, M., & Burdzy, D. (2011). The Brief RCOPE: Current psychometric status of a short measure of religious coping. *Religions. 2*(1), 51–76.

Pargament, K. I. (2007). *Spiritually Integrated Psychotherapy: Understanding and Addressing the Sacred.* New York, NY: The Guildford Press.

Pargament, K. I. (2013). Spirituality as an irreducible human motivation and process. *International Journal for the Psychology of Religion, 23*(4), 271–281. doi: 10.1080/10508619.2013.795815

Pargament, K. I., Koenig, H. G., & Perez, L. M. (2000). The many methods of religious coping: Development and initial validation of the RCOPE. *Journal of Clinical Psychology. 56*(4), 519–543.

Park, C. L., Edmondson, D., Hale-Smith, A., & Blank, T. O. (2009). Religiousness/spirituality and health behaviors in younger adult cancer survivors: Does faith promote a healthier lifestyle? *Journal of Behavioral Medicine. 32*(6), 582–591. doi: 10.1007/s10865–009–9223–6

Pesut, B. (2008). A conversation on diverse perspectives of spirituality in nursing literature. *Nursing Philosophy. 9*(2), 98–109.

Peterman, A. H., Fitchett, G., Brady, M. J., Hernandez, L., & Cella, D. (2002). Measuring spiritual wellbeing in people with cancer: The Functional Assessment of Chronic Illness Therapy–Spiritual Wellbeing Scale (FACIT-Sp). *Annals of Behavioral Medicine. 24*(1), 49–58.

Puchalski, C., Ferrell, B., Virani, R., Otis-Green, S., Baird, P., Bull, J., … Sulmasy, D. (2009). Improving the quality of spiritual care as a dimension of palliative care: The report of the Consensus Conference. *Journal of Palliative Medicine. 12*(10), 885–904. doi: 10.1089/jpm.2009.0142

Puig, A., Lee, S. M., Goodwin, L., & Sherrard, P. A. D. (2006). The efficacy of creative arts therapies to enhance emotional expression, spirituality, and psychological well-being of newly diagnosed Stage I and Stage II breast cancer patients: A preliminary study. *The Arts in Psychotherapy. 33*(3), 218–228.

Rawdin, B., Evans, C., & Rabow, M. W. (2013). The relationships among hope, pain, psychological distress, and spiritual well-being in oncology outpatients. *Journal of Palliative Medicine. 16*(2), 167–172. doi: 10.1089/jpm.2012.0223

Reker, G. T. (1992). *Life Attitude Profile-Revised.* Peterborough, ON: Student Psychologists Press.

Reker, G. T. (2005). Meaning in life of young, middle-aged, and older adults: Factorial validity, age, and gender invariance of the Personal Meaning Index (PMI). *Personality & Individual Differences. 38*(1), 71–85.

Reker, G. T., & Chamberlain, K. (2000). *Exploring existential meaning: Optimizing human development across the life span.* Thousand Oaks, CA: Sage Publications.

Romero, C., Kalidas, M., Elledge, R., Chang, J., Liscum, K. R., & Friedman, L. C. (2006). Self-forgiveness, spirituality, and psychological adjustment in women with breast cancer. *Journal of Behavioral Medicine. 29*(1), 29–36. doi: 10.1007/s10865–005–9038-z

Rosmarin, D. H., Wachholtz, A., & Ai, A. (2011). Beyond descriptive research: Advancing the study of spirituality and health. *Journal of Behavioral Medicine. 34*(6), 409–413. doi: 10.1007/s10865–011–9370–4

Sansone, R. A., & Sansone, L. A. (2010). Demoralization in patients with medical illness. *Psychiatry. 7*(8), 42–45.

Sawatzky, R., Ratner, P. A., & Chiu, L. (2005). A meta-analysis of the relationship between spirituality and quality of life. *Social Indicators Research. 72*(2), 153–188.

Schreiber, J., & Edward, J. (2014). Image of God, religion, spirituality, and life changes in breast cancer survivors: A qualitative approach. *Journal of Religion & Health.* 1–11. doi: 10.1007/s10943–014–9862-y

Schreiber, J. A. (2011). Image of God: Effect on coping and psychospiritual outcomes in early breast cancer survivors. *Oncology Nursing Forum. 38*(3), 293–301. doi: 10.1188/11.ONF.293–301

Schreiber, J. A., & Brockopp, D. Y. (2012). Twenty-five years later–what do we know about religion/spirituality and psychological well-being among breast cancer survivors? A systematic review. *Journal of Cancer Survivorship. 6*(1), 82–94. doi: 10.1007/s11764–011–0193–7

Selman, L., Harding, R., Gysels, M., Speck, P., & Higginson, I. J. (2011). The measurement of spirituality in palliative care and the content of tools validated cross-culturally: A systematic review. *Journal of Pain & Symptom Management. 41*(4), 728–753. doi: 10.1016/j.jpainsymman.2010.06.023

Sheard, T., & Maguire, P. (1999). The effect of psychological interventions on anxiety and depression in cancer patients: Results of two meta-analyses. *British Journal of Cancer. 80*(11), 1770–1780.

Sire, J. W. (2004). *Naming the elephant: Worldview as a concept.* Downers Grove, IL: IVP Academic.

Stanton, A. L., Danoff-Burg, S., & Huggins, M. E. (2002). The first year after breast cancer diagnosis: Hope and coping strategies as predictors of adjustment. *Psycho-Oncology. 11*(2), 93–102. doi: 10.1002/pon.574

Stark, R., Hamberg, E., & Miller, A.S. (2005). Exploring spirituality and unchurched religions in America, Sweden, and Japan. *Journal of Contemporary Religion 20*(1), 3–23. doi: 10.1080/1353790052000313882

Stroope, S., Draper, S., & Whitehead, A. (2013). Images of a loving God and sense of meaning in life. *Social Indicators Research. 111*(1), 25–44. doi: 10.1007/s11205–011–9982–7

Tarakeshwar, N., Vanderwerker, L. C., Paulk, E., Pearce, M. J., Kasl, S. V., & Prigerson, H. G. (2006). Religious coping is associated with the quality of life of patients with advanced cancer. *Journal of Palliative Medicine. 9*(3), 646–657.

Targ, E. F., & Levine, E. G. (2002). The efficacy of a mind-body-spirit group for women with breast cancer: A randomized controlled trial. *General Hospital Psychiatry. 24*(4), 238–248.

Taylor, E. J. (2003). Spiritual needs of patients with cancer and family caregivers. *Cancer Nursing. 26*(4), 260–266.

Thomas, J. C., Burton, M., Griffin, M. T., & Fitzpatrick, J. J. (2010). Self-transcendence, spiritual wellbeing, and spiritual practices of women with breast cancer. *Journal of Holistic Nursing. 28*(2), 115–122. doi: 10.1177/0898010109358766

Thune-Boyle, I. C., Stygall, J. A., Keshtgar, M. R., & Newman, S. P. (2006). Do religious/spiritual coping strategies affect illness adjustment in patients with cancer? A systematic review of the literature. *Soc Sci Med. 63*(1), 151. doi: 10.1016/j.socscimed.2005.11.055

True, G., Phipps, E. J., Braitman, L. E., Harralson, T., Harris, D., & Tester, W. (2005). Treatment preferences and advance care planning at end of life: The role of ethnicity and spiritual coping in cancer patients. *Annals of Behavioral Medicine. 30*(2), 174–179.

Tuck, I. (2004). Development of a spirituality intervention to promote healing. *Journal of Theory Construction & Testing. 8*(2), 67.

Underwood, L. G., & Teresi, J. A. (2002). The daily spiritual experience scale: Development, theoretical description, reliability, exploratory factor analysis, and preliminary construct validity using health-related data. *Annals of Behavioral Medicine, 24*(1), 22–33.

Underwood, S. M., & Powell, R. L. (2006). Religion and spirituality: Influence on health/risk behavior and cancer screening behavior of African Americans. *Association of Black Nurses Faculty Journal. 17*(1), 20–31.

Vail, K. E., Arndt, J., & Abdollahi, A. (2012). Exploring the existential function of religion and supernatural agent beliefs among Christians, Muslims, atheists, and agnostics. *Personality & Social Psychology Bulletin. 38*(10), 1288–1300. doi: 10.1177/0146167212449361

van Laarhoven, H. W., Schilderman, J., Vissers, K. C., Verhagen, C. A., & Prins, J. (2010). Images of God in relation to coping strategies of palliative cancer patients. *Journal of Pain & Symptom Management. 40*(4), 495–501. doi: http://dx.doi.org/10.1016/j.jpainsymman.2010.02.021

Van Ness, P. H., Kasl, S. V., & Jones, B. A. (2003). Religion, race, and breast cancer survival. *International Journal for Psychiatry & Medicine. 33*(4), 357–375.

Vehling, S., Lehmann, C., Oechsle, K., Bokemeyer, C., Krull, A., Koch, U., & Mehnert, A. (2011). Global meaning and meaning-related life attitudes: Exploring their role in predicting depression, anxiety, and demoralization in cancer patients. *Supportive Care in Cancer. 19*(4), 513–520. doi: 10.1007/s00520–010–0845–6

Vehling, S., Lehmann, C., Oechsle, K., Bokemeyer, C., Krull, A., Koch, U., & Mehnert, A. (2012). Is advanced cancer associated with demoralization and lower global meaning? The role of tumor stage and physical problems in explaining existential distress in cancer patients. *Psycho-Oncology. 21*(1), 54–63. doi: 10.1002/pon.1866

Vehling, S., & Mehnert, A. (2013). Symptom burden, loss of dignity, and demoralization in patients with cancer: A mediation model. *Psycho-Oncology. 23*(3), 283–290.doi: 10.1002/pon.3417

Vidal, C. (Ed.). (2008). *What is a worldview?* Acco, NL: Leuven.

Vidal, C. (2012). Metaphilosophical criteria for worldview comparison. *Metaphilosophy. 43*(3), 306–347. doi: 10.1111/j.1467–9973.2012.01749.x

Villagomeza, L. R. (2005). Spiritual distress in adult cancer patients: Toward conceptual clarity. *Holistic Nursing Practice. 19*(6), 285–294.

Weber, S. R., Pargament, K. I., Kunik, M. E., Lomax, J. W., 2 nd, & Stanley, M. A. (2012). Psychological distress among religious nonbelievers: A systematic review. *Journal of Religion & Health. 51*(1), 72–86. doi: 10.1007/s10943–011–9541–1

Wellen, M. (2010). Differentiation between demoralization, grief, and anhedonic depression. *Current Psychiatry Reports. 12*(3), 229–233. doi: 10.1007/s11920–010–0106-x

Whitford, H. S., & Olver, I. N. (2012). The multidimensionality of spiritual wellbeing: Peace, meaning, and faith and their association with quality of life and coping in oncology. *Psycho-Oncology. 21*(6), 602–610. doi: 10.1002/pon.1937

Wills, M. (2007). Connection, action, and hope: An invitation to reclaim the "spiritual" in health care. *Journal of Religion & Health. 46*(3), 423–436.

Wonghongkul, T., Dechaprom, N., Phumivichuvate, L., & Losawatkul, S. (2006). Uncertainty appraisal coping and quality of life in breast cancer survivors. *Cancer Nursing. 29*(3), 250–257.

Wood, M. J., Molassiotis, A., & Payne, S. (2011). What research evidence is there for the use of art therapy in the management of symptoms in adults with cancer? A systematic review. *Psycho-Oncology. 20*(2), 135–145. doi: 10.1002/pon.1722

Worthington, E. L. Jr., Lin, Y., & Ho, M. Y. (2012). Adapting an evidence-based intervention to REACH forgiveness for different religions and spiritualities. *Asian Journal of Psychiatry. 5*(2), 183–185. doi: http://dx.doi.org/10.1016/j.ajp.2012.04.005

Wright, M. C. (2002). The essence of spiritual care: A phenomenological enquiry. *Palliative Medicine. 16*(2), 125–132.

Zwingmann, C., Wirtz, M., Müller, C., Körber, J., & Murken, S. (2006). Positive and negative religious coping in German breast cancer patients. *Journal of Behavioral Medicine. 29*(6), 533. doi: 10.1007/s10865–006.9074–3

THE PEDIATRIC CANCER SURVIVOR

CHAPTER 6

PEDIATRIC/FAMILY CONCERNS POSTTREATMENT

"I live in anticipation that the cancer may come back and fear that day when it does."

—A childhood cancer survivor

Key Terms

pediatric cancer • childhood cancer • cancer survivors survivorship • late effects

Upon completion of this chapter, the reader will be able to:

1. Describe the differences in the experience of cancer between children and adults.
2. Describe the health and quality of life issues facing survivors of childhood cancer.
3. Explain the effect of childhood cancer survivorship on parents and families.
4. Describe the role of the nurse in long-term care of childhood cancer survivors.

Introduction

Survivorship for individuals who have experienced cancer as children has become an increasingly important concern for nurses and other healthcare professionals, not only those working in pediatrics, but also those who care for adult survivors. Due to the improvement in the treatment of pediatric cancers over the last 50 years, the number of children who have survived cancer has increased significantly. This, along with the potential of these children to live many decades beyond their initial cancer diagnosis, has made apparent the impact that survivorship can have on their health and wellbeing. Although all individuals diagnosed with malignancy, regardless of age, must deal with the effects of cancer and its treatment, there are additional dimensions that must be addressed in survivors of pediatric cancer. The first obvious reason for this is that when cancer strikes children, it does so in their formative years—the period of development when somatic growth and maturity in organ function is taking place. Concomitant with the physical growth and development, psychosocial and intellectual development progresses in a fairly predictable pattern. For infants and young children, in particular, the rate of change occurs quite rapidly, but even beyond the early years, steady change in size, function, and ability continues. This may result in lingering physical and psychosocial problems and pose additional long-term health risks for this population of survivors that will be highlighted in this chapter.

Overview of Childhood Cancer

History

In order to better understand survivorship in those who have had childhood cancer, it is important to review what has occurred in cancer treatment and management over the last several decades and how the experience of cancer in children differs from that of adults. First, it has taken many years to fully realize all of the potential long-term issues facing pediatric cancer survivors as it is only now that the earliest survivors are reaching their elder years. Until the 1960s, cancer in children was, for the most part, a fatal disease with death often coming months after diagnosis. Initial attempts to treat acute leukemia, the most common type of pediatric cancer, in the late 1940s and 1950s, only managed to extend life and did not effect a cure; with the addition of other chemical agents and therapies, the 5-year survival gradually increased to 50%, and then 75% in the 1960s and 1970s (Childhood Leukemias, 2013). More recently, cure rates for acute lymphoblastic leukemia are reported to be 90% (American Cancer Society, 2014). This trend is reflected in other pediatric cancers as well. While there are differences in the prevalence and survival rates of the most common types of pediatric cancers between children and adolescents, the overall 5-year survival rate for all childhood cancers was 83% in 2003 to 2009; this is an increase of 20% in the survival rates reported by the American Cancer Society (ACS) for children diagnosed in 1975 to 1979 (2014). The estimated incidence of child and adolescent cancers and the observed 5-year survival rates in two time periods are displayed in Table 6.1. Although a small increase in the incidence of pediatric cancer has been noted (American Cancer Society, 2014), less than 1% of cancers diagnosed each year are pediatric cancers; thus, children with cancer still comprise a small number of the total population of individuals with this diagnosis (National Cancer Institute, 2014). Nevertheless, the slight increase in incidence and significant improvement in survival rates that has occurred over the last 50 years, coupled with the potential for childhood cancer survivors to live 60 or more years after diagnosis, has resulted in a tremendous increase in the number of adults survivors of childhood cancer. This trend of increased survival is expected to continue with further development of cancer treatments. As the number of survivors grows, the healthcare system must take the necessary steps to effectively address the issues facing childhood cancer survivors.

Differences in Cancer and Its Effects between Children and Adults

The experience of cancer in children is different from that of adults on many levels. This adds to the issues of survivorship facing those successfully treated for cancer in their younger years. Although cancer is no less a serious disease in adults, for this population, skeletal growth is complete, and maturity of organ and body system function has been achieved. This is not the case in children diagnosed with cancer. Growth is quite rapid

Table 6.1 • Estimated Incidence of Pediatric Cancer and Observed 5-Year Survival Rates for Two Time Periods

	Incidence %		5-Year Survival Rates (%) by Year of Diagnosis	
Cancer Type	0–14	15–19	1975–1979	2003–2009
Leukemia	31	12	48	84
ALL	26	8	57	90
AML	5	4	21	64
Brain and CNS	21	10	59	75
Lymphoma	10	23	72	91
Hodgkin	4	15	87	97
Non-Hodgkin	6	8	47	85
Neuroblastoma	7	—	54	79

American Cancer Society, Surveillance Research, 2014.

in the first year of life with infants typically doubling their birth weight by 6 months and tripling this by the first birthday. Although growth rate slows after this time, children continue to demonstrate steady increases in height and weight until puberty when accelerated growth rate is again experienced. Changes in head circumference are also significant with rapid brain growth and thickening of the skull, which results in the head reaching 80% of its adult size by age 2 (Edelman, Kudzma & Mandle, 2014). The degree of growth requires adequate nutrition, which is usually impaired in those diagnosed with cancer. Utilization of available nutrients by the rapidly dividing cancer cells and the inability of children undergoing cancer treatments to consume and/or absorb nutrients usually results in nutritional intake that may be insufficient to support adequate growth. Within the body, there is growth and development of the organs as well; for example, the amount of lung tissue increases as the child ages along with further development and enlargement of the internal diameter of the airways. Some organs and body systems are not mature at birth; for example, the kidneys become functionally similar to adults by age 2 and continue to grow and develop through adolescence. The rate and timing of organ development varies; some are functionally mature by age 12, whereas maturation of the reproductive system begins with the onset of puberty. This development generally occurs in late school-age and early adolescent children, and although it progresses in an expected way, the age at which sexual maturity is achieved differs between genders and among adolescents. For these reasons, children treated for cancer are particularly vulnerable to possible alterations in growth and function of these developing organs and systems.

The difference between children and adults in psychosocial, cognitive, and emotional development also alters the experience of cancer based on age. While it is true that developmental changes continue to occur throughout a person's lifetime, the type, number, and rate of change is what is notably different in children. This concept is best illustrated with various theories of development. Erikson theory of psychosocial development identified eight successive stages that individuals go through during their life span in their development of self-identify (Edelman et al., 2014). In each of these eight stages of human development, the individual needs to successfully resolve the conflict between two opposing forces for the person to proceed to the next stage. The first five stages, which occur in childhood and adolescence, range in duration from 1 year for infants, 2 years for toddlers, 3 years for preschoolers, and 6 years for school-age children to adolescents. These stages are much shorter than that of the young, middle, and older adult stages, each of which lasts 20 years or more. Because the treatment of many childhood cancers extends over several years to achieve the survival rates currently reported, the potential to impact one or more stages of psychosocial development exists.

There are several other aspects of psychosocial development that change over the course of childhood. One of these is the development of self-concept. Successful resolution of the developmental tasks prior to progression to the next stage, achieving mastery in at least some of the challenges encountered, and receiving support and encouragement help children to develop a positive self-concept. These factors can be impacted in children with cancer, which may impair a child's perception of self. Another aspect of children's development that changes with age is awareness of the image they portray to others. Early in life, awareness of body image does not appear to exist, but it becomes evident beginning in the preschool years and increases in importance and becomes a prominent concern for adolescents as they develop their sense of identity. Under normal circumstances, adolescents need to adjust the physical changes to their body that occur with puberty; they tend to be very critical of their bodies and may feel dissatisfied with how they look (Pillitteri, 2014). Then to add to this, cancer treatment may cause alteration in appearance (hair loss) or disfigurement (amputation) that causes their bodies to be even further from the ideal image they imagine. Since body image is integrated into the process of developing a sense of identity, perceived negative body image may have a significant effect on the development of positive self-concept; this in turn may impact psychological well-being in survivors.

Children also differ from adults in cognitive development. Although infants are limited in their thought-processing ability initially, experiential learning, in which all senses are used, promotes steady increase in their capabilities that follows a predictable pattern. According to Piaget theory of cognitive development, children progress through four stages and reach an adult level of cognitive functioning at about age 15 (Edelman et al., 2014). As in the first stage of Erickson theory, the sensorimotor stage is the shortest in duration and begins at birth and ends at age 2. Through the use of their senses and reflexive, then more purposive activity, infants learn about their environment and recognize the concept of permanence in the people and objects around them (Pillitteri, 2014). After a transitional period in early toddlerhood, children enter the preoperational stage, when thinking is concrete and very present-oriented. Understanding in children in this stage is strongly influenced by their observations and experience, but drawing conclusions based on what is obvious to young children may not always be accurate. During the latter part of the stage of preoperational thought, preschool children use assimilation to make the information they obtain conform to their existing ideas and thereby define their own reality as evidenced by what is called magical thinking (Pilletteri, 2014). Children then progress into the stage the Piaget termed, concrete operational thought, usually by age 7. At this point, they are capable of systematic reasoning, and memory has developed well enough that it can be used to learn concepts and classify objects (Pillitteri, 2014). When children enter adolescence, they are able to reason and think abstractly and begin the final stage of cognitive development, the formal operations stage (Edelman et al., 2014). Although cognitive development does not end in adolescence, it is the rate at which it occurs in children that increases the risk of experiencing negative effects for those treated for cancer. Limitations in thinking can greatly influence children's ability to understand what is happening both during and after their illness, thus increasing the stress they experience. This, combined with the emotional immaturity that exists in children, loss of control experienced during their illness, and their diminished capacity to cope with adversity, may affect psychological well-being in childhood cancer survivors.

Another obvious difference between children and adults with cancer is that, at the time of cancer diagnosis, most adults have finished their formal education, at least on the primary and secondary level. This is not the case for children. Those who are very young when they are diagnosed will not have begun formal schooling, although learning is very much a part of what they do every day. For most children, age 4 to 5 and above, who are diagnosed with cancer, the interruptions they experience during cancer treatment may affect their progress in school. Adults have been noted to use terms such as "brain fog" and "Chemo brain" to describe that clouded thinking they experience when undergoing cancer treatment. Although children, particularly those who are younger, may not be able to describe this phenomenon, it is probable that they may be affected similarly. This, in combination with lapses in their education that occur when children are too ill to keep up with their school work, may lead to delays in their academic progress. In addition, some cancer treatments such as surgery or radiation to the brain or other therapies may delay or alter cognitive development and lead to the possible occurrence of neurocognitive problems.

Cognitive, psychosocial, and physical immaturity all contribute to the dependency inherent in childhood. Children need their parents and families not only to provide physical care, but also to make decisions for them. As children develop their ability to comprehend, link cause and effect, and reason, they gradually become more capable of making appropriate choices; usually it follows that they are then permitted to participate more in decision making. But when cancer is diagnosed in children, it is the parents/guardians who are ultimately responsible to make an informed decision regarding treatment. It can be very stressful for the parents to see their children experience physical and/or psychological problems, both during treatment and especially later, knowing that these children bear the burden of the parents' choices. Adults diagnosed with cancer, except in the case of individuals with cognitive impairment, decide for themselves among the cancer treatment options. The diagnosis of cancer is stressful for families regardless of the age of the individual who is diagnosed, but the impact on family dynamics is different for children and adults. All children need care, but children with cancer need additional care and resources during treatment. Many families find the physical and emotional toll draining. The treatment, travel, and other costs combined with the loss of income that occurs if a parent stops working to care for the sick child can create an economic burden for these families. In addition, some survivors may require continued parental care and support if they experience persistent health problems as a result of the cancer or treatment. This can put a tremendous strain on the family and impair effective functioning, which can have lasting effects on its members of the family. In contrast, adult cancer survivors manage their own lives and often are responsible to provide for other family members such as spouses or children. For adults, the impact of the cancer diagnosis is greater for their own families than their siblings or parents as is the case with children with cancer. Thus, while family stress exists when individuals have cancer, the family dynamics is different between children and adults with the disease.

The types of cancer that prevail in children are somewhat different from those that occur in adults. Although the exact cause of cancer has not been identified, current research indicates that interaction between genetics, individual, and, in some cases, environmental factors function in the development of cancer (National Cancer Institute, 2014). While many adult cancers are associated with certain behaviors or exposures, no environmental or lifestyle factors have been definitely linked to the development of cancer in children (National Cancer Institute, 2014). Hence, there are no actions or early screening tests available to reduce the risk or make early diagnosis easier. In addition, the most common childhood cancers are not localized but develop in the blood and lymph, so the disease is most often disseminated upon diagnosis. Because of this and the rapid cell division that occurs with childhood cancer, chemotherapy, either alone or with other therapies, is the primary way to treat these cancers.

Surviving Childhood Cancer

Issues Facing Childhood Cancer Survivors

It has been recognized for some time that cancer and its treatment can negatively affect the health and well-being of individuals years after therapy has been completed successfully. The nature and extent of the health problems of childhood cancer survivors has become more apparent as the number and age of these survivors increase. Recent estimates by the National Cancer Institute (2012) place the number of cancer survivors diagnosed before age 21 to be at least 328,000. To better understand and address the problems experienced by these individuals later in life, systematic inquiry was started in the 1970s by the groups actively involved in researching and treating childhood cancers. The need for collaboration was recognized in order to have sufficient numbers to better identify trends and draw conclusions. As part of its Long-term Follow-up Study (LTFU), the National Cancer Institute funded the Childhood Cancer Survivor Study (CCSS) in 1994, a multi-site study with 27 participating institutions in the United States and Canada. This initial study, coordinated by St. Jude Children's Research Hospital, used a retrospective cohort design to obtain health data from over 20,000 childhood cancer survivors who were diagnosed between 1970 and 1986; 4,000 of the siblings were also enrolled to serve the comparison group (2014). Recognizing that improvements in cancer treatment may result in differences in the long-term problems experienced by individuals more recently diagnosed, the CCSS, in 2007, began obtaining data from a second set of participants, those diagnosed with cancer between 1987 and 1999. The plan is to expand the LTFU by enrolling 15,000 cancer survivors diagnosed during this second time frame and an additional 4,000 of their siblings (St. Jude Children's Research Hospital, 2014). To date, much of the published research on the long-term effects used data from the first cohort (National Cancer Institute, 2012). But once enrollment of participants is complete, future studies are expected to report the long-term issues of the second cohort and compare the two. Evidence of the magnitude of the problems is reflected in the research; a current study that compared survivors treated for cancer from 1970 to 1987 with their siblings revealed that nearly two thirds developed long-term problems related to the cancer or its treatment (Oeffinger et. al., 2006). In addition to the research using the CCSS data, there are many studies conducted in the United States and in many other countries published in the literature.

Some of the problems that children experience following treatment are not unique to this age group, but may be experienced by adult cancer survivors as well. But it is the potential for childhood survivors to develop long-term complications that has garnered recent attention for several reasons. First, these complications often are not apparent immediately when treatment is finished and therefore do not need to be addressed at that time. Second, it is now evident that engaging in certain lifestyle behaviors, such as cigarette smoking or alcohol consumption may increase the risk of developing complications among cancer survivors (Children's Oncology Group, 2007). In addition, screening that adults are advised to have on a routine basis as they age may be particularly important or may need to be performed at different intervals for childhood cancer survivors. Initially any monitoring that is recommended as a follow-up to cancer treatment may be arranged for by parents, but eventually it is the survivors who are responsible for seeing that necessary screening tests are done. Survivors may not follow the recommendations appropriately, because the risk is not fully understood or recognized by those who have little or no recollection of their cancer treatment. Finally, the degree that complications affect survivors' education, career, and personal goals such as completing their desired level of education, pursuing careers, finding life partners, having children, and being able to support themselves and their families can significantly affect their future quality of life (QOL).

There are numerous physical complications that can occur at various points in time in children that have been diagnosed and successfully treated for cancer. The relative risk of developing these complications varies with the type of cancer and the type and intensity of the treatment. Treatment with surgery, radiation and combination therapies, and greater exposure from higher doses and/or longer treatment periods tend to increase the risk. Cardiac, pulmonary, neurological, renal, and thyroid problems have all been known to occur as a result of cancer treatment.

Effects of Surgery

Surgery, when used in the treatment of cancer, will, to some extent, result in a change in a child's body. Even when surgery does not have a long-term effect on the child's functioning, the presence of scarring may alter his or her body image particularly for older children and adolescents. Concerns for their appearance may lead children to feel self-conscious because they are different and this may affect their self-esteem. A child's well-being may also be affected if participation in activities is restricted as a result of surgery. A child, who has had a kidney removed following a diagnosis of Wilm tumor or one with an ocular prosthesis, may be precluded from playing certain sports. This may result in negative emotions and impact self-esteem.

This issue is magnified when surgery causes significant changes in structure and function that results with amputation or the removal of other tissue. In these cases, prostheses (eyes, limbs) or stomas may be required to maintain function and these will require special care. For children, as with adults, education regarding prosthesis or stoma care is needed and the child, when old enough, should be included in this process.

> ### Late Effects of Cancer Treatment for Survivors of Childhood Cancers
>
> - Cardiac, pulmonary, renal, and other organ dysfunction
> - Impaired growth and development
> - Altered sexual development, infertility, and impaired lactation
> - Neurocognitive problems
> - Increased risk of developing secondary cancers later in life

Similar issues in terms of altered function and body image can occur when osteosarcoma results in amputation. Although increasingly limb salvage techniques with endopros-thetic devices are being used in place of amputations and traditional prostheses with good outcomes, problems do occur (Gibson & Soanes, 2004). Alterations in movement may affect the ability to participate in certain activities leading to dissatisfaction with the device and QOL issues. The use of such devices in growing children may cause leg length discrepancies; loosening and other failures of the implants can result in impair-ment of function and necessitate surgical revision (Gibson & Soanes, 2004). As described before, the impact of disfiguring surgery on the child's body image can be significant, and this can alter the development of positive self-concept. In addition to education regard-ing physical care, it is important for nurses to address the social and emotional needs of these children and their families. Providing adequate support can assist them with the grieving process and help them cope effectively with the altered body image.

Effect on Growth

Another late effect of cancer treatment that is particularly a problem for children is alterations in skeletal growth and weight gain. There are certain cancers and treatments, those that involve the central nervous system (surgery, irradiation, and chemotherapy), for which disruption in growth seems more likely to occur. Cranial surgery or irradiation may cause pituitary gland dysfunction that alters levels of growth hormone, which then affects height (Gibson & Soanes, 2004). Approximately one third of the childhood brain tumor survivors have been reported to have significant growth reduction (Gurney, 2003). Also, total body irradiation or spinal radiation can affect growth of the spine causing skeletal disproportion (Gibson & Soanes, 2004).

But children with other cancers may also be affected to some extent; studies indi-cate that 10% to 15% of children being treated for leukemia have their growth similarly affected (Chow et al., 2007). Short stature may predispose individuals to problems of overweight and obesity as even modest weight gain can result in higher body mass index (BMI). A study that compared three different central nervous system (CNS) therapies for children with ALL, identified that regardless of the whether cranial irradiation was used, final height was compromised in children younger than 13 years when compared to the growth charts for children in the United States published by the Centers for Dis-ease Control (Dalton et al., 2003). The researchers also reported an increase in the BMI standardized scores in the same children, primarily as a result of shorter stature rather than excessive weight gain (Dalton et al., 2003).

Another factor that may affect growth in children is the use of corticosteroids. This group of medications is used as part of the treatment of childhood cancer, to manage nausea and cerebral edema. But extended corticosteroid use has been shown to have an adverse effect on long-term bone and joint health. There is concern that bone growth may be inhibited in children because corticosteroids decrease bone formation and the protein matrix of the bone (Prednisone, 2014). Prolonged use of these medications is also associated with the development of osteonecrosis, which can lead to joint damage particularly in older children (Bhatia, 2012). The adverse effects of long-term corticosteroid use that can lead to muscle weakness and osteoporosis may result in limitations in mobility in later life. Corticosteroids are also known to stimulate appetite and promote weight gain, which may contribute to the problem of excessive weight gain and obesity during and after treatment.

Issues with physical growth can lead to psychosocial problems related to altered body image due to dissatisfaction with height and weight and result in low self-esteem. Consistent monitoring of height and weight throughout the growth period is necessary to identify patterns and alterations in growth. Weight gain and assessment of BMI should continue so that appropriate dietary counseling can be provided throughout adult life. Good nutrition is an important component in the care of those with childhood cancers and survivors as it can optimize skeletal growth and reduce obesity, thus avoiding additional stress being placed on the individual's joints.

Effect on Neurocognitive Function

It has become evident, as a greater number of children treated for cancer survive, that serious, permanent deficits exist that affect neurological, neurosensory, and neurocognitive functioning of these individuals (Packer et al., 2003). As with other late effects, the impact of cancer treatment is usually greater in those who are younger and receive more intensive therapy (Gibson & Soanes, 2004). The rate of brain growth and the myelination of the nerves that occurs in younger children make them more susceptible to nervous system injury. The type of cancer and treatment are other factors associated with increased risk of developing these problems; children diagnosed with brain tumors and those treated with cranial radiation and intrathecal methotrexate are more likely to be affected (Zeltzer et al., 2009). Some of the neurological problems may be present at the time of diagnosis and persist or develop after treatment; often the problems that develop from surgery are evident earlier whereas those resulting from treatment with chemotherapy and radiotherapy are noted later (Packer et al., 2003). Some of the neurological problems include seizures, dysphagia, impaired coordination, and motor deficits, all of which can significantly disrupt function, activities of daily living, and educational activities (Gibson & Soanes, 2004). Neurosensory deficits including vision and hearing impairment occur more often in childhood cancer survivors as a result of cranial nerve damage or cataracts and damage to the cochlear (Packer et al., 2003). It is estimated that more than 60% of children who received platinum-containing chemotherapy have experienced bilateral hearing loss (Knight, Kraemer, & Neuwelt, 2005). These also impair daily and educational activities and increase the need for rehabilitative services and ongoing support for families caring for these children (Gibson & Soanes, 2004).

The risk of developing neurocognitive impairments is higher for those who were treated for cancer as children than those who were not (Krull, 2013). Nearly 40% of childhood cancer survivors develop some difficulty with various aspects of cognition ranging from processing speed, attention, and/or memory; these difficulties can impair learning and result in children's inability to maintain or advance in their cognitive development as would be expected for their age (Zeltzer et al., 2009). Inadequate academic achievement can alter future planning regarding career and life goals and prompt feelings of disappointment. Lack of success in goal attainment can affect self-esteem and promote the development of behavioral and emotional disorders. Intellectual and educational performance needs to be observed and monitored by all those who interact with the child, including parents, healthcare professionals, and teachers so that difficulties can be recognized and addressed early. Continued monitoring and support services for these children as they transition into adulthood and enter higher education and vocational training is recommended to improve future success and QOL (Krull, 2013).

Effect on Reproductive Function

One of the late effects that both male and female cancer survivors may face is disruption in reproductive system function. Depending on the type of treatment and the age at which it occurs, reproductive problems can range from inadequate development of the reproductive organs to arrest of sexual development and inability to produce viable oocytes or sperm (Gibson & Soanes, 2004). For those treated for cancer as young children, it may be years before this problem is apparent. Abnormal endocrine function is one of the main causes; this can occur at the level of the brain and/or the gonads. Injury to the hypothalamic–pituitary axis (HPA) from cranial irradiation or surgery can cause deficiency of the hormones secreted from the anterior pituitary including the gonadotropins (Gibson & Soanes, 2004). This, in turn, can impair normal gonadal function as the primary function of the gonadotropins is to stimulate the gonads to produce the sex steroids and adequate number of sperm in males and mature ova in females. In both sexes, various treatments can also affect gonadal function directly. For males, radiation, surgery, and chemotherapy can cause depletion of germ cells and gonadal endocrine dysfunction; the extent of dysfunction is related to dosage amount and, for chemotherapy, the agent used (Bhatia, 2012). In females, treatment at older ages, radiation to the abdomen or pelvis, and certain chemotherapeutic agents increase the risk of loss of ovarian function (Bhatia, 2012). Although some female survivors retain ovarian function once cancer treatment is completed, premature menopause before age 40 has been known to occur (Bhatia, 2012). Another late effect of cranial irradiation that has been noted to occur in female survivors is the ability to produce breast milk following the birth of an infant. This has been associated with prolactin deficiency, which, like derangement in other anterior pituitary hormone levels, is also thought to occur from injury to the HPA (Johnston, 2008).

Periodic assessment of a child's growth and pubertal development using the Tanner stages is necessary to monitor progression and identify deviations, so appropriate testing and treatment may be initiated. Prior to treatment, options to preserve fertility should be offered to families to consider. For male adolescents who have experienced pubertal changes, sperm banking is an accessible and low-cost method to preserve fertility and should be offered before treatment (Ogle, 2008). The process of fertility preservation for females and prepubescent children is more complicated. Techniques currently available include cryopreservation of embryos or oocytes, which requires hormonal stimulation and delays initiation of cancer treatment, or the freezing of testicular or ovarian tissue, which is still considered investigational (Kelvin, Kroon, & Ogle, 2012). For families with a child recently diagnosed with cancer, the concern that treatment may potentially affect fertility is usually foreshadowed by their fear of their child succumbing to the cancer. But as is the case with other late effects of cancer treatment, reproductive system dysfunction can result in psychological distress and affect QOL. When appropriate, referral to an endocrinologist or reproductive medicine specialist should be considered for adult survivors of childhood cancer who experience reproduction system dysfunction, infertility, or lactation failure.

Cardiac, Pulmonary, and Renal Effects

The therapies used to treat cancer are known to have adverse effects on other organs and body systems including the heart, lungs, kidneys, and thyroid. Cardiac problems including arrhythmia, heart valve dysfunction, heart failure, and coronary artery disease are reported to be more prevalent in individuals over 45 years of age who were treated for childhood cancer than those who were not (Armstrong, 2013). Use of particular chemotherapeutic agents and radiation has been noted to increase risk. Anthracyclines have been associated with the development of dysrhythmias and cardiomyopathy; children who were treated at younger ages, were female, and were exposed to higher dosage regimens or chest irradiation demonstrate the greatest risk (Bhatia, 2012). Limits in total cumulative doses of anthracyclines have been established to minimize the risk, but may also minimize effectiveness of this antineoplastic agent (Oeffinger et al., 2006). Long-term benefit of chemoprotective agents such as Dexrazoxane on the cardiac status in children has not been well documented (Gibson & Soanes, 2004). As cancer survivors age, it has been evident that the development of hypertension, which alone contributes significantly to this problem, as well as other cardiac risk factors (dyslipidemia, obesity) add to the risk of experiencing major cardiac events in these individuals (Armstrong, 2013).

Radiation and certain antineoplastic agents have also been associated with increased risk of developing problems of the lungs, kidneys, and thyroid. Several agents including Busulfan, cyclophosphamide, and carmustine have been noted to cause pneumonitis and pulmonary fibrosis, especially when given to children at young ages (Gibson & Soanes, 2004). Radiation to the lung is noted to have a similar effect with higher incidence and greater lung damage noted in children who were treated at younger ages and those receiving larger doses or having more lung area exposed (Bhatia, 2012). Nephrotoxicity, with either an acute or gradual onset, has also been noted in children with cancer and survivors. Several risk factors have been identified with this problem as well; these include cancer involving the kidney, exposure to higher-dose radiation, treatment with some chemotherapeutic agents, particularly ifosfamide or cisplatin in higher doses, and concomitant use of other nephrotoxic agents (Gibson & Soanes, 2004). Another problem that occurs with increased incidence in childhood cancer survivors is thyroid gland dysfunction and hypothyroidism; treatment with radiation to the thyroid, especially with higher doses and those who are younger when treated appear to be at highest risk (Bhatia, 2012).

Because of the risk for developing conditions that can seriously affect health, it is evident that all childhood cancer survivors need specific education about the risks and health promotion activities to address these risks. Periodic assessment of these individuals is paramount to promote early identification and treatment of complications. Conditions such as hypertension and hyperlipidemia, which may be asymptomatic, are more likely to be detected early with regular follow-up and treated appropriately, thereby, reducing morbidity in survivors. In addition, other testing (i.e., blood tests, pulmonary and kidney function tests) can be arranged as needed to monitor those at risk for complications of the lungs, kidney, and thyroid. In this way, survivors can be referred to specialists and appropriate treatment initiated. It is equally important to encourage childhood cancer survivors to maintain a healthy lifestyle and avoid the factors such as cigarette smoking, high calorie and high fat diets, inactivity, and obesity that increase the risk of developing heart disease and other chronic conditions (Children's Oncology Group, 2014).

Development of Secondary Malignancies

Another problem that has come to light as childhood cancer survivors have both increased in number and in age is the higher incidence of developing secondary malignant neoplasms (SMNs). While the risk of being diagnosed with cancer increases with age, research indicates that the risk is greater for survivors; the incidence of SNM is four to six times higher for those surviving 30 years past diagnosis when compared to those without this history (Bhatia et al., 2003). There is evidence that there is a relationship between treatment and the type of secondary cancer, with use of alkylating agents associated with the development of acute myeloid leukemia and radiation exposure associated with the development of solid malignant tumors (Bhatia, 2012). Although the risk is increased for all survivors, studies conducted at different times have demonstrated an increased risk in those who have been treated for Hodgkin disease, Ewing, and other sarcomas (Neglia et al., 2001; Neglia, et al., 2006; Friedman et al., 2010). Other factors related to increased risk include age, female gender, and treatment with radiation therapy; higher radiation doses and increased length of time since treatment have also been noted to modify risk (Friedman et al., 2010; Bhatia, 2012). Common sites for secondary malignancies include the hematopoietic and central nervous system, are breast, thyroid, colon, and lung (Friedman et al., 2010; Bhatia, 2012). Whether it is the treatment itself or other factors that increase the risk has been debated. It is thought that individuals previously diagnosed with cancer may be genetically predisposed to developing malignancy or increased surveillance in this population has increased detection, which is reflected in the higher incidence (Grothey et al., 2014). Those childhood cancer survivors with secondary cancers, who are now over 60, were obviously treated during an earlier era; the impact of current improvements in therapy and health management for those more recently diagnosed will not be seen for many years to come.

The best practices for managing the problem of SMNs in childhood cancer survivors are also under discussion. There is a need for continued research in this area, not only to examine outcomes for the newer treatment regimens, but also to improve the recommendations for follow-up that are effective in identifying secondary cancers earlier without overburdening the survivors. Despite the variations identified in the research, continued follow-up has been shown to benefit this population. Participation in LTFU programs specifically geared to childhood cancer survivors is one model that exists for these individuals. These programs are designed to perform risk assessment and periodic examinations as well as to provide education about late effects and recommend appropriate screening activities (Children's Oncology Group, 2007).

Despite the risks that exist with cancer treatment, in reality, these treatments are necessary in order for children with cancer to be able to survive this disease. Since the evidence indicates that often the risk of adverse effects increases with greater exposure, continued research is needed to identify effective treatments using the lowest possible doses. It is also of utmost importance to educate children with cancer and their families of these effects during treatment and follow up to promote adherence to healthy lifestyle practices and recommended cancer screenings as survivors age. Screening intervals in some cases are different for survivors of certain childhood cancers, but evidence indicates that the recommendations are not always followed. The survivorship guidelines for adult female childhood cancer survivors, considered at higher risk for developing breast cancer due to chest irradiation, include recommendations to consume a healthy diet, exercise regularly and maintain normal weight, and to have a yearly physical examination and mammogram starting at 25 years (Children's Oncology Group, 2014). In a study with a large sample of adult female childhood cancer survivors, less than half of women aged 25 to 39 reported obtaining a mammogram in the last 2 years; higher screening rates were observed for those reporting physician recommendations for mammogram (Oeffinger et al., 2009). The importance of early and continued education by healthcare providers about the importance of screening to manage the problem of SMN cannot be underestimated.

Psychosocial Issues

Children who have survived a serious and life-threatening illness such as cancer are likely to be significantly affected by the experience both during treatment and in survivorship. When cancer occurs during the formative years, not only can physical and cognitive development be disrupted, but normal childhood experiences are altered as well. Social activities such as play, parties, and even school attendance and participation in extracurricular activities provide opportunities for children to interact with others, especially their peers, and this is very important to their social and emotional development. Participation in such activities may be precluded based on a child's health status. This not only can affect children when it happens, but also may have a lasting effect on the psychological well-being of childhood cancer survivors. The evidence indicates that there is some variation in the psychological outcomes of survivors in the United States and other countries, with some studies reporting more negative and others more positive outcomes (Eilertsen, Rannestad, Indredavik, & Vik, 2011; Servitzoglou, Papadatou, Tsiantis, & Vasilatou-Kosmidis, 2009; Sundberg, Lampic, Björk, Arvidson, & Wettergren, 2009). Some of the inconsistencies in the findings may be related to the composition of the samples in the studies and/or sample size. Use of the CCSS has enabled researchers to examine psychological status of a large number of survivors and to compare them to their siblings, who served as the control group (St. Jude Children's Research Hospital, 2014). The evidence on the psychological QOL indicates that while many childhood survivors fared well when compared to their siblings, childhood cancer survivors were more likely to report impaired physical and mental health and psychological and emotional distress than their siblings when compared to national norms (Zeltzer et al., 2009). According to Zeltzer et al. (2009), those individuals experiencing psychological distress often report more depression, anxiety, somatization, and fatigue and sleep disturbances. Survivors who are female, unmarried, have low educational attainment and household income, are unemployed and who have chronic problems and have been treated with cranial surgery or radiation are at high risk for developing psychological stress (Zeltzer et al., 2009). Also, the evidence indicates that those experiencing psychological distress are more likely to engage in unhealthy behaviors such as smoking cigarettes and using alcohol (Zeltzer et al., 2009).

A cancer diagnosis can continue to affect the psychosocial functioning of survivors long after treatment has ended. In a study of adults with neurocognitive deficits after successful treatment for ALL, researchers identified a 5% increase in self-reported behavior problems each year after diagnosis and an association between impairment and declines in educational attainment and employment (Krull et al., 2013). There is also evidence that indicates that posttraumatic stress symptoms (PTSS) occur in both childhood cancer survivors and their parents, which in some cases may persist for long periods after treatment (Ozono, 2007). The incidence and factors related to this condition vary among family members, but PTSS were associated with higher trait anxiety scores for survivors having health conditions (Ozono, 2007). Suicide risk also has been reported to be modestly higher for adolescents and young adults with cancer, with the greatest risk of suicidal behavior noted within a year of being diagnosed with cancer (Lu et al., 2013). There are other factors that affect psychological functioning that have not been well studied. Outcomes such as social isolation can impact the psychosocial function in childhood cancer survivors, but few studies have investigated the onset and progression of this problem in childhood cancer survivors (Howard et al., 2014).

It can be seen that psychosocial and emotional issues may significantly impact the psychological well-being and the QOL of childhood cancer survivors, both soon after diagnosis and/or many years later. In addition, changes in health and conditions that occur with time may contribute to developing psychological distress later. The potential to develop neurocognitive problems through adulthood, which can affect educational attainment, career goals, and many other aspects of life, makes it important for healthcare professionals to continue to monitor survivors at risk and provide treatment as needed (Krull et al., 2013). Another aspect to consider is that survivors may perceive the increased risks for developing secondary cancers or heart disease as threats to their future health status, contributing to increased anxiety, the development of sleep disorders, or depression. Incorporating ongoing assessment of psychological well-being into LTFU programs can promote identification and treatment of these problems and potentially improve the survivors' QOL.

Issues for Parents

An important aspect of survivorship to consider is the experience of the parents and families of childhood cancer survivors. Because the incidence of childhood cancer is lower than that of older adults, parents when first learning of the cancer diagnosis often feel very alone. Their child is usually the only one in their circle of friends, their neighborhood, or school to have this disease. This may lead to social isolation and increase stress; research indicates that parents with adequate social support are less likely to have high stress levels (Pollock, Litzelman, Wisk, & Witt, 2013). Higher levels of parental stress are also noted for those whose children have neurocognitive deficits and demonstrate lower executive functioning and behavior issues (Patel, Wong, Cuevas, & Van Horn, 2013). Problems experienced by parents of cancer survivors are varied and may include posttraumatic stress disorder (PTSD), marital strain, anxiety, and uncertainty. Although it is not the norm for the childhood cancer survivors and their parents, PTSD does occur in survivors and, in higher incidence, in their parents; this condition may persist or develop long after treatment is completed (Taieb, Moro, Baubet, Revah-Levy, & Flament, 2003). Increased levels of stress can have can negatively affect parents resulting in more mental health issues and lower perceived health-related quality of life (Witt, et al., 2010).

Feelings of loss and anxiety also contribute to the psychological and emotional distress parents experience. The losses that parents report after their child is diagnosed with cancer are numerous and may persist into survivorship. Despite being relieved that their child survived, they feel they have lost the life that they had before diagnosis, lost time in their lives during their child's treatment, and lost the healthy child they had before diagnosis (Van Dongen-Melman, Van Zuuren, & Verhulst, 1998). As is the case with any loss, these parents need to mourn the loss to achieve resolution. Also, anxiety and uncertainty about developing secondary cancers or other late effects, which is experienced by childhood survivors, is reflected in their parents as well (Van Dongen-Melman et al., 1998). Because the parents have faced the possibility of losing their child once, they may be overly concerned for the child's well-being. As a result, they may be over protective while the child is still under their care or may continue to worry excessively about the possible consequences of the cancer and treatment as their child ages.

Parents face challenges both during treatment and in survivorship. Persistent issues with psychological and emotional distress, and marital, financial, or other problems that significantly affect parents, can disrupt family functioning. Extreme concern for the childhood cancer survivor's health may interfere with the parents allowing the child to fully participate in normal childhood activities or appropriately disciplining the child when needed. Parenting of their other children may be altered as well, both during and after treatment. Family units and family members experience the diagnosis in various different ways. The knowledge that every family and every family member experiences things differently should guide interactions with parents and families. It is important to incorporate the care of the parent and family into the plan of care for the child in order to promote well-being for all family members. The therapeutic relationship that nurses develop with parents of childhood cancer survivors is purposeful and can assist the parents and family in coping and adaptation. Ongoing assessment of parents to identify any physical and/or psychological needs, their coping style, and other aspects of the experience is necessary to be able to address these needs. Targeted strategies such as stress-reduction, respite care, and referrals to appropriate services can improve well-being and psychological QOL (Pollock et al., 2013).

The Role of the Nurse in Long-Term Care of Childhood Cancer Survivors

The needs of childhood cancer survivors and their families depend on their unique experiences and circumstances; thus the type and extent of the needs varies between clients and between families. To add to the complexity, their issues do not remain static but change over time. In some cases, problems may be apparent during or soon after treatment ends. But most of the time, health problems do not develop until much later in life and may lack significant symptoms; so the problem may go unrecognized for a long period of time. The ability to identify and treat problems early and promote better outcomes is one reason that LTFU needs to be maintained. It is apparent that high-quality care for this population includes both appropriate early management during cancer treatment as well as effective, evidence-based LTFU care, provided by a multidisciplinary team of professionals of which nurses are an integral part.

Several factors have been identified that affect the ability of survivors to obtain adequate LTFU care. These have been outlined in the *Long-term Follow-up Program Resource Guide* (Children's Oncology Group, 2007) and include lack of awareness in both survivors and professionals of survivorship issues that affect health and well-being and the need for LTFU, psychological factors that result in survivors avoiding follow-up, difficulties in reaching or navigating complex healthcare systems, and financial/insurance issues. Any or all of these barriers can erode the delivery of LTFU necessary to deal with complications as they arise. To best address these childhood cancer survivors' problems, the need for multidisciplinary, comprehensive, and coordinated long-term care has been identified. The Institute of Medicine (IOM) report, *Childhood cancer survivorship: improving care and quality of life* (2003), addresses several of these barriers to follow-up care in its recommendations. These include, developing clinical practice guidelines and setting standards for systems of multidisciplinary comprehensive follow-up care for childhood cancer survivors, educating survivors and families and professionals about the late effects of cancer treatment, improving programs that provide services to those with special needs and making resources more accessible for cancer survivors, and continuing research on survivorship issues (IOM, 2003).

Nurses are a key part of the healthcare team; they focus on the client as a whole as well as incorporate the family in the plan of care. Thus, they can provide care that is thorough and comprehensive. Nurses, whether they are providing direct care or functioning as care coordinators or in advance practice roles, can assist these clients to attain and maintain an optimal level of health and well-being. In all cases, nurses use the nursing process to assess each client and family and develop an individualized plan of care. Nursing actions frequently used in implementation when caring for these clients include providing education and support, and advocating for clients. Nurses in a variety of settings can address the needs of the population. Those that are caring for these children during the treatment phase can begin the education process on the effects of the treatments they are receiving and ensure that that families be given detailed printed information about the treatment, doses and so forth, which they can use to inform future healthcare providers. This education may also address fertility preservation when appropriate. Nurses in these settings can support these children and families directly and by including other members of the healthcare team, such as child life professionals, as needed. They may also participate in school re-entry programs and other endeavors designed to transition these children and families to life after treatment. Nurses who are working with clients and parents after treatment is completed need to continue the education about the late effects, the importance of avoiding lifestyle behaviors known to increase the risk of late effects, and following screening recommendations. Nurses can assist clients in their efforts to maintain health; one study demonstrated that telephone counseling by advanced-practice nurses increased the number of childhood cancer survivors who obtained recommended cardiac screening (Hudson et al., 2014). Assisting children and families to transition to adult healthcare providers for follow-up is also an important function for those nurses working in pediatric care settings. Appropriate assessment, recognition, and reporting of issues that require referral to specialists or other resources are ways in which nurses in long-term follow-up care can advocate for these clients and improve the quality of the care they receive. There are also ways that nurses can help childhood cancer survivors indirectly. Nurses who participate in research or quality improvement initiates can help to identify the problems of survivors and best practices to address these problems.

It can be seen that the health and well-being of childhood cancer survivors will continue to be a growing issue for the healthcare system as increasing numbers of children are successfully treated for cancer. Although many adult childhood cancer survivors are healthy both mentally and physically, there are a number of problems that may occur particularly as these survivors age. As time goes on, the type of problems they may experience may also change. Nurses working in a variety of roles and settings will likely encounter these individuals with greater frequency as their numbers increase. It will be very important that nurses, particular those working in pediatric oncology and childhood survivor follow-up, use evidence to keep their practice current to best serve this population. By using the nursing process and developing therapeutic relationships, nurses can assist clients to maintain their health, address the many health risks, and manage health problems when they occur.

CASE STUDY

Jamie had just turned 8 when she started not feeling well and noticed bruises all over her legs. Her mom brought her to the doctor, who examined her and took some blood from her arm. That night they got a call to go to the hospital immediately. There Jamie had more tests done and was diagnosed with acute lymphoblastic leukemia. Jamie is now 31 years old and works as a librarian at the local library.

Jamie underwent 2 years of treatment. She remembers having many tests and procedures done like spinal taps and receiving chemotherapy during that time. She has mixed memories of the years when she was being treated. She remembers how her mother and father cried when she was first diagnosed. Jamie also remembers the horror in her grandmother's face when she first learned that Jamie had cancer, and she will never forget it. She has some fond memories of the staff at the hospital who helped her through the difficult times like when her port was not working and when her mouth sores were so bad she could not even swallow water. She thinks of the friends she made at the clinic where she went every week, some survived and some did not.

She finished third grade from home and resumed attending school once her treatment was completed. She needed tutors and extra help because she struggled with school work after her diagnosis. Although it required extra time and effort, Jamie graduated both high school and college; it took her longer but she reached her goal. She married her college sweetheart. They have been together for 5 years.

Jamie's parents were divorced a few years after she finished treatment; she blames her cancer for this. She believes the strain of having a sick child was hard for them and their married life suffered. Jamie thinks she would like to have children but the thought scares her. She is not sure if she is able to get pregnant since she has never had a regular menstrual cycle and she also has mild cardio-myopathy. Jamie knows that her past treatments can affect her health and that there is possibility that she could develop a secondary malignancy.

Case Study Discussion Questions

1. What late effects of being a cancer survivor does Jamie face?
2. She mentioned her grandmother in the case study. Are there other people that could be affected by her diagnosis?
3. How well do you think Jamie understands the issues regarding being a cancer survivor?
4. As a cancer survivor, what health promotion practices would you recommend to her?
5. How can you help someone that needs support and resources as a cancer survivor?

References

American Cancer Society. (2014). *Cancer facts and figures.* Retrieved from http://www.cancer.org/acs/groups/content/@research/documents/webcontent/acspc-042151.pdf

Armstrong, G. T. (2013). Modifiable risk factors and major cardiac events among adult survivors of childhood cancer. *Journal of Clinical Oncology. 31*(29), 3673–3680.

Bhatia, S. (2012). Long-term complications of therapeutic exposures in childhood: Lessons learned from childhood cancer survivors. *Pediatrics. 130*(6), 1141–1143.

Bhatia, S. Y., Yasui, Y., Robison, L. L., Birch, J. M., Bogue, M. K., Diller, L., … Meadows, A. T; Late Effects Study Group. (2003). High risk of subsequent neoplasms continues with extended follow-up of childhood Hodgkin's disease: Report from the late effects study group. *Journal of Clinical Oncology. 21*(23).

Childhood Leukemias. (2013). Retrieved from Science Connections: http://www.science-connections.com/profiles/pinkel/leukemia.html

Children's Oncology Group. (2007). *Long-term follow-up program resource guide.* Retrieved from http://www.survivorshipguidelines.org/pdf/LTFUResourceGuide.pdf

Children's Oncology Group. (2014). *Long-term follow-up guidelines for survivors of childhood, adolescent, and young adult cancers.* Retrieved from http://www.survivorshipguidelines.org/

Chow, E. J., Friedman, D. L., Yasui, Y., Whitton, J. A., Stovall, M., Robison, L. L., & Sklar, C. A. (2007). Decreased adult height in survivors of childhood acute lymphoblastic leukemia: A report from the Childhood Cancer Survivor Study. *Journal of Pediatrics. 150*(4), 370–375.

Dalton, V. K., Rue, M., Silverman, L. B., Gelber, R. D., Asselin, B. L., Barr, R. D., … Cohen, L. E. (2003). Height and weight in children treated for acute lymphoblastic leukemia: Relationship to CNS Treatment. *Journal of Clinical Oncology. 21*(15), 2953–2960.

Edelman, C. E., Kudzma, E. C., & Mandle, C. L. (2014). *Health promotion through the life span* (8th ed.). St Louis, MO: Elsevier Mosby.

Eilertsen, M. E., Rannestad, T., Indredavik, M. S, & Vik, T. (2011). Psychosocial health in children and adolescents surviving cancer. *Scandanavian Journal of Caring Sciences. 25*(4), 725–734.

Friedman, D. L., Whitton, J., Leisenring, W., Mertens, A. C., Hammond, S., Stovall, M, … Neglia, J. P. (2010). Subsequent neoplasms in 5-year survivors of childhood cancer: The Child hood Cancer Survivor Study. *Journal of the National Cancer Institute. 102*(14), 1083–1095.

Gibson, F., & Soanes, L. (2004). *Cancer in children and young people.* West Sussex, England: John Wiley & Sons, Ltd.

Grothey, A., Kalaycio, M., Morris, L. G. T., Neugut, A. I., & Robinson, L. L. (2014). Guidelines, predictive models needed to improve understanding of secondary primary malignancies. *HemOnc today. 15*(8).

Gurney, J. G. (2003). Final height and body mass index among adult survivors of childhood brain cancer: Childhood cancer survivor study. *Journal of Clinical Endocrinological Metabolism. 85*(10), 4731–4739.

Howard, A. F., Tan de Bibiana, J., Smillie. K., Goddard, K., Pritchard, S., Olson R., & Kazanjian, S. (2014). Trajectories of Social Isolation in adult survivors of childhood cancer. *Journal of Cancer Survivors. 8*, 80–93.

Hudson, M. M., Leisenring, W., Stratton, K. K., Tinner, N., Steen, B. D., Ogg, S., … Cox, C. L. (2014). Increasing cardiomyopathy screening in at-risk adult survivors of pediatric malignancies: A randomized controlled trial. *Journal of Clinical Oncology. 32*(35), 3974–3981.

Institute of Medicine. (2003). Childhood cancer survivorship: Improving care and quality of life. Retrieved from Institute of Medicine: http://books.nap.edu/openbook.php?record_id=10767&page=R1

Johnston, K. V. (2008). Failure to lactate: A possible late effect of cranial radiation. *Pediatric Blood and Cancer. 50*(3), 721–722.

Kelvin J. F., Kroon, L., & Ogle, S. K. (2012). Fertility preservation for patients with cancer. *Clinical Journal of Oncology Nursing. 16*(2), 205–210.

Knight, K. R., Kraemer, D. F, & Neuwelt, E. A. (2005). Ototoxicity in children receiving platinum chemotherapy underestimating a commonly occurring toxicity that that may influence academic and social development. *Journal of Clinical Oncology. 23*(34), 8588–8596.

Krull, K. R., Brinkman, T. M., Li, C., Armstrong, G. T., Ness, K. K., Srivastava, D. K., … Hudson, M. M. (2013). Neurocognitive outcomes decades after treatment for acute lymphoblastic leukemia: A report from St. Jude lifetime cohort study. *Journal of Clinical Oncology. 31*(35), 4407–4418.

Lu, D., Fall, K., Sparén, P., Ye, W., Adami, H. O., Valdimarsdóttir, U., & Fang, F. (2013). Suicide and suicide attempt after a cancer diagnosis among young individuals. *Annals of Oncology. 24*, 3112–3117.

National Cancer Institute. (2012). *The childhood cancer survivor study: An overview.* Retrieved from http://www.cancer.gov/cancertopics/coping/survivorship/ccss

National Cancer Institute. (2014). *Cancer in children and adolescents fact sheet.* Retrieved from http://www.cancer.gov/cancertopics/factsheet/Sites-Types/childhood

Neglia, J. P., Friedman, D. L., Yasui, Y., Mertens, A. C., Hammond, S., Stovall, M. … Robison, L. L. (2001). Second malignant neoplasms in five-year survivors of childhood cancer: Childhood cancer survivor study. *Journal of the National Cancer Institute. 93*, 618–629.

Neglia, J. P., Robison, L. L., Stovall, M., Liu, Y., Packer, R. J., Hammond, S., … Inskip, P. D. (2006). New primary neoplasms of the central nervous system in survivors of childhood cancer: A report from the childhood cancer survivor study. *98*(21), 1528–1537.

Oeffinger, K. C., Mertens, A. C., Sklar, C. A., Kawashima, T., Hudson, M. M., Meadows, A. T., Robison, L. L; Childhood Cancer Survivor Study. (2006). Chronic health conditions in adult survivors of childhood cancer. *New England Journal of Medicine. 355*(15), 1572–1582.

Oeffinger, K. C., Ford, J. S., Moskowitz, C. S., Diller, L. R., Hudson, M. M., Chou JF, … Robison, L. L. (2009). Breast cancer surveillance practices among women previously treated with chest radiation for childhood cancer. *Journal of the American Medical Association. 301*(4), 404–414.

Ogle, S. K. (2008). Sperm banking with adolescents with cancer. *Journal of Pediatric Oncology Nursing. 25*(2), 97–101.

Ozono, S. S. (2007). Factors related to posttraumatic stress in adolescent survivors of childhood cancer and their parents. *Support Cancer Care. 15*, 309–317.

Packer, G. P., Gurney, J. G., Punyko, J. A., Donaldson, S. S., Inskip, P. D., Stovall, M., ... Robison, L. L. (2003). Long-term neurological and neurosensory sequela in adult survivors of a childhood brain tumor: Childhood cancer survivor study. *Journal of Clinical Oncology. 21*(17), 3255–3261.

Patel, S. K., Wong, A. L., Cuevas, M., & Van Horn, H. (2013). Parenting stress and neurocognitive late effects in childhood cancer survivors. *Psycho-Oncology. 22*, 1774–1782.

Pillitteri, A. (2014). *Maternal & child health nursing: Care of the childbearing & childrearing family* (7th ed.). Philadelphia, PA: Lippincott, Williams & Wilkens.

Pollock E. A., Litzelman, K., Wisk, L. E., & Witt, W. P. (2013). Correlates of physiological and psychological stress among parents of childhood cancer and brain tumor survivors. *Academic Pediatrics. 13*(2), 105–112.

Prednisone. (2014). Retrieved from Drugs.com: http://www.drugs.com/pro/prednisone.html

Servitzoglou, M., Papadatou, D., Tsiantis, I., & Vasilatou-Kosmidis, H. (2009). Quality of life of adolescent and young adult survivors of childhood cancer. *Journal of Pediatric Nursing. 24*(5), 415–422.

St. Jude Children's Research Hospital. (2014). *The childhood cancer survivor study.* Retrieved from https://ccss.stjude.org/

Sundberg, K. K., Lampic, C., Björk, O., Arvidson, J., & Wettergren, L.(2009). Positive and negative consequences of childhood cancer influencing the lives of young adults. *European Journal of Oncology Nursing. 13*, 164–170.

Taieb, O., Moro, M. R., Baubet, T., Revah-Lévy, A., & Flament, M. F. (2003). Posttraumatic Stress symptoms after childhood cancer. *European Child & Adolescent Psychiatry. 12*, 255–264.

Van Dongen-Melman, J. E., Van Zuuren, F. J., & Verhulst, F. C. (1998). Experiences of parents of childhood cancer survivors: A qualitative analysis. *Patient Education and Counseling. 34*, 185–200.

Witt, W. P., Litzelman, K., Wisk, L. E., Spear, H. A., Catrine, K., Levin, N., & Gottlieb, C. A. (2010). Stress-mediated quality of life outcomes in parents of childhood cancer and brain tumor survivors: A case-controlled study. *Quality of Life Res. 19*, 995–1005.

Zeltzer, L. K., Recklitis, C., Buchbinder, D., Zebrack, B., Casillas, J., Tsao, J. C., ... Krull, K. (2009). Pyschological status in childhood cancer surviviors: A report from the childhood cancer survivor study. *Journal of Clinical Oncology. 27*(14), 2396–2424.

NURSING THEORIES

CHAPTER 7

THEORY OF UNCERTAINTY

"Initially [it was] just overwhelming not being able to sleep and feeling like my heart was pounding. I was trying to make plans all the time as to how to deal with everything. I had two fairly young children at the time, so my thoughts were constantly preoccupied with keeping things running for them, keeping my job, and so forth. I just was in a perpetual state of anxiety, and I keep worrying about what the outcome is going to be; I found that it's an ever-changing landscape" (Brisbois, 2014).

Key Terms

affect-control strategies • event congruence • event familiarity • illusion • inference • mobilizing strategies • probabilistic thinking • self-organization • stimuli frame • structure providers • symptom pattern • uncertainty

Upon completing this chapter, you will be able to do the following:

1. Identify key concepts and processes in the uncertainty in illness theory.
2. Describe concepts and processes in the reconceptualized uncertainty in illness theory.
3. Consider the role of the uncertainty in illness theory in guiding research with cancer survivors.
4. Discuss the role uncertainty in illness theory plays in guiding care for cancer survivors.

Nearly 14.5 million people living in the United States today have a medical history that includes cancer (American Cancer Society, 2014). This number is projected to grow to 19 million by 2024 due to improvements in cancer detection and treatment. Well after cancer treatment is completed, survivors have concerns about recurrence, treatment-related side effects, and long-term health outcomes. Therefore, persons with many types of cancer-related sequelae will require multidimensional nursing care (Sammarco, 2009).

Uncertainty is the inability to determine the meaning of an illness-related event and may occur if patients are unable to determine the meaning or predict the outcome of cancer-related stimuli (Hall, Mishel, & Germino, 2014). Nurses can anticipate that some level of uncertainty will persist for the remainder of a cancer survivor's life, making this an important concept of interest to oncology nurses.

Middle-range theories provide a conceptual basis for nursing practice and research and can be useful to nurses because they focus on a limited set of concepts that explain or predict human responses to illness (Smith & Liehr, 2014). Mishel's (1988; 1990) middle range theory of uncertainty in illness is useful in describing and explaining the experience of uncertainty that occurs in persons undergoing diagnosis and treatment of cancer. The reconceptualized uncertainty in illness theory retains the concepts of the original theory; however, this was expanded to include the concept of reformulated thinking, making it particularly relevant to cancer survivorship. The theory of uncertainty in illness and the reconceptualized uncertainty in illness theory include antecedent conditions, appraisal of uncertainty, and the outcome of coping (Mishel, 1988; Mishel, 1990). Guided by this theory, oncology nurses can assess a patient's level of uncertainty, intervene and evaluate the effectiveness of interventions in reducing uncertainty in cancer survivors.

This chapter will review the uncertainty in illness theory and the reconceptualized uncertainty in illness theory. Existing research that used the uncertainty in illness theory or theory-based measures of uncertainty as a framework to examine phenomena related to cancer survivorship will then be reviewed. Finally, two case studies will be presented to facilitate application of the theory to nursing care of the cancer survivor.

Uncertainty in Illness Theory

Major Concepts

Mishel (1988) developed the uncertainty in illness theory to explain how a person with acute illness cognitively processes illness stimuli and derives meaning from the event. Later, Mishel (1990) reconceptualized her theory to better explain uncertainty in chronic illness. As noted in Figure 7.1, the major concepts presented in the uncertainty in illness theory and the reconceptualized uncertainty in illness theory are (a) antecedent conditions; (b) appraisal of uncertainty; and (c) coping with uncertainty.

Antecedent conditions. The major antecedent variable of the theory, *stimuli frame*, represents the nature of the stimuli that the person with cancer perceives (Mishel, 1988). Three components make up the stimuli frame: symptom pattern, event familiarity, and event congruence. *Symptom pattern* is the consistency of symptoms that enables a person to determine that an illness is present and the meaning of the symptoms (Mishel, 1988). *Event familiarity* means that the situation is familiar or contains recognized cues that enables the person to associate it with some earlier event or condition (Mishel, 1988). Meaning of the illness event can be determined by comparing it with a previous illness episode and symptoms. In the event that a person cannot discern a pattern due to inconsistency in symptom number, type, or character, uncertainty can occur. *Event congruence* refers to a match between expected and actual events (Mishel, 1988). In an illness episode, event congruence occurs when an expected symptom can be classified based on a previous experience and leads to proper interpretation and understanding

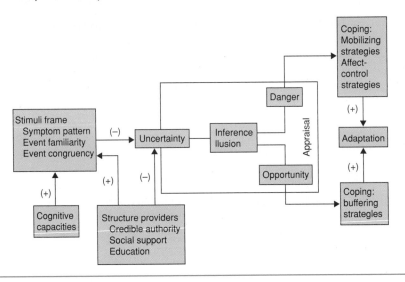

Figure 7.1 • Mishel's model of perceived uncertainty in illness.

of the illness experience. Severity of illness can lead to uncertainty especially when a symptom pattern cannot be classified (Mishel, 1997). These three components constitute the thinking process that a person with cancer will engage in to determine the meaning of their illness-related event. These components are posited to reduce uncertainty if the stimuli are familiar, recognized, and correctly classified.

Antecedent factors that influence the stimuli frame include cognitive capacity and structure providers. *Cognitive capacity,* the information processing ability of the person, directly influences the stimuli frame (Mishel, 1988). In those with limited information processing ability due to cognitive alterations or stimuli overload, uncertainty can develop. *Structure providers* positively influence stimuli frame by assisting with interpretation of illness events and also with minimizing uncertainty. *Structure providers* exist in three forms: (a) credible authority, (b) social support, and (c) education. *Education* provides understanding of the illness event by assisting with interpretation of the event. The level of education of the person influences the meaning of the illness event and the ability to more rapidly classify the event (Mishel, 1988). *Social support,* in the form of another person with whom to share your illness perceptions, assists to lower uncertainty levels. Social support also provides the person with the assurance through education, validation, and assistance with household tasks (Mishel & Braden, 1988). Healthcare providers assume the role of *credible authority* by providing education and support to the person with cancer. The person with cancer will seek out credible authorities for advice related to treatment decisions, diagnosis, and assistance with developing event congruence (Mishel, 1988; Mishel & Braden, 1988).

Appraisal of uncertainty. Uncertainty is a neutral experience until appraised by the person with an illness. The appraisal process results in either a positive or negative perception of the illness experience. During appraisal, two processes can occur: *inference* and *illusion. Inference,* influenced by personality, knowledge, and contextual cues, is the process of negatively evaluating the illness experience resulting in heightened uncertainty (Mishel, 1988). In contrast, *illusion* is a positive outlook based on appraisal of the illness-related situation as an opportunity (Mishel, 1988). The outcome of the appraisal processes is the perception that the illness is viewed as a danger or as an opportunity. Subsequent coping is based on the outcome of the appraisal process.

Coping with uncertainty. Danger, opportunity, coping, and adaptation are all coping reactions in response to the appraisal of uncertainty. The perception of an illness event as dangerous results in mobilizing strategies in response to the perceived threat (Mishel, 1988). *Mobilizing strategies* such as direct action, vigilance, and information seeking are all employed to reduce the experience of uncertainty during an illness event (Mishel, 1988). Information is sought from healthcare providers or social networks and reduces uncertainty by assisting to clarify the stimuli frame. If these active strategies are not successful in reducing uncertainty, *affect-control strategies* are employed to manage the emotional responses to illness events (Mishel, 1988). If coping strategies are effective, adaptation is the end result.

Reconceptualized Uncertainty in Illness Theory

In 1990, Mishel published a reconceptualized uncertainty in illness theory in response to the appraisal of uncertainty that occurs in the presence of chronic illness. The reconceptualized theory is similar to the original except for the gradual reappraisal of continual uncertainty as an opportunity. Self-organization and probabilistic thinking are antecedent conditions present when continual uncertainty exists. *Self-organization* occurs when uncertainty continues and is a daily part of a person's life, such as that which is seen in a chronic illness. This results in *probabilistic thinking* or a change in the expectation of certainty within the illness experience (Mishel, 1990). The person maintains this new view of life through support from healthcare providers and other resources.

Nurses' Roles within the Theory

As structure providers, nurses play an important role in the theory of uncertainty. Nurses provide comprehensive education to assist cancer survivors to make sense of the stimuli frame and support reformulated thinking related to living with daily uncertainty (Mishel, 1999). Uncertainty is a perception based on appraisal of an illness situation rather than the situation itself. Concerns about symptoms, treatments, or illness expectations can be perceived as stressful when uncertainty levels are high. Nurses assume a major role in assisting patients to recognize physical and emotional cues throughout the illness trajectory and in providing support to resume normalcy. Current research assists nurses to recognize those at risk for uncertainty and to provide interventions to reduce uncertainty.

Use of the Uncertainty in Illness Theory in Cancer Survivor Research

A search of the electronic database PubMed was conducted using the keywords "uncertainty in illness theory and cancer survivor" yielding 10 articles; "uncertainty in illness theory and cancer survivorship" yielding 3 articles; "uncertainty in illness and cancer survivor" yielding 46 articles; and "uncertainty in illness and cancer survivorship" yielding 41 articles. One hundred articles published between 1993 and 2014 were retrieved.

Of these, 24 were excluded for being published outside the last 10 years and 13 articles were duplicates. Titles and abstracts were reviewed for relevance in the remaining 63 articles. A final sample of 16 articles met the criteria for inclusion: utilization of the uncertainty in illness theory, or reconceptualized theory, as a framework for research or instrumentation specific to addressing cancer survivor–related phenomena. Authors described uncertainty in survivors of breast cancer, childhood cancer, prostate cancer, brain cancer, and cancer survivorship in general.

Hall et al. (2014) addressed the relationship between cancer-related uncertainty and disease- or treatment-related outcomes in the increasingly prevalent population of young breast cancer survivors (≤50 years old). A sample of 313 African-American and Caucasian breast cancer survivors (2 to 4 years posttreatment) self-reported their cancer-related uncertainty using Mishel's Uncertainty in Illness Scale (MUIS)-Survivor Version in addition to completing scales of fatigue, insomnia, and affect. Hierarchical regression analysis demonstrated that higher cancer-related uncertainty was significantly associated with ongoing elevated levels of fatigue, insomnia, and mood disorders years after completion of treatment.

Similarly, in a cross-sectional descriptive study of 252 young (mean age 47.5) Korean breast cancer patients, 51.6% undergoing treatment and 48.4% who had completed treatment, Kim, Lee, and Lee (2012) noted a correlation between symptom experience and uncertainty. In this study, women currently undergoing treatment reported more severe symptoms and higher levels of uncertainty on MUIS than women who had completed treatment. Symptom patterns also differed between in-treatment and posttreatment groups. In women who had completed treatment, symptoms of dyspnea, insomnia, systemic treatment side effects, and arm discomfort were significantly positively correlated with uncertainty. However, in women currently undergoing treatment, the symptoms were more severe and included the symptoms experienced by the posttreatment group with the addition of fatigue, gastrointestinal (GI) disturbance, and pain. Again, it is clear that uncertainty persists beyond the treatment phase, although in this study, the level of uncertainty differed based on where the patient was on the treatment trajectory. The symptom pattern subcomponent of the stimuli frame of the uncertainty in illness model was the prominent antecedent to uncertainty in these studies. These patients would benefit from nursing interventions directed at understanding and managing both current and potential symptoms.

Germino et al. (2013) also investigated uncertainty in younger breast cancer survivors. In this intervention study, 312 (mean age 44) African-American and Caucasian breast cancer survivors were randomly assigned to either the Younger Breast Cancer Survivor Uncertainty Management Intervention (YS-UMI) or a control group. The intervention group received an investigator-developed topic guide on treatment side effects and cancer-survivor issues, a professionally produced compact disc introducing participants to cognitive and behavioral strategies to reduce uncertainty and promote positive life changes, and weekly phone follow-up for a month. The control group received only standard weekly follow-up phone calls for a month. Breast cancer survivors who received the intervention demonstrated a reduction in uncertainty, and significant improvements in behavioral and cognitive coping strategies, better utilization of resources, and improved cognitive reframing. This intervention allowed survivors to access information, resources, and strategies to manage uncertainty in the present and in the future (before a follow-up mammogram or oncology visit). This study follows up on a similar intervention by the lead authors (Gil et al., 2006) conducted in 483 cancer survivors 5 to 9 years posttreatment. A 20-month follow-up outcome assessment of that intervention trial indicated that the uncertainty management training resulted in reduced uncertainty and also yielded improvements in cognitive framing, knowledge, coping, and personal growth. The results of these interventional studies highlight the impact of the cognitive capacity and structure provider variables of Mishel's model in mediating uncertainty in a positive direction.

Cultural (Sammarco & Konency, 2010) and age differences (Sammarco, 2009) variability in social support, quality of life (QOL), and uncertainty was the focus of two comparative studies. In these studies, uncertainty (MUIS) was investigated as a mediator of QOL. Analysis revealed the presence of a higher level of perceived total social support in Caucasian participants ($n = 182$), although Hispanic participants ($n = 98$) reported higher levels of spousal and family support. This is consistent with the cultural value Hispanics place on family relationships. Significantly higher levels of uncertainty was reported by Hispanic participants, fueled by the coexistence of comorbidities, treatment side effects, fear of death, and health-related financial concerns in this subset. Lower educational levels of Hispanics, compared to their Caucasian counterparts, also contributed to this finding. These factors resulted in a reported significantly poorer QOL by Hispanic breast cancer survivors. Differences on the dimension of age were significant only for the variable of social support, with younger women perceiving more total social support and spousal support.

Wonghongkul, Dechaprom, Phumivichuvate, and Losawatkul (2006) also investigated uncertainty and QOL with the additional variable of appraisal coping. Hierarchical multiple regression revealed that survival time, uncertainty (MUIS), and harm (stress appraisal) were statistically significant in predicting QOL. The overall level of uncertainty was found to be moderate in this sample, but decreased as survival time increased. As noted in the previously described intervention studies, the importance of social support in mediating uncertainty cannot be underestimated. Patient-centered, culturally informed assessments of patient support needs should be conducted and appropriate resources provided to promote successful adaptation.

The concept of uncertainty related to fertility, reproduction, and motherhood in a young adult woman was explored by Halliday and Boughton (2011) who concluded that the "importance of fertility to young female cancer survivors cannot be underestimated" (p. 139). The impact of uncertain motherhood on younger women's psychosocial health needs to be addressed by healthcare providers, and appropriate education, management, and support provided, as delineated in the uncertainty in illness model.

Childhood Cancer

Childhood cancer survivors have unique concerns and challenges. Survivors of childhood cancers have a higher risk of being diagnosed (again) with cancer than their cancer-free peers. They also experience a high rate (70%) of treatment-related complications that occur well beyond the treatment period (Lee, Gau, Hsu, & Chang, 2009). In addition, developmental challenges occur across transition points, but especially during emerging adulthood as the young adult struggles with independence, self-management of health, and risk-behavior temptations. Lee et al. (2009) and Santacroce and Lee (2006) presented proposed models to describe the relationship between uncertainty, posttraumatic stress symptoms, and health behaviors. They posit that survivors living with prolonged uncertainty are at risk for developing posttraumatic stress symptoms and subsequently engaging in high-risk health behaviors. A comparative study (Decker, Haase, & Bell, 2007) of uncertainty across the cancer trajectory of young adults found that survivors >5 years continued to report uncertainty (MUIS) related to diagnosis, symptoms, and treatment success. They also reported having many unanswered questions about their illness course. Survivors reported high levels of uncertainty regarding ambiguous communication from physicians. Based on these findings, and consistent with the uncertainty model, young adults may benefit from individualized health education, self-management training, coping skill development, frequent clinical monitoring, improved health care provider communication, ongoing social support from adults and anticipatory guidance to reduce uncertainty, promote a positive life view and improve health behaviors.

Prostate Cancer

Prostate cancer, the male counterpart of breast cancer, is the most common male gender-specific cancer. Diagnosis and treatment of both these cancers are riddled with body image and intimacy concerns in addition to general cancer-related psychosocial issues in survivors. In prostate cancer, uncertainty fluctuates in relationship to prostate specific antigen (PSA) monitoring in the posttreatment period. Uncertainty surrounding treatment decisions is also high in this population. In a longitudinal study of surgically treated prostate cancer patients, three trajectory patterns (stable, unstable, and mixed) were identified based on PSA value and psychosocial measure scores. Results revealed high levels of cognitive reframing, QOL, and positive mood as well as stable levels of uncertainty (MUIS) in patients with stable PSA levels over time. Conversely, patients with unstable or fluctuating PSA levels demonstrated poor or fluctuating scores on all these measures (Bailey, Wallace, Polascik, & Roberston, 2014).

Because disease recurrence in prostate cancer is insidious, and physical side effects of treatment are complex, ongoing psychosocial support and strong patient–provider communication is of particular importance in this population. Patients need assistance with cognitive reframing and achieving a new view of life in which uncertainty is viewed as normal. Nurse-led support groups, patient-centered education, formal stress management, and health promotion programs may be of value in assisting patients to achieve this new life view (Weber, Roberts, Chumbler, Mills, & Algood, 2007). Assessment of patient's "certainties and uncertainties" will provide insight for nurses when developing interventions aimed at reframing cognitive structures, solving issues, and nurturing relationships aimed at attaining a new perspective of life (Yu Ko & Degner, 2008).

Brain Cancer

An integrative review of brain tumor symptoms as antecedents to uncertainty was conducted by Cahill, LoBiondo-Wood, Bergstron, and Armstrong (2012). Twenty-one studies described a range of diverse symptoms among brain tumor patients that persisted beyond the treatment phase. The presence of fatigue, altered mental status, and neurological symptoms were consistent across brain tumor patients, with fatigue being most strongly correlated with uncertainty in the treatment and posttreatment period. In addition, the appearance of new, irregular, or exacerbated symptom patterns in the posttreatment period perpetuated an ongoing state of uncertainty by raising questions about treatment effectiveness and prognosis. Fortunately, as symptoms stabilized uncertainty was reduced. These findings suggest that interventions aimed at symptom interpretation and management and ongoing support may be warranted in this population.

Across Cancer Types

Miller (2012) conducted a qualitative study to investigate the sources of uncertainty in survivors of a broad range of cancer types, and their partners. Participants described medical, personal, and social sources of uncertainty that persisted long after they had completed cancer treatment, and that were unique from a cancer illness context. For survivors and their partners, knowing the common sources of anxiety may allow adjustment to an "uncertain survivorship trajectory." Healthcare providers should be focused on management of chronic uncertainty throughout survivorship. The uncertainty in illness theory provides a structure for thoughtful, individualized patient interventions.

Implications for Nursing with Cancer Survivors

Nurses, as structure providers, provide comprehensive education and support to assist cancer survivors to make sense of the stimuli frame and support reformulated thinking related to living with the daily uncertainty of survivorship. Concerns about symptoms, treatments, or illness recurrence can be perceived as stressful when uncertainty levels are high. Nurses assume a major role in assisting patients to recognize physical and emotional cues throughout the illness trajectory and in providing support to resume normalcy. Current research assists nurses to recognize those at risk for uncertainty and to provide interventions to reduce uncertainty. Survivors benefit from frequent clinical monitoring, improved healthcare provider communication, ongoing social support, and anticipatory guidance to reduce uncertainty, promote a positive life view, and improve health behaviors.

CASE STUDY 1

Rose is a 64-year-old breast cancer survivor. She received her diagnosis 16 years ago. On that day she was a 48-year-old wife, mother of two teenage daughters, a critical care nurse, and a devoted friend. Rose's mother had been diagnosed with breast cancer at the age of 47, and died a year later at the young age of 48. Since that day, Rose has been fearful, yet almost certain that she too would be diagnosed with breast cancer. Rose had fibrocystic breasts, so frequently found lumps. Year after year she faithfully had her screening mammogram, and held her breath until she got her "all is normal" results. In the summer of 1997, hours after having her yearly examination the phone rang. The voice on the other end of the call stated "we have scheduled an ultrasound and biopsy for you tomorrow." Rose did not need the biopsy results to reveal her fate, "I knew I had cancer." Her greatest fear was realized.

Rose had an oncology consult scheduled the following week. Three options were presented, each with a cure rate attached. The opportunity to be in a blinded study was also offered. However, she quickly declined that opportunity because the outcome was uncertain. In the end, she chose the option that she believed provided her with the greatest chance of cure: radical mastectomy, chemotherapy, radiation, and Tamoxifen for 5 years. "It would kill me or cure me." The motivator behind her aggressive choice was to live long enough for her youngest daughter to graduate from high school. However, she remained "in constant fear of cancer recurring or metastasizing for years." With every new lump, or unusual symptom, Rose was sure she had cancer again. Her constant worrying was beginning to drain her family, as they were ready to move on to a "normal" life again. Her relationship with her eldest daughter became "distanced."

Six years later, while on a spa weekend away with friends everything changed. Rose was scheduled for a therapeutic massage and Reiki session and was remarkably energized after this session. Upon returning home she sought out a local center to have additional sessions. Eventually she enrolled in classes to be trained in massage therapy, and alternative healing modalities. She has since retired from her nursing position and now practices holistic healing full-time. She has a steady clientele of breast cancer survivors.

• Critical Thinking **Questions**

1. Identify specific stimuli frame components that were antecedents to Rose's uncertainty.
2. Describe how the variables of cognitive capacity and structure providers positively and negatively impacted Rose's level of uncertainty.
3. Discuss how Rose's illness appraisal and coping shifted over time.
4. How would you label Rose's chronic uncertainty outcome?
5. Develop an intervention plan that you would have implemented at the time of Rose's initial diagnosis. How might that have changed her uncertainty trajectory?

CASE STUDY 2

Mark is a 51-year-old prostate cancer survivor. He was diagnosed 5 years ago, after visiting his healthcare provider for symptoms of urinary frequency, and reduced urine stream. His physical examination that day revealed an irregularly shaped prostate. Laboratory work was completed and the Prostate Serum Antigen was abnormally elevated. A biopsy and urology consult was recommended. Mark's father had prostate cancer diagnosed at age 68, and underwent a radical prostatectomy. Mark remembers the embarrassing incontinence his father experienced after the surgery. Recently remarried after being widowed for 10 years, Mark is concerned about the impact potential cancer treatment would have on his sexual and urinary function. Mark was very anxious and unable to sleep in the following days waiting for his biopsy procedure and results. His anxiety impacted his performance at work.

Mark finally underwent ultrasound and biopsy, which revealed adenocarcinoma in a single area. Treatment options were discussed and included surgical management, brachytherapy, external-beam radiotherapy (EBRT), and delayed treatment (active surveillance). Given his young age, small mass, and PSA value, a wait and see option was recommended. Mark had frequent PSA monitoring and urology follow-ups. Mark would become extremely anxious and sleepless in the weeks prior to each scheduled PSA monitoring test, but symptoms would quickly abate when results were known to be stable.

After a year of monitoring, Mark's PSA level began to climb steadily. His mass also increased in size by 50%. Additional treatment was recommended, and options were again discussed. Mark's worry and anxiety was once again exacerbated. He worried about his treatment being unsuccessful and dying from cancer, as his wife of 16 years had 10 years before. He also worried about treatment complications, most prominently sexual dysfunction. In the following weeks, Mark researched new treatment options for prostate cancer. He decided to investigate the possibility of EBRT with proton therapy at a major metropolitan medical center, and scheduled a consult. After meeting with the team, that included a social worker and support groups, Mark decided to have the treatment. His treatment was successful and he is free of cancer and complications.

• Critical Thinking **Questions**

1. Identify specific stimuli frame components that were antecedents to Mark's uncertainty.
2. Discuss how the variables of cognitive capacity and structure providers altered Marks's level of uncertainty.
3. Describe Mark's illness appraisal and coping strategy during the diagnosis period and during the final treatment decision period.
4. How would you label Mark's chronic uncertainty outcome?
5. Develop an intervention plan that you would have implemented at the time of Mark's initial diagnosis. How might that have changed his uncertainty trajectory?

References

American Cancer Society. (2014). *Cancer treatment and survivorship facts and figures 2014–2015.* Retrieved from http://www.cancer.org/acs/groups/content/@research/documents/document/acspc-042801.pdf

Bailey, D. E., Jr., Wallace Kazer, M., Polascik, T. J., & Robertson, C. (2014). Psychosocial trajectories of men monitoring prostate-specific antigen levels following surgery for prostate cancer. *Oncology Nursing Forum. 41*, 361–368. doi: 10.1188/14.ONF.361–368

Brisbois, M. D. (2014). An interpretive description of chemotherapy-induced premature menopause among Latinas with breast cancer. *Oncology Nursing Forum. 41*, E282–E289.

Cahill, J., LoBiondo-Wood, G., Bergstrom, N., & Armstrong, T. (2012). Brain tumor symptoms as antecedents to uncertainty: An integrative review. *Journal of Nursing Scholarship. 44,* 145–155. doi: 10.1111/j.1547–5069.2012.01445.x

Decker, C. L., Haase, J. E., & Bell, C. J. (2007). Uncertainty in adolescents and young adults with cancer. *Oncology Nursing Forum. 34,* 681–688.

Germino, B. B., Mishel, M. H., Crandell, J., Porter, L., Blyler, D., Jenerette, C., & Gil, K. (2013). Outcomes of an uncertainty management intervention in younger African American and Caucasian breast cancer survivors. *Oncology Nursing Forum. 40,* 82–92. doi: 10.1188/13. ONF.82–92

Gil, K. M., Mishel, M. H., Belyea, M., Germino, B., Porter, L. S., & Clayton, M. (2006). Benefits of the uncertainty management intervention for African American and White older breast cancer survivors: 20-month outcomes. *International Journal of Behavioral Medicine. 13,* 286–294.

Hall, D. L., Mishel, M. H., & Germino, B. B. (2014). Living with cancer related uncertainty: Associations of fatigue, insomnia, and affect in younger breast cancer survivors. *Journal of Psychosocial Oncology. 22,* 2489–2495. doi: 10.1007?s00520–014–2243-y

Halliday, L. E., & Boughton, M. A. (2011). Exploring the concept of uncertain fertility, reproduction, and motherhood after cancer in young adult women. *Nursing Inquiry. 18,* 135–142. doi: 10.1111/j.1440–1800.2011.00532.x

Kim, S. H., Lee, R., & Lee, K. S. (2012). Symptoms and uncertainty in breast cancer survivors in Korea: Differences by treatment trajectory. *Journal of Clinical Nursing. 21,* 1014–1023. doi: 10.1111/j.1365–2648.2011.05888.x

Lee, Y. L., Gau, B. S., Hsu, W. M., & Chang, H. H. (2009). A model linking uncertainty, post-traumatic stress, and health behaviors in childhood cancer survivors. *Oncology Nursing Forum. 36,* E20–E30. doi: 10.1188/09.ONF.E20-E30

Miller, L. E. (2012). Sources of uncertainty in cancer survivorship. *Journal of Cancer Survivorship. 6,* 431–440. doi: 10.1007/s11764–012–0229–7

Mishel, M. H. (1988). Uncertainty in illness. *Image: The Journal of Nursing Scholarship. 20,* 225–232. doi: 10.1111/j.1547–5069.1988.tb00082.x

Mishel, M. H. (1990). Reconceptualization of the uncertainty in illness theory. *Image: The Journal of Nursing Scholarship. 22,* 256–262. doi:10.1111/j.1547–5069.1990.tb00225.x

Mishel, M. H. (1997). Uncertainty in acute illness. *Annual Review of Nursing Research. 15,* 57–80.

Mishel, M. H. (1999). Uncertainty in chronic illness. *Annual Review of Nursing Research. 17,* 269–294.

Mishel, M. H., & Braden, C. J. (1988). Finding meaning: Antecedents of uncertainty in illness. *Nursing Research. 37,* 98–127.

Sammarco, A. (2009). Quality of life of breast cancer survivors: A comparative study of age cohorts. *Cancer Nursing. 32,* 347–56. doi: 10.1097/NCC.0b013e31819e23b7

Sammarco, A., & Konency, L. M. (2010). Quality of life, social support, and uncertainty among Latina and Caucasian breast cancer survivors: A comparative study. *Oncology Nursing Forum. 37,* 93–99. doi: 10.1188/10.ONF.93–99

Santacroce, S. J., & Lee, Y. L. (2006). Uncertainty, posttraumatic stress, and health behavior in young adult childhood cancer survivors. *Nursing Research. 55,* 259–266.

Smith, M. J., & Liehr, P. R. (2014). *Middle range theory for nursing* (3rd ed.). New York, NY: Springer Publishing Company.

Weber, B. A., Roberts, B. L., Chumbler, N. R., Mills, T. L., & Algood, C. B. (2007). Urinary, sexual, and bowel dysfunction and bother after radical prostatectomy. *Urology Nursing. 27,* 527–533.

Wonghongkul, T., Dechaprom, N., Phumivichuvate, L., & Losawatkul, S. (2006). Uncertainty appraisal coping and quality of life in breast cancer survivors. *Cancer Nursing. 29,* 250–257.

Yu Ko, W. F., & Degner, L. F. (2008). Uncertainty after treatment for prostate cancer: Definition, assessment, and management. *Clinical Journal of Oncology Nursing. 12,* 749–755. doi: 10.11.88/08.CJON.749–755

CHAPTER 8
THEORY OF UNPLEASANT SYMPTOMS

"Every day I experience fatigue that does not go away. It is there when I go to sleep and when I wake up. Some days I can barely function. My husband tells me that I use fatigue as an excuse; he just doesn't understand."

—*A cancer survivor*

Key Terms

influencing factors • middle-range nursing theory • performance outcomes • physiologic factors • psychologic factors • situational factors • symptoms

Upon completing this chapter, you will be able to do the following:

1. Describe the purpose of the Theory of Unpleasant Symptoms.
2. Differentiate between the basic concepts of the theory: symptoms, influencing factors, and performance outcomes.
3. Discuss patient management situations in which an understanding of the Theory of Unpleasant Symptoms assists in improving patient care.

History of the Theory of Unpleasant Symptoms

The origin of the Theory of Unpleasant Symptoms (TOUS) stems from the work of four nurses who were simultaneously working on their PhD dissertations while attending the same program (Elizabeth Lenz, Audrey Gift, Renee Milligan, and Linda Pugh; 1995). Each researcher was looking at a specific "unpleasant symptom" and collaborated in dyads or triads using the same studies and theoretical articles to expand on the "unpleasant symptom," which was their focus. Fatigue for the childbearing cycle, being studied by both Pugh and Milligan, was common to the fatigue an individual experienced with dyspnea, as looked at by Gift and Pugh. The nurses determined that while physiological problems have both acute and chronic symptoms, the psychological aspects must be considered due to their direct and indirect influence. In addition, the nurses recognized that each patient experienced distress related to the fatigue or dyspnea because it had impact on their lives. As their investigations continued, they realized that they had found a common thread; they were all using a common vocabulary and descriptors to describe phenomena that were occurring in totally different areas of patient care.

> "The mainstay of nursing research must increasingly become the development of the regularities between such identified descriptors with enough precision to enable them to guide nursing practice" (Lenz, Suppe, Gift, Pugh, & Milligan, 1995; p. 4).

As a result of this work, the researchers realized that they had the beginnings of a middle-range theory, one that used real experiences in an attempt to investigate a real problem that is encountered daily in every nurse's world.

Basic Concepts

Collectively, the researchers examined three concepts: symptoms, influencing factors, and performance outcomes and then each of these concepts was broken down further. The theory's overall structure asserts that "three interrelated categories of factors (physiologic, psychologic, and situational) influence predisposition to and manifestation of a given symptom or multiple symptoms and the nature of the symptom experience" (Lenz & Pugh, 1997; p. 163). The model they developed (Fig. 8.1) demonstrates the physiological, psychological, and the situational factors influencing the symptom(s) and this in turn influences the performance of the patient.

Symptoms

Symptoms, their intensity or severity, the degree of associated distress to the individual, their timing, and the quality of the unpleasant symptoms were studied using fatigue, dysp-

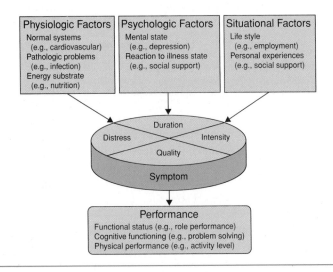

Figure 8.1 • Middle-range theory of unpleasant symptoms.

nea, and pain either experienced singularly or together as a cluster to better understand the subjective experience of the individual. It is possible for one symptom to give rise to other symptoms (Lenz & Pugh, 1997). Also when more than one symptom are experienced, it can make all the symptoms seem worse as stated by Sarna, Evangelista, Tashkin, Padilla, Holmes, and Brecht in their study in 2004. When a postpartum patient is tired from caring for a new infant, the pain she is experiencing from either the cesarean section or the episiotomy incision can be perceived as more intense than if the new mother had several hours of sleep. The same can be said of a cancer patient who has been vomiting postchemotherapy; the degree of fatigue can be perceived to be more intense the more he vomits.

In the TOUS, all symptoms can vary in their intensity or severity, associated distress, timing, and quality (Lenz & Pugh, 1997). The intensity dimension is the most frequently measured subjective experience, using tools such as the Numeric Pain Scale, with 0 being no pain and 10 being the worst pain ever, as this is something that a patient can explain verbally to another. In the pediatric setting, children are asked to pick a face from the Faces Pain Assessment Tool that matches the degree of pain that they are feeling at the moment. This tool can also be used by patients who are intubated, but awake enough to pick a "face."

How much a patient is bothered by the symptom is the "distress factor." The distress factor can be modified by outside influences, as well as the individual patient's degree of tolerance. When one individual might need a narcotic for his/her pain, another individual might only want an aspirin. Tolerance for any unpleasant symptom varies from individual to individual and can vary within the individual depending on many external and internal factors. It is very important to realize that while some patients may find one symptom mildly bothersome, the addition of a symptom that a patient finds distressful, may make the first symptom unbearable (Lenz & Pugh, 1997).

Timing of the symptom can include duration and frequency (Lenz & Pugh, 1997). For example, the patient in the first trimester of pregnancy may experience acute episodes of nausea and vomiting and although not a pleasant experience, the individual knows that this problem will most likely stop during the second trimester. A patient with hyperemesis of pregnancy who continues to vomit until the end of her pregnancy will attach a totally different meaning to the experience. Most people can tolerate discomfort once in a while for a short period of time. It becomes debilitating and can affect other symptoms with increasing frequency and duration. Along with the timing of the unpleasant symptom, an emotional component is attached to it; the more frequent and the longer the problem continues the more unpleasant the symptom becomes until it is all that the patient may think about and verbalize to others.

Quality is the way the symptom(s) are experienced, or "the nature of the symptom or the way in which it is manifested or experienced, that is, what it feels like to have the symptom" (Lenz & Pugh, 1997; p. 166). As nurses, we always assess how a pain feels. Is it burning, aching, throbbing, dull, and so forth? "By including this dimension, the TOUS acknowledges that in addition to reflecting characteristics that are common across all symptoms, each symptom has unique aspects and characteristics" (Lenz & Pugh, 1997; p. 166). How does it feel to be unable to take a deep breath or finish a sentence without losing your ability to speak because you do not have enough air to finish that sentence? Only the individual can describe this and the terms that are used or descriptors can change as the problem progresses. This is important as it can help those around the patient to track the progression of the medical problem. If the patient is experiencing dyspnea, how he describes it; for example as a tightness or feeling of suffocation, will assist those around the patient to understand that experience and to assist the patient as needed.

Influencing Factors

While the patient may go through a variety of unpleasant symptoms during the course of their illness, there are different factors influencing these symptoms and the patients' perception of their degree of unpleasantness. The influencing factors may be physiological, psychological, or situational. What is happening outside the individual that adds to the experience of unpleasant symptoms? The three categories identified in TOUS are "physiologic factors, psychologic factors, and situational factors" (Lenz & Pugh, 1997; p. 167). The "combination and/or interaction of multiple influencing factors can impact the symptom experience differently from any given influencing factor alone" (Lenz & Pugh, 1997; p. 167). One of these factors can influence another factor to make the first issue more intense. For example, the patient is experiencing extreme fatigue from the vomiting that has kept him up all night after his chemotherapy treatment (the physiological factor). On top of that, his wife is having surgery in a week (the psychological factor) and he is behind on his mortgage because he has been unable to work (situational factor). All of these together will make his fatigue, his unpleasant symptom, much more intense.

Physiologic factors include "anatomical/structural, physiological, genetic, and treatment-related variable" (Lenz & Pugh, 1997; p. 167). All the internal mechanisms that make each one of us the unique being that we are and how the specific disease process affects each different body system to produce the symptoms that are being experienced make up the physiological factors. The symptoms that are experienced are usually the first indication that there might be a problem that could use further investigation. When a problem is discovered, the effect on the body can then be made more noticeable to the patient because of the treatment chosen. A patient who has been diagnosed with cancer of the stomach might first notice a feeling of extreme fullness after a cup of coffee in the morning. This rather vague symptom might become more uncomfortable as time passes to the feeling of nausea after only eating several bites of a meal to belching without eating anything. No pain, which most of us assume, is an early symptom. Yet these symptoms can be uncomfortable to the patient. Weight loss would be a common early symptom, but many individuals pass this off as "I am trying to lose weight—thanks for noticing" and again, not put all of the symptoms together. Many times a patient will see the doctor and in passing mention these symptoms, but unless there is a possible family history of stomach cancer, the doctor may not put these symptoms together either.

Once the diagnosis has been made of stomach cancer and treatment has begun, the patient may complain more about the original symptoms, even though the severity of the symptoms has not changed. This change in the level of distress is due to the psychological factors that then come into play; psychological factors may be difficult to understand or control. Prior to the diagnosis, the patient was only experiencing vague, and to him/her, unrelated symptoms. Now they are a major medical issue that has the potential to turn into a medical crisis. How he/she responses to this are in part his/her personality; whether the patient is an upbeat individual or a depressed individual; and his/her affective response to the problem, such as fear, anger, and bitterness.

The psychological factors "represent one of the most complex components of the model. They include both affective and cognitive variables" (Lenz & Pugh, 1997; p. 167). The cognitive variables would include patient knowledge of his condition, his personal coping skills, and what the prognosis is. Again, these cognitive variables are as unique as the patient and can change as time and the cancer progress. It is difficult to separate the psychological and physiological factors as they are intertwined with each other (Lenz & Pugh, 1997).

Situational factors are the patient's environment and the environment includes the physical environment as well as the social and cultural environment of the patient. Examples of social/cultural environment include age, marital status, and family availability for support while cultural environment can include how an individual reacts to pain, whether physical or emotional, as there is a "learned component to interpreting and expressing symptoms" (Lenz & Pugh, 1997; p. 168). The individual's background also comes into play when discussing situational factors. Examples can include smoking and drinking history, prior drug use, and the amount of exercise prior to the diagnosis. The physical environment includes temperature, lighting, and noise level, in other words, everything that makes up the physical environment that the patient now finds themselves in that can affect how they experience symptoms.

Performance Outcomes

The last major concept of the TOUS is performance outcomes. Performance outcomes refer to the consequences of the symptom experience. The individual's ability to function with the symptoms or the impact of the symptoms on the day-to-day activities is what is being examined here. Again the concept of performance has several components. These components are "physical activity and impairment; functional role performance, including ADLs, cognitive, including comprehension, learning, concentration, and problem solving; and social interaction" (Lenz & Pugh, 1997; p. 167). An example of this might again be the patient who has been diagnosed with cancer, his wife having surgery the following week, and no money for the mortgage. He might have been an active man prior to the diagnosis, but now he is unable to go running as he did prior to his diagnosis. He is having increased difficulty being the "man of the house" because he cannot work due to the effects of chemotherapy and he is having increasing difficulty in thinking clearly because of the pain medications. His performance outcome has decreased because he can no longer do what he could in the past.

The one area that TOUS does not examine, in relationship to outcomes, is aspects of quality of life (QOL). The rational for not looking at QOLs is explained in the theory as there is a "high degree of overlap with functional status in many of the QOF measures" (Lenz & Pugh, 1997; p. 169). Many other studies such as Fox & Lyon in 2006 and Francocur in 2005, Gift & McCrone in 1993 and Redeker, Lev, & Ruggiero in 2000 have researched this aspect of unpleasant symptoms and their impact on the QOLs, although there is a possibility that this area of research might be included in future revisions of the TOUS theory; in the present model, the QOL issues are "…handled by the feedback loop from the symptom experience to psychologic factors rather than as an explicit outcome" (Lenz & Pugh, 1997; p. 169).

Implication for Nursing

Many studies have utilized the TOUS to guide our practice for the many different "unpleasant symptoms" that our patients present. Farrell and Savage (2010) investigated inflammatory bowel disease and their conclusion was "with consideration to all three concepts (symptoms, influencing factors, and performance) the TOUS is a complex interactive model of symptom experience. However, despite its complexity, the theorist have stated that for both researchers and practitioners, the dimensions of unpleasant symptoms are measurable" (Farrell & Savage, 2010; p. 439). Other studies include *Application of the Theory of Unpleasant Symptoms in Bariatric Surgery* (Tyler & Pugh, 2009) and the study by Lenz and Gift (1998) *Response to "The Theory of Unpleasant Symptoms and Alzheimer's Disease"* where the authors of the original theory have utilized the information that they gained and applied it to other "unpleasant symptoms." Other studies have utilized the original work and compared and contrasted the findings with other theories. In a discussion paper by Myers (2009), she compares the TOUS with the Conceptual Model of Chemotherapy-Related Changes in Cognitive Function. Myers (2009) states for implications for nursing, "Blending of the TOUS (TUS) and the Conceptual Model of Chemotherapy-Related Changes in Cognitive Function may provide an enhanced framework for further research about the physiologic and psychological aspects of chemotherapy-related cognitive impairment."

Middle-range nursing theories are applicable at the bedside where our care is administered. Singularly, these theories can help the nurses to help the patients with their medical issues and needs. Together, the theories can add an additional dimension to the care that we administer and improve the overall QOL for our patients.

CASE STUDY

Z. R., a 68-year-old male, was diagnosed with Stage IV lung cancer 6 months ago. He is currently undergoing aggressive chemotherapy treatments for the cancer. He is using nasal oxygen at 2 L/min and has been complaining of increasing shortness of breath and fatigue even with the oxygen therapy. His wife reports that he is experiencing increasing confusion and can no longer be left alone at home. He has a history of severe depression, approximately 20 years ago, that required inpatient care and has been on an antidepressant with good results since that time. Currently, besides the chemotherapy and the antidepressant, he has no other significant medical history.

Z. R. has lost approximately 66 kg (30 lb) and does not have an appetite, complaining of a dry mouth because he is mouth-breathing and a metallic taste in his mouth. Even when his wife offers his favorite foods, he refuses to eat.

• Critical Thinking Questions

1. The TOUS theory discusses the concept of situational influencing factors. Using Z. R.'s case study, what are the situational factors and how can the nurse improve his day-to-day environment?

2. With Z. R.'s past psychological history, how can his current situation be compounded?

3. Using the TOUS, how can the nurse help Mrs. R to help her husband through this journey that they both are on?

References

Armstrong, T. (2003). Symptoms experience: A concept analysis. *Oncology Nursing Forum. 30*(4), 601–606.

Brant, J. M., Beck, S., & Miaskowki, C. (2010). Building dynamic models and theories to advance the science of symptom management research. *Journal of Advance Nursing. 66*(1), 228–240. doi: 10.1111/j.1365–2648.2009.05179.x

Farrell, D. & Savage, E. (2010). Symptom burden in inflammatory bowel disease: Rethinking conceptual and theoretical underpinnings. *International Journal of Nursing Practice. 16*, 437–422.

Good, M. (1998). A middle-range theory of acute pain management: Use in research. *Nursing Outlook. 46*, 120–124.

Kim, H., McGuire, D., Tulman, L. & Barsevick, A. (2005). Symptoms clusters; Concept analysis and clinical implications for Cancer nursing. *Cancer Nursing. 28*(4), 270–282.

Lenz, E. & Gift, A. (1998). Response to "The Theory of Unpleasant Symptoms and Alzheimer's Disease." *Scholarly Inquiry for Nursing Practice: An International Journal. 12*(2), p. 160.

Lenz, E., Suppe, F., Gift, A., Pugh, L. & Milligan, R. (1995). Collaborative development of middle-range nursing theories: Toward a theory of unpleasant symptoms. *Advance Nursing Science. 17*(3), 1–13.

Lenz, E. R., & Pugh, L. C. (2008). Theory of Unpleasant Symptoms. In M. J. Smith, & P. R. Liehr (Eds.), *Middle Range Theory for Nursing.* (2nd ed., pp. 159–182). New York: Springer.

Liehr, P. & Smith, M. (1999). Middle range theory: Spinning research and practice to create knowledge of the new millennium. *Advance Nursing Science. 21*(4), 81–91.

Myers, J. (2009). A Comparison of the theory of unpleasant symptoms and the conceptual model of chemotherapy-related changes in cognitive function. *Oncology Nursing Forum. 36*(1), E1–E10.

Nightingale, F. (1859). *Notes on Nursing.* United States: Barnes and Noble Publishing, Inc.

Smith, M & Liehr, P. (2008). *Middle range theory for nursing.* chapter 9. New York, NY: Springer Publisher Company.

Tyler, R., & Pugh, L. (2009). Application of the Theory of unpleasant symptoms in bariatric surgery. *Bariatric Nursing and Surgical Patient Care. 4*(4), 271–276. doi: 10.1089/bar.2009.9953

CHAPTER 9
TRANSITIONS

"Nothing ever becomes real till it is experienced."
—*John Keats*

Key Terms

transition • middle-range theory • theorizing • types and patterns of transitions • properties of transition experiences • transition conditions • patterns of response • nursing therapeutics

Upon completing this chapter, you will be able to do the following:

1. Define transition.
2. Describe types and patterns of transitions.
3. Discuss the role of nursing within transition theory.
4. Identify patient populations for which transitions theory may be in used in nursing practice.

Oncology nurses frequently find themselves involved in various transitions that cancer patients and their families are experiencing throughout the process of cancer diagnosis, treatment, and survivorship, and attest changes in nursing care needs that such transitions bring about in the lives of cancer patients and their families.

Nursing Theories—Transitions

Over 13 million cancer survivors are currently residing in the United States, which is about 4% of the US population (de Moor et al., 2013). Among them, about 64% has reportedly survived over 5 years, 40% has survived over 10 years, and 15% has survived over 20 years (de Moor et al., 2013). Also, it is projected that the number of cancer survivors would increase by 31% by 2022 (de Moor et al., 2013). With the drastically increasing number of cancer survivors, there is an urgent need for nursing care for this specific population.

To provide systematic and integrated nursing care for cancer survivors, nurses have tried to develop theoretical bases that could be easily used to describe, explain, and predict nursing phenomenon. Throughout nursing history, several different types of nursing theories have been proposed and used (Meleis, 2011). Among them, middle-range theories were relatively recently proposed and have been widely used in nursing. Because middle-range theories could directly explain research phenomena and generate hypotheses for research projects, they have gained acceptance in the past decade (Meleis, 2011). Nevertheless, middle-range theories have been critiqued because they basically aim at hypothesis generation, which cannot be applicable to qualitative studies (Im & Meleis, 1999).

Among the middle-range theories, transitions theory could be easily applicable to nursing care for cancer survivors. Since nursing phenomenon related to cancer survivors frequently involve different types of transitions such as situational transitions, health–illness transitions, developmental transitions, or organizational transitions, transitions theory can be easily adopted and used in nursing research, education, and practice. Indeed, oncology nurses frequently find themselves involved in various transitions that cancer patients and their families are experiencing throughout the process of cancer diagnosis, treatment, and survivorship, and attest changes in nursing care needs that such transitions bring about in the lives of cancer patients and their families. Therefore, transitions theory could provide an outstanding theoretical perspective through which cancer survivors' transition experience could be systematically and comprehensively explained and understood.

The most updated version of transitions theory is the middle-range transitions theory (Meleis, Sawyer, Im, Hilfinger Messias, & Schumacher, 2000; Fig. 9.1). The middle-range transitions theory was developed using an integrative approach based on previous theoretical works and five different studies on different types of transitions. This version has been widely used in nursing research, education, and practice, and will benefit oncology nursing care by providing directions for research, education, and practice. This chapter will focus on the most recent middle-range transitions theory and its implications for nursing care with cancer survivors. First, the middle-range transitions theory will be concisely described by reviewing its sources for theorizing, major concepts, and usages in nursing in general. Then, the roles of nurses within the theory are discussed, and the existing research studies on cancer survivors using transitions theory are described. Finally, implications for nursing care with cancer survivors are proposed with two case studies and their related critical questions.

The Middle-Range Transitions Theory

Sources for Theorizing

The sources for theorizing included (a) the findings and experience from research projects, educational programs, and/or clinical practice in hospital and/or community settings; (b) a systematic and integrated literature review; and (c) collaborative efforts among researchers who used the transition theoretical framework in their studies.

Major Concepts

The major concepts of the middle-range transitions theory are (a) types and patterns of transitions; (b) properties of transition experiences; (c) transition conditions; (d) patterns of response; and (e) nursing therapeutics.

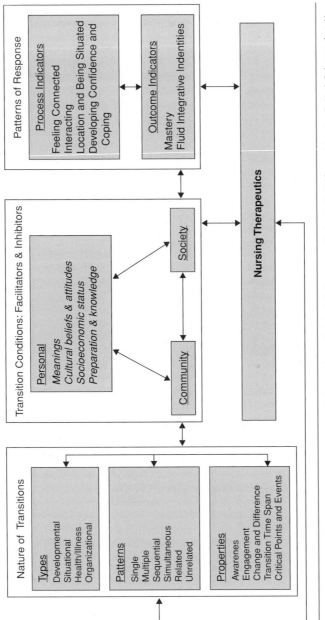

Figure 9.1 • The middle-range transitions theory. (Adapted from Meleis, A. I., Sawyer, L. M., Im, E. O., Hilfinger Messias, D. K., & Schumacher, K. (2000). Experiencing transitions: an emerging middle-range theory. *Advances in Nursing Science. 23*(1), pp. 12–28.)

Types and patterns of transitions. The major concept of *types of transitions* includes several subconcepts. *Developmental transitions* are transitions due to developmental process such as birth, adolescence, menopause, elderly, and death (Im, 2009). *Health and illness transitions* are those due to recovery process, hospital discharge, and diagnosis of chronic illness (Im, 2009). *Organization transitions* are those in institutions/organizations that influence their members' and their clients' lives (Im, 2009). *Patterns of transitions* include two subconcepts of *multiplicity* and *complexity* (Im, 2009). The transitions that people experience are not necessarily single transitions. Rather, they are frequently experiencing *multiple* transitions at the same time. Also, their transitions could be sequential or simultaneous, and some transitions could be overlapped with others. In other words, interrelationships among the transitions could be characterized by *complexity.*

Properties of transition experience. The major concept of *properties of transition experience* includes four subconcepts. These subconcepts are not mutually exclusive, but interrelated as a whole. *Awareness* refers to "perception, knowledge, and recognition of a transition experience" (Im, 2009; p. 420). *Engagement* means the degree to which a person demonstrates involvement in the process inherent in the transition (Im, 2009; p. 420). *Changes* mean "changes in identities, roles, relationships, abilities, and patterns of behavior, and transitional changes are supposed to bring a sense of movement or direction to internal processes as well as external processes" (Im, 2009; p. 421). Confronting *differences* as a property of transitions could be explained by "unmet or divergent expectations, feeling different, being perceived as different, or seeing the world and others in different ways" (Im, 2009; p. 421). Transitions are also characterized as *time spans* "with an identifiable end point, extending from the first signs of anticipation, perception, or demonstration of change; through a period of instability, confusion, and distress; and to an eventual 'ending' with a new beginning or period of stability" (Im, 2009; p. 421). *Critical points and events* mean "identifiable marker events, such as birth, death, the cessation of menstruation, or the diagnosis of an illness" (Im, 2009; p. 421). All these subconcepts of the properties of transitions interrelate each other. For example, the level of awareness could influence the level of engagement; engagement may not begin without awareness. Also, the level of engagement of people in transitions who are aware of changes would be different from that of people who are not aware of the changes.

Transition conditions. Another major concept of the middle-range transitions theory is *transition conditions.* *Transition conditions* refer to "the conditions that influence the way a person moves through a transition and that facilitate or hinder progress toward achieving a healthy transition" (Im, 2009; p. 421). The middle-range transitions theory conceptualized transition conditions as "personal, community, or societal conditions that may facilitate or constrain the processes of healthy transitions and the outcomes of transitions" (Im, 2009; p. 421). *Personal conditions* refer to "meanings, cultural beliefs and attitudes, socioeconomic status, preparation and knowledge" (Im, 2009; p. 421). Personal conditions include the subconcept of *cultural beliefs and attitudes* (e.g., Chinese stigmatization of cancer), *socioeconomic status,* and *anticipatory preparation or lack of preparation* (Im, 2009). *Community conditions* refer to conditions of specific communities (e.g., community resources, community environments, etc.) that facilitate or inhibit transitions. *Societal conditions* refer to conditions of specific society (e.g., sociopolitical issues, societal expectations, etc.) that facilitate or inhibit transitions.

Patterns of response. A major concept of the middle-range transitions theory is *patterns of response*. The concept of patterns of response includes two subconcepts—*process indicators* and *outcome indicators*. *Process indicators* refer to indicators of "moving clients either in the direction of healthy or toward vulnerability and risk that could allow early assessment and interventions by nurse to facilitate healthy outcomes" (Im, 2009; p. 422). The subconcept of process indicators includes "feeling connected, interacting, being situated, and developing confidence and coping" (Im, 2009; p. 422). These indicators could be easily used by nurses working with cancer survivors in determining if the cancer survivors are in healthy transitions or not. For example, feeling and staying connected may indicate a healthy transition. If a cancer survivor makes new contacts related to her/his disease (e.g., healthcare providers, peers, etc.) and continues old connections with her/his family and friends, she/he is usually in a healthy transition. *Outcome indicators* refer to the indicators of "if a transition is a healthy one or not" (Im, 2009; p. 422). The subconcept of outcome indicators includes *mastery* and *fluid integrative identities*. The extent to which people demonstrate mastery of the skills and behaviors required to manage their changes due to transitions may indicate healthy or unhealthy transitions. The extent to which people in transitions develop and reformulate their identity may also indicate if their transitions are healthy or unhealthy.

Nursing therapeutics. The last major concept of the middle-range transitions theory is *nursing therapeutics*. Nursing therapeutics refer to "nursing measures that are widely applicable to therapeutic intervention during transitions" (Im, 2009; p. 422). The concept of nursing therapeutics includes three subconcepts. *Assessment of readiness* refers to "assessment through multidisciplinary endeavor to obtain a comprehensive understanding of the patient that requires assessment of each of the transition conditions in order to create an individual profile of client readiness and to enable clinicians and researchers to identify various patterns of the transition experience" (Im, 2009; p. 422). *Preparation of transition* means "education as the primary modality for creating optimal conditions in preparation for transition" (Im, 2009; p. 422). *Role supplementation* refers to "any deliberative process whereby role insufficiency or potential role insufficiency is identified by role incumbent and significant others, and the conditions and strategies of role clarification and role taking are used to develop a preventive or therapeutic intervention to decrease, ameliorate, or prevent role insufficiency" (Im, 2009; p. 422).

Usages in Nursing in General

Because of its comprehensiveness, applicability, and affinity with health, the middle-range transitions theory has been translated into several different languages and used internationally. Transitions theory has also been used in nursing practice with diverse groups of people including geriatric populations, psychiatric populations, maternal populations, family caregivers, menopausal women, Alzheimer patients, immigrant women, and people with chronic illness. Also, the middle-range transitions theory has been used in graduate and undergraduate education throughout the world. There is a growing international interest on integrating transitions theory into nursing curricular across countries. The middle-range transitions theory was also used as a curriculum framework or for a course development in a number of places including the University of Connecticut and the University of California, San Francisco.

Nurses' Roles within the Theory

The roles of nurses are reflected in the concept of *nursing therapeutics* within transitions theory. The concept of nursing therapeutics is included as a major concept in transitions theory although this concept is the least developed concept within the theory. The subconcepts under the concept of nursing therapeutics (assessment of readiness, preparation of transitions, and role supplementation) specifically provide directions for nurses' roles in oncology care for cancer survivors. For example, by adopting these three subconcepts, oncology nurses could help patients go through specific diagnosis and/or treatment procedures by assessing the patients' readiness for the procedures (assessment of readiness), preparing the patients by providing education on the procedures (preparation of transitions), and providing role models to deal with anxiety related to the procedures (role supplementation). Furthermore, transitions theory can help develop nursing therapeutics that are congruent with the unique transition experience of patients and their families in transitions by providing a comprehensive and systematic understanding of the transitions that patients and their families are going through.

Research on Cancer Survivors Using Transitions Theory

When the PUBMED was searched with keywords of "transitions theory," or "transition theory," and "cancer survivor" for the period from 1966 to 2014, only 10 articles were retrieved. Among them, 8 articles were published during the past 10 years, and only 1 study on cancer survivors actually used transitions theory as the theoretical basis. The study is by Rancour (2008) on the transition process of cancer patients from active treatment to survivorship. Through the study, the transition from active treatment to survivorship was classified into three stages including endings, the neutral zone, and beginnings. Each transition was characterized by its own unique qualities and challenges, and nurses were the ones who could help facilitate the transition through assisting survivors to be aware of emotional experiences from the transition process, to accept the emotions as normal, and to develop compassion for others.

Although the theoretical basis was not transitions theory, the remaining studies that were retrieved through the PUBMED were dealing with transitions that cancer patients go through due to the diagnosis and treatment of cancer. Cancer survivors' transition experience could be easily explained by the middle-range transitions theory. For example, Mollica and Nemeth (2014) conducted a grounded theory study to explore African-American women's experience and coping throughout their transition from being a breast cancer patient to a breast cancer survivor. They found four main themes reflecting the women's transition experience, which included "perseverance through struggles supported by reliance on faith," "persistent physical issues," "anticipatory guidance needed after treatment," and "emotional needs as important as physical needs." They concluded that the transition from cancer patient to survivor was filled with stress, loss of safety net, and significant coping measures, which would require support from peers as they complete treatment. The findings of this study could be easily applied to several major concepts of transitions theory very well. For instance, "anticipatory guidance needed after treatment" could be easily linked to the subconcept of *preparation for transitions* under the major concept of *nursing therapeutics.*

Taylor, Richardson, and Cowley (2011) also conducted a qualitative study to explain the relationship between fears of recurrence and individuals' recovery from curative colorectal cancer surgery. They found that many patients reported anxiety about cancer recurrence despite their successful treatment for early-stage colorectal cancer and this fear made some adopt new health behaviors to pursue a "more dependable and controllable" body. However, they also found that other patients did not perceive the risk of cancer recurrence, could manage any such concerns, and found "a sense of resolution" in their recovery. These findings could be easily linked to the properties of transitions in the middle-range transitions theory. Furthermore, their conclusion on nursing therapeutics (e.g., providing opportunities to openly discuss the possibility of cancer recurrence, assessing individual fears, and offering suggestions on possible coping strategies to lessen the associated distress) could also be easily linked to the concept of nursing therapeutics of the middle-range transitions theory.

Roundtree, Giordano, Price, and Suarez-Almazor's (2011) study could also be easily linked to the middle-range transitions theory. They conducted a qualitative study using focus group discussions to explore breast cancer survivors' perceptions and attitudes about their current healthcare utilization, screening, and information needs. They found that participants' perceptions and attitudes about care were circumscribed in terms of personal experiences, personal attitudes, and social influences. This finding could be linked to the major concepts of Transition conditions within the middle-range transitions theory. Based on the findings, they proposed nursing therapeutics that included providing a cancer treatment summary, switching from provider to provider, and implementing communication changes in healthcare providers' interactions with patients, and enhancing social influences.

Implications for Nursing with Cancer Survivors

Transitions that cancer survivors go through can be influenced by multiple factors as depicted in transitions theory, and transitions theory could provide an excellent perspective to comprehensively understand the multiple influencing factors. Thus, nurses could use this theory in their research and practice to understand the multiple influencing factors that may influence cancer survivors' transition experience, and consider them in program designs and treatment plans for cancer survivors. As discussed above, studies related to the transition from active treatment to cancer survivorship are emerging in the literature. Researchers working with cancer survivors could use the middle-range transitions theory to theoretically guide their studies, and they could use their study findings to further develop and refine the middle-range transitions theory or to develop situation specific theories derived from transitions theory that could be easily adopted to guide nursing research and practice with the specific populations of interests (e.g., breast cancer survivors). As mentioned by Meleis et al. (2000), transitions theory is an emerging framework that could be further developed through future endeavors in nursing research, education, and practice. Thus, oncology nurses could contribute to further development of major concepts and subconcepts of transitions theory, through which they could adequately explain the transition experience that cancer survivors go through. Further development of the theory in actual oncology care practice would certainly strengthen the linkages among theory, practice, and research by providing a strong explanatory power. This chapter concludes with the following case studies and their related critical questions.

CASE STUDY 1: Breast Cancer

Jennifer is a 33-year-old woman working as a fund manager in New York City. She graduated from one of the top universities in the United States and has been successful in her work. Her friends and colleagues describe her as a perfectionist, having few friends and seldom sharing her life story. Jennifer has been living alone in a small apartment since she was diagnosed with breast cancer as she does not want others to know about her health condition. She received a bilateral mastectomy with breast reconstruction and became a breast cancer survivor 3 years ago. She is very careful about following the diet and exercise recommendations for breast cancer survivors. She never misses doctors' appointments and is open to health education; however, she has never attended a meeting for breast cancer survivors (e.g., a breast cancer support group). Jennifer's fiancé recently proposed to her, and she answered "yes". However, she is worried about how her marriage will change her lifestyle and affect her health condition. Also, she is not sure whether she can get pregnant, how her healthcare plan would change in the event of a pregnancy, and whether her health condition might negatively affect her future baby (e.g., genetically). Jennifer has discussed her worries with her fiancé, but she does not have anyone else to talk to or ask about her worries. You are the nurse who is taking care of Jennifer. You find that Jennifer is becoming more anxious and starting to feel that she is not a normal woman.

• Critical Thinking Questions

1. What types and patterns of transition(s) is Jennifer experiencing?
2. What kinds of transition properties can you identify from Jennifer's case?
3. Which personal, community, and societal transition conditions may have influenced Jennifer's experience?
4. What are the process and outcome indicators in Jennifer's case?
5. How could Transition Theory aid in your nursing assessment and care for Jennifer?
6. Please describe your plan of nursing care for Jennifer.

CASE STUDY 2: Colorectal Cancer

Jim is a 50-year-old man working as the CEO of a computer company in California. He has been active and successful in his work. In his free time, he enjoys jogging with his friends and gardening with his wife. Jim's company recently launched a branch company in Boston. Jim is planning to fly to Boston and work for a year at this new company. However, he is worried about how this decision could influence his health condition. He had colorectal cancer when he was 42 and underwent a colectomy and a series of chemotherapy and radiotherapy treatments. He has been a colorectal cancer survivor for over 5 years. He tries not to miss doctors' appointments, manages his colostomy care well, and regularly

participates in an online cancer survivors' community to seek health information. His wife is very supportive and cares about his diet and health condition;
however, she cannot move to Boston with him. You are the nurse who is taking
care of Jim. You find that while Jim is excited about moving to Boston, he is also
worried about the continuity of his care, how stress from this life change could
affect his health condition, and the possibility of cancer recurrence. He often
experiences stomach cramping, fatigue, and sleep difficulties.

• Critical Thinking **Questions**

1. What types and patterns of transition(s) is Jim experiencing?
2. What kinds of transition properties can you identify from Jim's case?
3. Which personal, community, and societal transition conditions may have influenced Jim's experience?
4. What are the process and outcome indicators in Jim's case?
5. How could Transition Theory aid in your nursing assessment and care for Jim?
6. Please describe your plan of nursing care for Jim.

References

de Moor, J. S., Mariotto, A. B., Parry, C., Alfano, C. M., Padgett, L., Kent, E. E., ... Rowland, J. H.
(2013). Cancer survivors in the United States: Prevalence across the survivorship trajectory
and implications for care. *Cancer Epidemiology Biomarkers & Prevention. 22*(4), 561–570.
doi:10.1158/1055–9965.EPI-12–1356

Im, E.O. (2009). Meleis Transition Theory. In M.R. Alligood & A. M. Tomey (Eds.), *Nursing theorists and their work* (7th ed., pp. 416–433). St. Louis, MO: Mosby.

Im, E. O., & Meleis, A. I. (1999). Situation-specific theories: Philosophical roots, properties, and
approach. *Advances in Nursing Science. 22*(2), 11–24.

Meleis, A. I. (2011). *Theoretical nursing: Development and progress* (5th ed.). Philadelphia, PA:
Lippincott Williams & Wilkins.

Meleis, A. I., Sawyer, L. M., Im, E. O., Hilfinger Messias, D. K., & Schumacher, K. (2000).
Experiencing transitions: An emerging middle-range theory. *Advances in Nursing Science.
23*(1), 12–28.

Mollica, M., & Nemeth, L. (2014). Transition from patient to survivor in African American breast
cancer survivors. *Cancer Nursing. 38*, 16–22. doi:10.1097/NCC.0000000000000120

Rancour, P. (2008). Using archetypes and transitions theory to help patients move from active treatment to survivorship. *Clinical Journal of Oncology Nursing. 12*(6), 935–940. doi:10.1188/08.
CJON.935–940

Roundtree, A. K., Giordano, S. H., Price, A., & Suarez-Almazor, M. E. (2011). Problems in transition and quality of care: Perspectives of breast cancer survivors. *Supportive Care in Cancer.
19*(12), 1921–1929. doi:10.1007/s00520–010–1031–6

Taylor, C., Richardson, A., & Cowley, S. (2011). Surviving cancer treatment: An investigation of
the experience of fear about, and monitoring for, recurrence in patients following treatment for
colorectal cancer. *European Journal of Oncology Nursing. 15*(3), 243–249.

CHAPTER 10

ADAPTATION

> "He who loves practice without theory is like a sailor who boards ship without rudder and compass and never knows where he may cast."
>
> *—Leonardo da Vinci*

Key Terms

stress • stressor • adaptation • maladaptation

After reading this chapter, you will be able to do the following:

1. Discuss the philosophical assumptions underlying the Roy Adaptation Model.
2. Discuss the theoretical assumptions underlying the Stuart Adaptation Model of psychiatric nursing care.
3. Describe Selye's stress–adaptation theory.
4. Discuss the implications of stress and adaptation theories and models in psychosocial adjustment related to surviving from cancer.
5. Discuss the effects of stress and cancer diagnosis on individual and family.
6. Discuss stress management and coping strategies.

Introduction

One of the most unpredictable sources of stress that a family can encounter is when a loved one is diagnosed with a catastrophic illness such as cancer. Cancer is the second most common cause of death in the United States and exceeds only by heart disease accounting for nearly one of every four deaths (American Cancer Society, 2013). Sudden onset of cancer and intense stress reaction is considered as an acute stress. Cancer is also a chronic stressor because treatment effects may prolong for years, and the terror sensation of recurrence and death is constantly experienced. The ways an individual and the family communicate and deal with cancer are important indicators of family health and function. Stress includes not only a wide range of environmental events, but also reactions to nerve-wracking life events (Fontaine, 2009; p. 116).

To deepen one's understanding about cancer and its effects on the person's life course, it is crucial to acknowledge person–environment interactions as well as changes in the condition of life processes for the human adaptive system. In this section the major stress and adaptation theories and/or models, and their implications in relation to surviving from cancer are reviewed. For this purpose, stress and adaptation theories and models with emphasis on nursing theories are introduced and the relationships among stress, adaptation, cancer, and family role are explored.

Stress and Adaptation Theories and Models

As indicated in the literature, the traditional view of stress as a merely biological phenomenon is replaced by a biopsychosocial model, that is, stress is a product of a complex interaction of biologic, psychological, and sociocultural factors. Several elements are involved in understanding stress (Kneisl & Trigoboff, 2013). They include personality factors (such as how we handle anger), cognitive factors (such as whether we perceive an event as a threat), physical factors (such as how the body responds to stress), environmental factors (such as flood, fire, or tornado), cultural factors (such as our beliefs about religion, health, and family), and coping strategies (how we handle or manage stress). See Figure 10.1 (Kneisl & Trigoboff, 2013; p. 141).

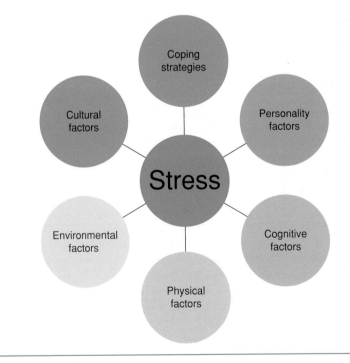

Figure 10.1 • Factors involving stress.

The Roy Adaptation Model: A Nursing Model

Sister Callista Roy, RN, Ph.D., is professor and influential and visionary nurse theorist at the William F. Cornell School of Nursing, Boston College, Massachusetts. Her work, Roy Adaptation Model (RAM) is known worldwide. Her model has had a profound impact on theory, research, and professional practice. She is involved in teaching, innovative and scholarly research, and writing related to the development of nursing knowledge. Her conceptual work embraces philosophical conceptualization of the nature of knowledge as Universal Cosmic Imperative and how this worldview impacts the development of nursing knowledge and nursing practice (Roy & Jones, 2007). In collaboration with colleagues, she established the Boston-Based Adaptation Research in Nursing Society, now called the Roy Adaptation Association. Roy developed measurement of coping (Roy & Chayaput, 2004). To discuss the applications of RAM for constructing nursing theory, Roy and Roberts (1981) wrote *Theory Construction in Nursing: An Adaptation Model* and offered 74 propositions related to the theory. In addition, Roy is the author, coauthor, and contributing author of numerous works, including *Roy Adaptation Model-Based Research: Twenty-Five Years of Contributions of Nursing Science* (Roy & Andrew, 1999) and *Nursing Knowledge Development and Clinical Practice* (Roy & Jones, 2007).

In 1964, Roy introduced the RAM as part of her graduate work and credited the works of von Bertalanffy's (1968) general system theory and Helson's (1964) adaptation that served as a foundation for creating the original basis of her scientific assumptions underpinning the Roy Adaptation Model (RAM). The philosophical assumptions were originated from humanistic perspectives of creativity, holism, purposefulness, and interpersonal process leading to the RAM concept of veritivity, comprising purposefulness of existence, activity and creativity, unity of purpose, and the value and meaning of life (Roy & Andrew, 1999). In 1970, Roy first published her views about adaptation and the RAM was adopted as the conceptual framework of the undergraduate nursing curriculum at Mount Saint Mary's College in Los Angeles (Roy, 1970).

Roy (1976) defined adaptive responses as behavior that sustains the integrity of the individual. Adaptation is regarded as positive and is correlated with a healthy response. When a behavior interrupts the integrity of the person, it is perceived as maladaptive. Adaptation is defined as "the process and outcome whereby thinking and feeling persons, as individuals or in groups, use conscious awareness and choice to create human and environmental integration" (Roy & Andrew, 1999; p. 30). The four major concepts of RAM are "humans as adaptive systems as both individuals and groups; the environment; health; and the goal of nursing" (Roy & Andrew, 1999; p. 35). Roy conceptualizes the human system in a holistic perspective. Holism is the aspect of unified meaningfulness of human behavior in which the human system is greater than the sum of individual parts (Roy & Andrew, 1999; p. 35). It is noteworthy to indicate that any of the individual, groups, organizations, communities, and societies may be viewed as human system and each is considered as a holistic adaptive system. Roy and Jones (2007) have also listed their most recent scientific assumptions related to RAM that include: (1) integration of human and environment meanings results in adaptation; (2) system relationships include acceptance, protection, and fostering of interdependence; (3) thinking and feeling mediate human action; (4) and human decisions are accountable for the integration of creative process.

The Stuart Stress Adaptation Model of Psychiatric Nursing Care

Adaptation/maladaptation continuum is distinct from heath/illness continuum and it comes from nursing worldview. The Stuart Stress Adaptation Model is one of the conceptual nursing models that serve as a framework to describe and address patients, environment and health statuses, and nursing practice (Stuart, 2010). The model consists of theoretical assumptions and focuses on how the individual relates to the whole and its existence must be considered in a social hierarchy from the simplest unit to the most complex (Fig. 10.2; Stuart, 2010; p. 45). The model emphasizes that although each level

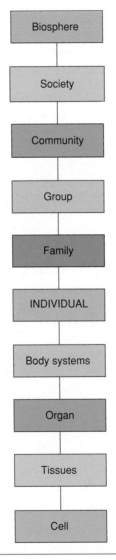

Figure 10.2 • Levels of organization. (Stuart, G. W. (2010). *Principles and Practice of Psychiatric Nursing* (5th ed., p. 45). Oxford: Elsevier.)

of the social hierarchy has a distinct property, it is an integral part of the next higher level. The model assumes that the nursing care is provided within a biological, psychological, sociocultural, environmental, and legal-ethical context. It is crucial that the nurse understands each of them in order to provide holistic nursing care (Stuart, 2010).

Selye's Stress–Adaptation Theory

Selye developed a response-oriented framework for understanding the effects of stress on human body (1956). He believed that any emotion or activity requires a response to change in individual and life itself is stressful because it entails a process of adaptation to constant change. Stressors can be chemical, physical, developmental, physiological, or emotional (Selye, 1956). Selye argued that stress can be objectively measured by the structural and chemical changes that it produces in the body and these changes are called general adaptation syndrome (GAS). In Selye's theory stress affects the whole person and the whole person must adjust to the changes. It is noteworthy that response-based models such as Selye's are criticized for the current view that each individual is unique and people respond differently in similar situations. Since the publication of Selye's novel research, it is evident that "fight or flight" syndrome of symptoms happens in response to physical stimuli as well as psychological or emotional stimuli.

Implications of Stress and Adaptation Theories

It is essential to study the human adaptation to major life events, and more specifically major threats to human health stress and gain better understanding about the processes related to surviving from cancer. In a number of theories the focus is on adaptive/coping/defensive responses and some discuss the nature of central concepts or components related to stress and adaptation theories. One of these components is the appraisal of stress and/or the experience of distress that stimulates adaptive, coping, or defensive responses. Coping patterns directly influence the appraisal process and lead to the development of certain adaptive/defensive patterns, such as sensitizing the person to the disvalued life circumstances (Kaplan, 1996). Effects of unsuccessful coping include hopelessness, fatigue, and passivity that would interfere with health maintenance. A number of factors contribute to dysfunctional coping responses, including past experience of the usefulness of coping responses, and the experience of distress. When people are diagnosed with a chronic disease, they adjust to their new reality and the stress process is interpreted based on social identity and self-evaluation (Kaplan, 1996).

To mitigate distress and help the patient to adjust to his or her new reality, it is asserted that nurses understand what the patients with cancer are going through. Philosophically, "nurses should see persons as coexistence with their physical and social environments" (Roy, 1997; p. 42). The theoretical basis for mental health nursing practice is originated from nursing science as well as from biological, social, and behavioral sciences (Stuart, 2010) and nurses need to know that no one theory is applicable to all patients.

Stress and Cancer: The Effects on Individual and Family

A cancer diagnosis imposes a number of stressors and has many unfavorable effects on patients, partners, family members, and friends. One of the greatest stressors in patient's experience is the initial cancer diagnosis that results in shock, surprise, fear, and—for some—hope (Weber & Solomon, 2010). Cancer diagnosis means death for some. Metastatic cancer diagnosis leads to a traumatic stressor that involves continuous, imminent life threat which affects patient's life expectancy and subsequent physical and emotional symptoms such as traumatic stress symptoms, depression, and anxiety (Badr, Carmack., Kashy, Cristofinili, & Revenson, 2010). Other problems include posttraumatic stress disorder (re-experiencing the events and symptoms through intrusive thoughts and nightmares), sleep disturbances, irritability, and avoidance related to the topic (Brown et al., 2007).

When cancer treatment has begun, patients encounter additional stressors, including bodily changes related to treatment, career and financial difficulties, changes in their intimate relationship and social network, and dealing with adverse effects of treatment modalities. Stress resumes during the posttreatment period due to fear of recurrence, physical and mental limitations, and diagnostic-related problems with family and others. If the patient's diagnosis is metastatic cancer, his/her partner may encounter imminent loss of the loved one and should prepare for the end-of life discussion (Badr et al., 2010).

Stress, Coping, Resources, and Family Role

The environmental influence on the developmental process varies among individuals with regard to size and type of consequence. Of particular interest in this relation is the occurrence of single events that may have profound impact on the life course of a person. A stressor event could produce positive or negative stress in the family system, and the effects of the stressor event could be short and/or long term.

In considering the relationship between life circumstances and the experience of distress, there are subjective constructs such as evaluation of threat and adaptive/coping/defensive responses, and resources (Kaplan, 1996). Individuals differ in their reaction to life events because the individual's perception of the event or threat varies due to the degree to which the change is perceived stressful. Kaplan (1996) stated that "coping patterns directly influence the experience of stress by managing emotional responses to the appraisal of stress, and indirectly influence the experience of stress by changing life circumstances that are appraised as stressful" (p. 9). Positive coping mechanisms and strong familial and social support can reduce the intensity of the stressful life change and foster a more adaptive response. Patterson and Garwick (1994) recommend that families try to make meaning of stressful or crisis situations that "reduce guilt and blame and include shared responsibility for managing the condition" (p. 300) to increase a family's chance of adapting successfully to a family crisis.

Families have a number of coping resources to help them through cancer journey. Social support and family communications are two particular coping resources that would help family cope with cancer. The number one source of support is usually the partner. Kayser, Watson, and Andrade (2007) have indicated that couples can communicate the process of reciprocal coping with cancer through awareness (what is happening in their relationship in the illness situation), authenticity (sharing genuine feeling with their partners), and mutuality (connecting in a way that permits each partner to take part in the shared journey). In a research study of a breast cancer survivor, Weber and Solomon (2010) revealed that participants appraised their dialogues with their partners about identity and intrapersonal concerns as helpful and supportive during the coping process. The importance of contact with others for physical health has been underscored in the increasing number of reports from research on social network (Willis, 1984; Wortman & Dunkel-Schetter, 1987).

Conceivably it should be recognized that people differ in the demands made on them, and in the resources available to them. They differ further in their capacity to achieve certain kinds of valued or disvalued outcomes. From family systems perspective, it may be more helpful to make acknowledgments that refrain from blaming a specific family member for stress in the family but instead permit the family to accept responsibility for the situation and take action (Maguire, 2012).

Research on Psychological Treatments for Cancer-Related Distress

One of the largest samples utilized a database of over 4,000 cancer patients who had completed the Brief Symptom Inventory as part of their comprehensive cancer care and found an overall prevalence rate for distress of 35% (Zabora, Brintzenhofeszoc., Curbow, Hooker, & Piantadosi, 2001). Moorey (2013) stated that researchers explored the effects of cancer treatment such as colostomy or mastectomy on psychological adjustment. They uncovered that up to a quarter of women remained depressed 1 year after mastectomy (Morris, Greer, & White, 1977; Maguire et al., 1978) and that 25% to 50% postcolostomy experienced psychological distress (Devlin, Plant, & Griffin, 1971; Eardley et al., 1976).

A range of pharmacological and psychological interventions for alleviating psychological distress has been established. The effectiveness of psychological treatments including cognitive behavior therapy, both as individual sessions and in groups, has been shown to be helpful for people with cancer (Moorey, 2013). Interestingly, researchers have found complex links between the body and the mind, and mind–body therapy is used as a means of cost-effective self-care and an adjunct to medical care to promote emotional wellness. "The goal of mind–body techniques is to regulate the stress–response system so that balance and equilibrium can be maintained and sustained, to restore prefrontal cortex activity, to decrease amygdala activity, and to restore the normal activity of the HPA axis and locus coeruleus-sympathetic nervous system (Selhub, 2007; p. 5). Healthcare professionals including counselors and nurses should embrace preventive approach to help individuals achieve mental, physical, and emotional wellness and improve the quality of life in proactive and positive ways. It is noteworthy that psychoeducational groups that include programs such as relaxation, stress management, cognitive restructuring, and problem solving have shown positive therapeutic outcomes (Moorey & Greer, 2012).

A meta-analysis result indicated that preintervention significantly moderated effects with most distressed participants showing better adjustment (Schneider et al., 2010). Groarke, Curtis, and Kerin's (2013) findings demonstrated reduction in global stress, and enhancement benefit finding with breast cancer participating in a shorter cognitive-behavioral stress management (CBSM) intervention. A substantial body of research has investigated the association between stress-related psychosocial factors and cancer outcomes. Chida, Hamer, Steptoe, and Wardle (2008) evaluated longitudinal associations between stress and cancer using meta-analytic methods. Their analyses suggest that stress-related psychosocial factors have adverse effects on cancer incidence and survival, although there is evidence of publication bias and results should be interpreted with caution.

Psychological Treatments: Stress Management and Coping Strategies

Stress management involves use of adaptive coping strategies in response to stressful situations. Coping mechanisms or strategies are attempts directed to managing stress. Coping strategies are the behaviors one uses to manage one's stress and protect oneself from psychological harm. Three general coping strategies have been identified: problem-focused coping; cognitively focused coping; and emotion-focused coping (Kaplan, 1996; Stuart, 2010). Problem-focused coping mechanisms are attempts to do something actively to alleviate stressful situations. Cognitively focused strategies are efforts to control the meaning of the problem and counteract it. Emotion-focused coping involves attempts to regulate or moderate the emotional distress and consequences (Stuart, 2010). Adaptive coping strategies include awareness, relaxation, meditation, interpersonal communication with caring people, problem solving, pet therapy, and music therapy (Townsend, 2009).

Summary

The diagnosis and treatment of cancer are sources of noticeable psychological stress for patients and their families. The positive and negative effects of stress on biopsychological development are highlighted in the literature. Stress may reduce/deplete a person's physiologic, social, and economic capacity and increase vulnerability to illness or injury (Stuart, 2010). In this section you read about stress and adaptation theories and/or conceptual models with the emphasis on nursing theories. In general, all of the theoretical frameworks draw analytical distinction between similar components: life circumstances, that is, the subjective evaluation of life circumstances; adaptive/coping/defensive responses; and consequences of outcomes. You were also introduced to adaptive/coping/defensive strategies or mechanisms; the ways families might make sense of stressful situations or life-threatening events; the importance of coping resources and stress management strategies; and family functioning during the coping process.

CASE STUDY

Mrs. K is a 35-year-old single mother with two school-age children. Mrs. K suffered from facial burn as a result of fire in her kitchen several months ago. The injuries have healed without complications, but she has moderate residual scarring. Ms. K. tries to avoid social occasions or gatherings, and wears dark glasses and big hats.

• Critical Thinking Questions

The nurse decides to use Roy's adaptation model in the nursing care of Mrs. K. Please respond to the following questions using the Roy's adaptation model.
1. How does the nurse begin to assess Mrs. K?
2. Which nursing diagnosis(es) should the nurse identify in relation to adaptation?
3. What would be the goal for each nursing diagnosis?

• Critical Thinking **Exercise**

1. Develop a plan for the identified problem/nursing diagnosis using Roy's theory as the basis for practice, while considering at least one of the four major concepts/adaptive modes.

References

American Cancer Society. (2013). *Cancer facts and figures for 2014.* Surveillance Research, Cancer Facts Statistics. Retrieved on August 10, 2014 from http://www.cancer.org/acs/groups/content/@research/documents/webcontent/acspc-042151.pdf

Badr, H., Carmack, C. L., Kashy, D. A., Cristofinili, M., & Revenson, T. A. (2010). Dyadic coping in metastatic breast cancer. *Health Psychology. 29*, 169–180.

Brown, R. T., Fummeler, B., Anderson, D., Jamieson, S., Simonian, S., Hall, R. K., & Brescia, F. (2007). Adjustment of children and their mothers with breast cancer. *Journal of Pediatric Psychology.* 32, 297–308.

Chida, Y., Hamer, M., Steptoe, A., & Wardle, J. (2008). Do stress-related psychosocial factors contribute to cancer incidence and survival? *Nature Clinical Practice Oncology.* 5(8), 466–475.

Devlin, H. B., Plant, J. A., & Griffin, M. (1971). Aftermath of surgery for ano-rectal cancer. *British Medical Journal. 3*, 413–418.

Eardley, A., George, W. D., Davis, F., Schofield, P. F., Wilson, M. C., Wakefield, J., & Sellwood, R. A. (1976). Colostomy: The consequences of surgery. *Clinical Oncology. 22*, 277–283.

Fontaine, K. L. (2009). *Mental health nursing.* New Jersey: Pearson.

Groarke, A., Curtis, R., & Kerin, M. (2013). Cognitive-behavioral stress management enhances adjustment in women with breast cancer. *British Journal of Health Psychology. 18*, 623–641.

Helson, H. (1964). *Adaptation level theory.* New York, NY: Harper & Row.

Kaplan, H. B. (1996). *Psychosocial stress: Perspectives on structure, theory, life-course, and methods.* New York, NY: Academic Press.

Kayser, K., Watson, L. E., & Andrade, J. T. (2007). Cancer as a "we-disease": Examining the process of coping from a relational perspective. *Family Systems & Health.* 25, 404–418.

Kneisl, C. R., & Trigoboff, E. (2013). *Contemporary psychiatric-mental health nursing.* New York, NY: Pearson.

Maguire, K. C. (2012). *Stress and coping in families.* UK: Polity Press.

Maguire, G.P., Lee, E. G., Bevington, D. J., Küchemann, C. S., Crabtree, R. J., & Cornell, C. E. (1978). Psychiatric problems in the first year after mastectomy. *British Medical Journal.* 1, 963–965.

Moorey, S. (2013). 'I know they are distressed. What do I do now?'. *Psycho-Oncology. 22*, 1946–1952.

Moorey, S., & Greer, S. (2012). *The Oxford guide to CBT for people with cancer.* Oxford: Oxford University Press.

Morris, T., Greer, H. S., & White, P. (1977). Psychological and social adjustment to mastectomy: A two-year follow-up study. *Cancer. 77*, 2381–2387.

Patterson, J. M., & Garwick, A. W. (1994). Levels of meaning in family stress theory. *Family process. 33*, 287–304.

Roy, C. (1970). Adaptation: A conceptual framework for nursing. *Nursing Outlook. 18*, 43–45.

Roy, C. (1976). *Introduction to nursing: An adaptation model.* New Jersey: Prentice Hall.

Roy, C. (1997). Future of the Roy Model: Challenge to redefine adaptation. *Nursing Science Quarterly. 10*, 42–48.

Roy, C., & Andrew, H. (1999). *The Roy adaptation model* (2nd ed.). Stamford, CT: Appleton & Lange.

Roy, C., & Chayaput, P. (2004). Coping and adaptation processing scale—English and that versions. *RAA Review Newsletter. 6*(2), 4–6.

Roy, C., & Jones, D. A. (2007). *Nursing knowledge development and clinical practice.* New York, NY: Springer.

Roy, C., & Roberts, S. (1981). *Theory construction in nursing: An adaptation model.* Upper Saddle River, NJ: Prentice Hall.

Schneider, S., Moyer, A., Knapp-Oliver, S., Sohl, S., Cannella, D., & Targhetta, V. (2010). Pre-intervention distress moderates the efficacy of psychosocial treatment for cancer patients: A meta-analysis. *Journal of Behavioral Medicine. 33,* 1–14.

Selhub, C. (2007). Mind-body medicine for treating depression. *Alternative & Complementary Therapies. 2,* 4–9. doi: 10.1089/act2007.13107

Selye, H. (1956). *The stress of life.* New York, NY: McGraw-Hill.

Stuart, G. W. (2010). Stress and Adaptation. In *Principles and practice of psychiatric nursing* (5th ed.). Oxford: Elsevier.

Townsend, M. C. (2009). *Psychiatric Mental Health Nursing.* Philadelphia, PA: F.A.Davis Company.

von Bertalanffy, L. (1968). *General system theory.* New York, NY: Braziller.

Weber, K. M., & Solomon, D. H. (2010). Understanding challenges associated with breast cancer: A cluster analysis of intrapersonal and interpersonal stressors. In M. Miller-Day (Eds.), *Going through this together: Family communication, connection, and health transitions* (pp. 77–100). New York, NY: Peter Lang.

Willis, T. A. (1984). Supportive function of interpersonal relationships. In S. Cohen & L. Syme (Eds.). *Social support and health* (pp. 61–82). New York, NY: Academic Press.

Wortman, C. B., & Dunkel-Schetter, C. (1987). Conceptual and methodological issues in study of social support. In A. Baum & J. E. Singer (Eds.), *Handbook of psychology and health* (Vol. 5, pp. 33–67). New Jersey: Erlbaum.

Zabora, J., Brintzenhofeszoc, K., Curbow, B., Hooker, C., & Piantadosi, S. (2001). The prevalence of psychological distress by cancer site. *Psycho-Oncology. 10,* 19–28.

RESILIENCE

Upon completing this chapter, you will be able to do the following:

1. Define resilience.
2. Discuss the history of the theory of resilience.
3. Describe ways in which nurses can promote resilience.

When confronted with a diagnosis such as cancer, many patients display a fighting spirit, a willingness to persevere, and a belief that the cancer can be "beaten." What makes these individuals approach their illness in this manner while other people do not? The concept of resilience assists in explaining the ability to bounce back and deal with an adversity, the proverbial "pull oneself up by one's bootstraps."

What is resilience? Resilience is defined as the ability to become strong, healthy, or successful again after something bad happens. In her discussion of the middle-range theory of resilience, Haase (2009) defined resilience as "positive adjustment in the face of adversity" as well as "the process of identifying or developing resources and strengths to gain a positive outcome, a sense of confidence/mastery, self-transcendence, and self-esteem" (p. 326). However, within the nursing literature, a consistent definition of resilience remains elusive (Haase, 2009).

History of the Theory of Resilience

The concept has predominantly been studied by psychologists and psychiatrists (Earvolino-Ramirez, 2007). The earliest studies of resilience examined children considered to be at risk due to their mothers' diagnosis of schizophrenia (Garmezy, 1974). The major finding from these early studies was that the children continued to grow and develop despite their parents' mental illness. This finding was consistent with observations by child development theorists that some children did well in spite of some of the most negative of circumstances. Other studies have focused on trying to understand the individual differences and factors in response to adversity. Rutter (1979) researched socioeconomic adversity and found that attitudes and educational practices could develop resiliency and healthy development for youths at risk. Wells and Schwebel (1987) researched resilience among chronically ill children who were no more likely to have psychological issues than normally developing children given the same degree of stress and family dysfunction.

Nursing began exploring the concept of resilience only as far back as the 1980s, so nursing research on resilience is still in its infancy. Early nursing studies included examining resilience in children with cancer (Hockenberry-Eaton, Kemp, & Dilorio, 1994), homeless adolescents (Hunter, 2001), families with an ill child (McCubbin & McCubbin, 1993), school-aged children with asthma (Vinson, 2002), and older adults (Wagnild & Young, 1990). A sample of recent studies included examining resilience in children with cancer (Rishel, 2013), parents of children with cancer (Jones, 2012), older adults with cancer (Hughes, Closs, & Clark, 2009), and nurses themselves (Sherman, Edwards, Simonton, & Mehta, 2006). Several studies by Earvolino-Ramirez (2007) and Gillespie, Chaboyer, and Wallis (2007) began analyzing the concept of resilience and documenting their conclusions in journal articles. A concept analysis assists in developing the nurse's understanding of the concept and summarizes what is known about the phenomenon in the literature. Surprisingly, a review of the CINAHL database, a database containing many nursing journals and other nursing related resources, revealed only 32 studies on resilience from 2006 to 2013 when the search words "resilience, cancer, and nursing" were entered in the search box. Ten of these were published in foreign language journals and 12 focused on children with cancer. A second search of the Nursing and Allied Health database using the same search words revealed only four studies from 2009 to 2013 which included one on childhood cancer, one on nurses, and one on end-of-life. This is an area in need of future research since examining other populations with cancer may be beneficial in understanding the relationship between resilience and a life-threatening illness with consideration of gender, age, and different cultures.

Description of the Theory of Resilience

Resilience is a complex concept, partially due to the psychological realm for which it belongs. Due to the complexity of the concept, as with the definition, there continues to be a lack of agreement in the nursing literature (as in other disciplines) on exactly what the antecedents, characteristics, and to some degree, what outcomes are anticipated. In terms of this chapter, a general presentation of the concept will be presented. The reader is referred to Petersen and Bredow's *Middle Range Theories: Application to Nursing Research*, 2nd edition (2009) for a more complete explanation of the theory of resilience.

Critical Attributes of Individuals Demonstrating Resilience

Critical attributes or characteristics of individuals who demonstrate resilience have included the ability to rebound and carry on, a sense of self, determination, and the ability to interact with those around in order to elicit social support (Dyer & McGuinness, 1996). Other attributes reported in the literature include confidence, self-esteem, and self-transcendence (Haase, Heiney, Ruccione, & Stutzer, 1999), having a sense of hope (Gillespie et al., 2007), being flexible, and having a sense of humor (Earvolino-Ramirez, 2007).

Antecedents to Resilience

Another name for antecedents is experiences or precursors. Antecedents are events that must be present for the concept to occur. Adversity (Kadner, 1989), interpretation of an event as traumatic, the ability to recognize that adversity or a traumatic event has occurred, and having a "realistic worldview" (Gillespie et al., 2007; p. 127) as well as having a least one caring person in the individual's life (Dyer & McGuinness, 1996) have also been reported.

Outcomes or Consequences of Resilience

Having resilience, being able to bounce back from adversity results in being able to cope or adapt to an issue or in simpler terms, being able "to roll with the punches." Other outcomes include integration, control, adjustment, and growth. Individuals possessing resilience may view cancer as an opportunity to look at life differently:

> "My cancer scare changed my life. I'm grateful for every new healthy day I have. It has helped me prioritize my life."
>
> *—Olivia Newton-John*

Implications for Nursing

The important question for nurses is how to promote resilience for survivors of cancer. Six characteristics of individuals who display resilience have been identified and they include rebounding/reintegration high expectancy/self-determination, positive relationships/social support, flexibility, a sense of humor, and self-esteem/self-efficacy (Earvolino-Ramirez, 2007). Other characteristics of resilience include pre-existing social support, family support, intelligence, education level, communication and reading skills, and ability to self-regulate emotions and behaviors. An early study of resilience in children identified poverty, parental psychopathology, parental criminality, family conflicts or violence, family disruptions such as divorce or abandonment of child, large family size of more than four children, or living in a high crime area as risk factors for failure to develop resilience (Werner & Smith, 1982).

A review of the literature of studies from 1993 to 2012 (Molina et al., 2014) concluded that identification of baseline characteristics and recognition coping mechanisms would assist nurses in encouraging "positive psychosocial outcomes among patients and survivors" (p. 99). In order to promote positive psychosocial outcomes, a thorough psychosocial assessment would be beneficial. The assessment should include available social support, family relationships, and the patient's past experience(s) with adversity in order to develop a holistic plan of care.

Recently, a study examined the role of the autonomic nervous system and hypothalamic—pituitary–adrenal axis in resilience and survivorship (Edward, 2013). Advances in science such as the functional MRI (magnetic imaging) may one day demonstrate how resilience develops in an individual (Edward, 2013) and may assist in developing a valid and reliable tool to measure resilience across the life span.

The nurse should assess for these protective or risk factors on initial contact to assist in developing a plan of care with appropriate patient-centered interventions. Individuals diagnosed with cancer as children who display resilience have frequently reported that they found at least one adult they were able to view as support to them during their cancer experience. These characteristics and risk factors would be referred to as "baseline traits" (Molina et al., 2014).

Possessing resilience has been looked at as a "mechanism" of positive adjustments that changes over time and protects against psychological distress (Mancini & Bonanno, 2009). Coping strategies developed during and after diagnosis would be a "mechanism." All patients would benefit from nurses who engage in therapeutic communication, who offer themselves as professional support, and who include the psychosocial dimension in the plans of care. Examples of nursing interventions that may assist the patient are stress management, coping skills, mindfulness, and goal setting.

Summary

Resilience is a complex, multidimensional concept that is important to consider when caring for patients with cancer. Despite the lack of agreement concerning the definition of resilience as well as antecedents and identifiable characteristics, nurses will benefit from having a general understanding of what resilience is. Consider that not all patients demonstrate resilience outwardly but may still possess resilience. A patient who possesses resilience may be unable or unwilling to verbalize feelings that reflect the presence of resilience.

Since most of the research on resilience has been in children, additional research examining resilience in adults and older adults would increase nursing's knowledge about the concept. Do individuals retain resilience with age? Do other factors affect the ability to remain resilient? Do individuals learn to become resilient with age? Is resilience only innate or can it be learned from watching others, for example, parents. These are just some of the questions that additional research might be able to answer and clarify.

CASE STUDY

F.M., a 45-year-old female, is diagnosed with Stage II breast cancer. She is an executive in a large investment firm and she plans on working through her treatments. She lives with her husband and two teenage sons who have all been supportive. Her three siblings have offered to help her with anything that she needs. The patient has scheduled her chemotherapy and radiation treatments around her work schedule but she is concerned about how the change in appearance will be perceived by her coworkers and clients. In conversations with the oncology nurse, she has voiced her concern about dying but feels she "can beat this thing if I continue to do what I do and maintain a positive outlook. I am a strong woman and I have dealt with adversity before."

• Critical Thinking **Questions**

1. What critical attributes related to resilience are noted in F.M.?
2. What antecedents of resilience are identifiable in this scenario?
3. How can the nurse promote resilience in the patient described in the scenario?
Please see **Appendix: Nursing Diagnosis** at the end of the book.

References

Dyer, J. G., & McGuinness, T. M. (1996). Resilience: Analysis of the concept. *Archives of Psychiatric Nursing. 10*(5), 276–282.

Earvolino-Ramirez, M. (2007). Resilience: A concept analysis. *Nursing Forum. 42*(2), 73–82.

Edward K. (2013). Chronic illness and well being: Using nursing practice to foster resilience as resistance. *British Journal of Nursing. 22*(13), 741–746.

Garmezy, N. (1974). The study of competence in children at risk for severe psychopathology. In C. Koupernik (Ed.): *The child in his family: Children at psychiatric risk* (pp. 77–97). New York, NY: Wiley.

Gillespie, B., Chaboyer, W., & Wallis, M. (2007). Development of a theoretically derived model of resilience through concept analysis. *Contemporary Nurse. 25*(1–2), 124–135.

Haase, J. E. (2009). Resilience. In S. J. Petersen, & T. S. Bredow (Eds.), *Middle range theories: Application to nursing research* (pp. 326–362). Philadelphia, PA: Wolters Kluwer.

Haase, J. E., Heiney, S. P., Ruccione, K. S., & Stutzer, C. (1999). Research triangulation to derive meaning-based quality-of-life theory: Adolescent resilience model and instrument development. *International Journal of Cancer Supplement. 12*, 125–131.

Hockenberry-Eaton, M., Kemp, V., & Dilorio, C. (1994). Cancer stressors and protective factors: Predictors of stress experienced during treatment for chidhood cancer. *Research in Nursing & Health. 17*(5), 351–361.

Hughes, N., Closs, S., & Clark, D. (2009). Experiencing cancer in old age: A qualitative systematic review. *Qualitative Health Research. 19*(8), 1139–1153.

Hunter, A. J. (2001). A cross-cultural comparison of resilience in adolescents. *Journal of Pediatric Nursing. 16*(3), 172–179.

Jones, B. L. (2012). The challenge of quality care for family caregivers in pediatric cancer care. *Seminars in Oncology Nursing. 28*(4), 213–220.

Kadner, K. D. (1989). Resilience: Responding to adversity. *Journal of Psychosocial Nursing & Mental Health Services. 27*(7), 20–25.

Mancini A. D., & Bonanno, G. A. (2009). Predictors and parameters of resilience to loss: Toward an individual differences model. *Journal of Personality. 77*(6), 1805–1832.

McCubbin, M., & McCubbin, H. (1993). Family coping with health crisis: The resiliency model for family stress, adjustment and adaptation. In P. Winstead-Fry (Ed.), *Families, health, and illness* (pp. 3–63). St. Louis, MO: Mosby.

Molina, Y., Yi, J. C., Martinez-Gutierrez, J., Reding, K. W., Yi-Frazier, J., & Rosenberg, A. R. (2014). Resilience among patients across the cancer continuum: Diverse perspectives. *Clinical Journal of Oncology Nursing. 18*(1), 93–101.

Rishel, C. J. (2013). Tough courage: Oncology Nursing Forum addresses childhood cancer then and now. *Oncology Nursing Forum. 40*(4), 308–310.

Rutter, M. (1987). Psychosocial resilience and protective mechanisms. *American Journal of Orthopsychiatry. 57*(3), 316–331.

Sherman, A., Edwards, D., Simonton, S., & Mehta, P. (2006). Caregiver stress and burnout in an oncology unit. *Palliative & Supportive Care. 4*(1), 65–80.

Vinson, J. A. (2002). Children with asthma: Initial development of the child resilience model. *Pediatric Nurse. 23*(5), 149–158.

Wagnild, G., & Young, H. M. (1990). Resilience among older adults. *Journal of Nursing Scholarship. 22*(4), 252–255.

Wells, R., & Schwebel, A. (1987). Chronically ill children and their mothers: Predictors of resilience and vulnerability to hospitalization and surgical stress. *Developmental & Behavioral Pediatrics. 2*(2), 83–89.

Werner, E. & Smith, R. (1982) *Vulnerable but invincible: A longitudal study of resilient children and youth.* New York, NY: McGraw-Hill.

SECTION VI

UNDERSTANDING THE NURSE'S ROLE IN CANCER SURVIVORSHIP

CHAPTER **12**

ONCOLOGY CLINICAL NURSE SPECIALISTS

"It takes a leader with vision to see the future leader within the person."

—*John C. Maxwell*

Key Terms

survivorship • oncology practice settings • oncology clinical nurse specialist

Upon completing this chapter, you will be able to do the following:

1. Describe how the oncology clinical nurse specialists play an integral role in the healthcare team.
2. Describe what the role of oncology clinical nurse specialists are in cancer survivorship.
3. Describe the interventions that oncology clinical nurse specialists carry out in order to assist patients.

Oncology Practice Settings

Nurses across all practice settings foster patient discovery. There are countless scenarios depicting the role of nurses as they walk alongside their patients and families during illness. Nurses learn from their patients that their needs are in a constant state of change and they play a vital role in the cancer care continuum addressing what is important to patients and their families at any given point in the disease trajectory. The Cancer Control Care Continuum (Grant & Economou, 2010) encompasses care from health maintenance and prevention, screening, patient counseling upon diagnosis, treatment settings (surgical oncology, radiation therapy, and infusion centers for chemotherapy), and survivorship issues including surveillance, management of late effects, rehabilitation, coping, and health promotion after cancer treatment through end-of-life care.

Practice settings include ambulatory outpatient services, inpatient care, and specialized end-of-life care consequently; oncology care takes place in primary, acute or secondary, and tertiary care settings. Nursing roles in these various practice settings are as diverse and unique as cancer itself and the individualized needs of oncology patients. Therefore, care of oncology patients extends beyond comprehensive cancer centers or community hospitals. Recalling the cancer care continuum, practice settings may initiate as preventive health in the primary care environment, screening and diagnosis in the acute care setting, while some cancer treatments may be seen in a tertiary or hospital setting.

Often patients experience care across numerous settings within an oncology program. Each transition across care settings offers a distinct patient care focus offering opportunities for nurses to provide education, support, and/or treatment pertaining to the patients' and their families' needs at that moment in time. For example, oncology outpatient services ensure ongoing patient assessment, communication, and modification of the patient's treatment plan based on how the patient is responding to current treatment. The primary goals of outpatient services are to ensure patients understand who the members of the oncology team are, and how they are involved in their care, mutually agreed upon treatment options, and a realistic understanding of the goals of therapy: cancer cure, control, or palliative (American Cancer Society, 2013). Outpatient services work with patients to promote compliance with the recommended treatment plan, addressing concerns or questions, and responding to any physical, psychological, or spiritual changes throughout visit encounters. Additional outpatient services include physician office visits, community health centers, mobile clinics, infusion centers, radiation therapy, pain management clinics, and psychosocial, spiritual, and nutritional support services.

Another practice setting includes inpatient services. When patients require a higher level of care as a result of disease progression or symptom management, patients will be referred to inpatient care by their oncologist, or if the patient arrives in the emergency department, the admitting physician may determine inpatient level of care. Nursing care essentially maintains the same focus as outpatient services: accurate patient assessment, effective communication with the patient and healthcare providers, education, treatment, and support. However, inpatient care focuses on an acute problem or multiple complications of cancer and adverse effects of cancer therapy as well as comprehensive supportive care. Inpatient care addresses multifocal complications such as infection/sepsis; oncological emergencies; life-threatening electrolyte imbalances; alterations in hemodynamics, pain, and organ toxicity; and/or failure. Supportive care addresses physical well-being; psychosocial, spiritual, and nutritional support; and pain management. The oncologist will determine the appropriateness of resuming treatment during periods of hospitalization, or if the treatment plan needs to be modified or delayed. Patients may require surgical intervention to correct an acute problem during their inpatient hospitalization such as creation of an ostomy, or supportive surgery for port placement or PEG feeding tube. Nurses, in collaboration with the oncology team, keep the patient and family informed of any changes, provide explanations of the plan of care, and continuously advocate for patient care needs.

To ensure quality care across the cancer continuum, patients with advanced cancer may require end-of-life care. When treatment options have been exhausted and patients succumb to irreversible disease progression or organ failure, palliative or hospice care would be the essential specialized care provided to manage the multitude of distressing symptoms. Inpatients as well as outpatients may be referred to a palliative or hospice program. Some programs are within the hospital setting, others may require a transfer to a tertiary facility specializing in palliative or hospice care. Patients and families may request home hospice services. Nurses play a pivot role in advocating for patients' wishes during end-of-life care, in addition to referring support services to assist families with decision making during this difficult time.

Survivorship Planning

Program Development

"A pessimist sees the difficulty in every opportunity, an optimist sees the opportunity in every difficulty."

—Winston Churchill

There is no doubt cancer survivors often face lifelong challenges. Each cancer patients' experience is unique as one's fingerprints. We remember each of our patients fondly leaving footprints in our hearts as we had the privilege of sharing the joys of remission and the sorrows of disease progression. Oncology nurses endearingly wished patients well as they transitioned away from the clinical setting. Each past patient experience offers learning opportunities for nurses to grow both personally and professionally, ultimately making nurses better care providers for future patients. The relationships and connections shared with past patients become lost, often leaving nurses feeling empty and contemplating if they have survived years later. Fortunately, research has identified patient transitions as "gaps" in care. This research was published by the Institute of Medicine (IOM) in 2005, "From Cancer Patient to Cancer Survivor: Lost in Transition" (Hewitt, Greenfield, & Stovall, 2005). This report finally put a long overdue voice to the growing needs of cancer survivors. Implications for driving healthcare costs astronomically as a direct result of poorly managed long-term effects of cancer as well as negative overall survival outcomes resulting from noncompliance with comorbid management and/or screening for secondary cancers or cancer recurrence. Healthcare systems finally understood the disturbing realization that cancer patients do not return to the person they were before the cancer diagnosis, but evolve into a survivor with specific healthcare needs that cannot be ignored.

The American College of Surgeons Commission on Cancer, a professional organization dedicated to improving survival and quality of life for cancer patients (American College of Surgeons Commission on Cancer, 2012), announced a new cancer program standard (Standard 3.3 Survivorship Care Plan) specifying that a survivorship program must be in effect by 2015. The requirement finally answers the needs of cancer patients while striving for quality patient-centered cancer care. Approaching a decade after the publication of the IOM report, what have we done to improve care? A national call to action campaign commenced among oncology professional organizations. Organizations including but not limited to the American Society of Clinical Oncology (2014), National Comprehensive Cancer Network (Denlinger et al, 2014), National Cancer Institute (2012), Oncology Nursing Society (2008), American Cancer Society (2013), National Coalition of Oncology Nurse Navigators (2013) and the Commission on Cancer (2012) recognized and continue to recognize the challenges of redefining survivorship, developing guidelines for new survivorship processes, and addressing interventions for survivorship care implementation. Cooperation from experts among various oncology fields in collaboration with national organizations focused on efforts to apply survivorship research findings into practice. The collaborative effort generated years of guideline planning, publications, and educational conferences, ultimately facilitating the disbursement of the concept of survivorship planning among healthcare professionals, in addition to offering structural guidance for survivorship programs and recommendations for regulatory compliance.

The role of oncology nurses is evolving as patients' needs evolve in terms of survivorship care planning. Patients deserve seamless comprehensive care before, during, and after cancer treatment, which is achievable through dedicated care providers. Nurses' participation on hospital-based cancer committees, revising policy and procedures, and implementing recommended practice changes to address survivorship issues are a few examples highlighting the evolving role of oncology nurses. Nurses, regardless of practice settings, share a vision with oncology patients that extend beyond the here-and-now and immediate treatment and are actively involved in survivorship care with each patient encounter as well as becoming integral members of interprofessional collaboration. Active participation in survivorship planning involves engaging patients and families by educating about long-term effects of cancer, promoting awareness of support resources, advocating for referrals when applicable, reviewing treatment summaries to communicate pertinent oncology focused information, and promoting healthy behaviors for management of pre-existing comorbidities or preventative behavior.

Interprofessional Collaboration

"Empathy shines its light on our deepest needs, never allowing us to forget that our very survival depends on our ability to accurately understand and sensitively respond to each other."

—Arthur P. Ciaramicoli and Katherine Ketcham

Clinical Nurse Specialist

"Problems almost always create opportunities to learn, grow, and improve."
—John C. Maxwell

The Oncology Clinical Nurse Specialist (OCNS) is an expert clinician who provides direct care for patients with cancer. The OCNS's role extends beyond clinical expertise, making a significant impact on nursing practice. The OCNS is involved with advancing nursing practice by utilizing evidence-based practice to influence nursing practice changes within an organization (Oncology Nursing Society, 2008). OCNSs work in leadership positions in a variety of clinical settings including hospital inpatient units, outpatient centers, community clinics, or hospice programs. Graduate programs that prepare OCNSs include advanced pathophysiology, pharmacology, and advanced physical assessment (American Association of Colleges of Nursing, 1996).

The Oncology Nursing Society published core competencies for the OCNS' role in 2008. The core competencies identified three spheres of influence: patient focus, nurse and practice focus, and organizational focus. OCNS applies advanced nursing knowledge and skills to assess and manage cancer-related illness. Advocating for patient-centered care, the OCNS is an active participant in ensuring the provision of quality nursing care. The OCNS influences nurses and practice issues by revising nursing policies, provides leadership through change processes, and implements educational opportunities on evidence-based practice and best practice guidelines. Finally, the OCNS influences healthcare systems by communicating effectively, leading interprofessional groups, and participating in organizational leadership forums to advocate for innovative patient care programs.

Another variation of the Clinical Nurse Specialist derives from organizational need. Organizations may choose to develop master's prepared nurses into "Clinical Nurse Specialists" in role definition. An organizational appointed CNS nurse brings years of clinical oncology experience, often certified in their specialty, with a master's degree in nursing science. Although the MSN degree differs from a CNS academic program, the MSN degree offers a strong foundation of nursing leadership, administration, and education, contrary to the CNS degree program that offers a clinical concentration in oncology care that is not offered in an MSN program. As organizations adapt to meet the changing needs of oncology patients, utilizing CNS either by degree preparation or role definition complements the oncology team and functions as an advanced practitioner in care. Similar to the core competencies outlined by the ONS in 2008, organizations outline job responsibilities for the Clinical Nurse Specialist. Role responsibilities may vary among institutions based on patient and organizational needs; therefore it is important for master's prepared nurses to remain flexible in efforts to contribute effectively. Five domains of the Clinical Nurse Specialist concentrate on the roles as educator, clinician, researcher, administrator, and consultant.

CNS as Educator

The CNS as educator has a strong presence in designing and implementing educational programs. The educational programs may include but not limited to unit-based in-services of new products or procedures, organizational wide educational seminars, updating nursing orientation programs, providing content review courses, and promoting continuous learning through professional literature. The CNS prioritizes educational content based on an educational needs assessment of the nursing team as well as identifying trends in patient outcomes. Once the needs assessment is evaluated, the CNS reflects on the mission and philosophy of the organization, ensuring consistency with standards of nursing practice and code of ethics. The CNS as educator also performs ongoing evaluation of nurses' progress and compliance with skilled competencies. Continuous monitoring ensures compliance with safety standards and policy and procedures as well as facilitating the nurses' professional development. In collaboration with the oncology nurse manager, the CNS will make recommendations regarding opportunities for clinical nurses to develop into preceptor positions or progress to the next level in their professional development program. The CNS as educator promotes the profession of nursing through offering continuous learning opportunities, contributing to a culture of lifelong learning, and support for staff development ultimately shaping the future of the nursing profession.

CNS as Clinician

The CNS as clinician directs clinical practice to include expertise in advanced assessment, implementing nursing care, and evaluating patient outcomes. In this role, the

CNS assesses patient needs, identifies educational needs of patients and families, and participates in plan of care and discharge planning (if applicable). In addition, the CNS as clinician assists with planning realistic goals and interventions with nursing staff. The CNS participates in ongoing collaboration with physicians and the interdisciplinary team, focuses on unit based initiatives, and mentors clinical nurses toward professional development.

CNS as Consultant

The CNS as consultant provides expert knowledge and skill in a specialized area of practice and represents nursing by keeping teams informed of nursing projects, objectives, and outcomes. They are responsible for providing timely and accurate information within and across organizational systems. Clinical Nurse Specialists participate in various committees, lead discussions regarding practice concerns, and identify issues that impact staff or workflow. The CNS serves as a resource, assists with identifying patient care problems, and takes initiative to develop innovative solutions and continuous improvements that add value to the work environment. The CNS also empowers nurses to become active participants in change and improvement processes.

CNS as Researcher

The CNS as researcher disseminates current information and theories to ensure the provision of quality care. The CNS evaluates evidence for practice, understands, interprets, and utilizes research models when applying research into practice. Through this process, the CNS advances nursing practice by integrating evidence-based interventions and best practice guidelines into nursing practice. The CNS provides leadership in assessment, revision, and implementation of policies to improve outcomes. Furthermore, as researcher, the CNS leads performance improvement activities, collects and analyzes data for benchmarking, and identifies relevant researchable clinical nursing themes.

CNS as Administrator

The CNS as administrator, in partnership with nursing management, provides unit focus and direction in the practice setting. Educating, monitoring, and updating staff on unit performance measures and outcomes allows the nursing team to quickly identify clinical practice issues in need of improvement. The CNS serves as patient advocate in the administrator role, addressing patient and family concerns and complaints efficiently. As administrator, the CNS leads interprofessional teams to solve specific patient problems and identify existing or potential system barriers. The CNS also participates enthusiastically with the organizations' nursing recognition and reward programs.

The CNS contributes to the facility's survivorship program fundamentally by providing survivorship education to the oncology nurses. Remaining abreast of new regulatory requirements and literature offers opportunities to provide evolving information to organization leaders as well as oncology nurses. Knowledgeable of the oncology healthcare environment, the CNS serves as consultant, participates on an organizational survivorship taskforce or committee, advocates for oncology patient needs, contributes in designing workflow improvements, and monitors compliance and effectiveness of survivorship care plans. The CNS as researcher investigates evidence-based literature for survivorship program implementation and participates in developing survivorship educational material for patients. As researcher, the CNS is responsible for revising existing policies, and creating policies for new processes including survivorship care. The CNS as administrator participates in planning survivorship community events and survivorship educational seminars.

Summary

The OCNS is a master's prepared practitioner whose expertise in oncology provides evidence-based learning, guidance, and advocacy for patients, families, and the cancer care team. The multi-role responsibilities as educator, clinician, consultant, researcher, and administrator offer not only a unit-focused perspective, but demonstrate a global perspective of healthcare issues, organizations, and collaborative patient-focused care. As a member of the nursing team, the Clinical Nurse Specialist is an integral change agent, impacting people, processes, and the healthcare environment through investing in nursing professional development, policy change, and process implementation (such as a Survivorship Program) to yield optimal patient outcomes. As a fundamental lifelong learner, the Clinical Nurse Specialist essentially evolves their role to achieve organizational goals and address effectively the evolving needs of cancer patients ensuring that patients receive quality comprehensive care.

CASE STUDY

G.G. is a 27-year-old female who has been diagnosed with Hodgkin disease, Stage II. She is married with one son aged 2 years and she is a first grade teacher who recently started working in a new school district. She is being discharged from the hospital and she will be undergoing chemotherapy and radiation as part of her treatment regimen as an outpatient. The nurse assigned to her on the inpatient unit is a new graduate from a baccalaureate program.

• Critical Thinking **Questions**

1. In what capacity do you see the OCNS working with this patient?
2. How can the OCNS assist the new nurse in caring for this patient?
3. How will the clinical nurse specialist participate in the discharge plan for this patient and assist her in her transition to survivor?

References

American Association of Colleges of Nursing. (1996). The essentials of masters education for advanced practice nursing. Retrieved from http://www.aacn.nche.edu/education-resources/masessentials96.pdf

American Cancer Society. (2013). *Goals of chemotherapy*. Retrieved from http://www.cancer.org/treatment/treatmentsandsideeffects/treatmenttypes/chemotherapy/chemotherapyprinciplesanin-depthdiscussionofthetechniquesanditsroleintreatment/chemotherapy-principles-goals-of-chemo

American College of Surgeons Commission on Cancer. (2012). *Cancer program standards 2012: Ensuring patient-centered care* [v.1.2.1]. Retrieved from https://www.facs.org/~/media/files/quality%20programs/cancer/coc/programstandards2012.ashx

American Society of Clinical Oncology. (2014). ASCO cancer survivorship compendium. Retrieved October 12, 2014 from http://www.asco.org/practice-research/cancer-survivorship

Denlinger, C. S., Ligibel, J. A., Demark-Wahnefried, W., Dizon, D., Goldman, M., Jones, L., Kvale, E., Montoya, J., Syrjala, K. L., Urba, S. G., Zee, P., et. al. , NCCN Clinical Practice Guidelines in Oncology (NCCN Guidelines®) for Survivorship V.2.2014. © 2014 National Comprehensive Cancer Network, Inc. Retrieved October 13, 2014 from NCCN.org.

Grant M, Economou D. (2010). Survivorship education for quality cancer care. *Oncology Issues*. 48–49. Retrieved from http://accc-cancer.org/oncology_issues/articles/mayjune10/MJ10-Grant.pdf

Hewitt, M., Greenfield, S., & Stovall E. (Eds.). (2005). *From cancer patient to cancer survivor: Lost in transition*. Washington, DC: The National Academies Press. National Cancer Policy Board. Institute of Medicine and National Research Council of the National Academies. Retrieved from http://www.iom.edu/Reports/2005/From-Cancer-Patient-to-Cancer-Survivor-Lost-in-Transition.aspx

Institute of Medicine. (2005). *From cancer patient to cancer survivor: Lost in transition*. Retrievedfromhttp://www.iom.edu/Reports/2005/From-Cancer-Patient-to-Cancer-Survivor-Lost-in-Transition.aspx

National Cancer Institute. (2012). *Cancer survivorship conference highlights research for survivor care: Biennial conference aims to improve quality and length of life for cancer survivors*. Retrieved October 13, 2014.

National Coalition of Oncology Nurse Navigators. (2013). *Oncology nurse navigator core competencies*. Retrieved from http://www.nconn.org

Oncology Nursing Society. (2008). *Oncology clinical nurse specialist competencies*. Retrieved from https://www.ons.org/sites/default/files/cnscomps.pdf

CHAPTER **13**

ONCOLOGY NURSE NAVIGATORS

"Before I started working here, I wonder how many patients slipped through the cracks in terms of needing financial assistance and not receiving the appropriate referrals. Cancer treatment is very expensive and even having insurance does not cover all of the expenses that arise."

—An oncology nurse navigator

Key Term

nurse navigator

Upon completing this chapter, you will be able to do the following:

1. Identify five essential functions of the oncology nurse navigator.
2. Describe barriers to care that impact on oncology patients.
3. Describe how the oncology nurse navigators play an integral role assisting oncology patients overcoming barriers to care.
4. Discuss why oncology nurse navigators are essential members of the healthcare team.

Nurse Navigation

Patients are almost never prepared to hear the words "You have cancer." Before they have time to process the news, they are thrust into a whirlwind of oncology consultations and more diagnostic testing, and required to make treatment decisions often involving surgery, chemotherapy, and radiation therapy. Many struggle to cope with the news of their new diagnosis that not only affects them, but also their families. In addition to this, many patients struggle to keep financially afloat as they are faced with multiple co-pays and other out-of-pocket medical expenses, including costly prescriptions, transportation to medical appointments, and the need to take time off work for medical care (Freeman & Reuben, 2013). The challenge of maneuvering through a complex healthcare system during a stressful time in a patient's life has not gone unnoticed. Patient navigation has evolved over several decades and has become increasingly relevant and is now considered a vital service of most oncology centers.

The original goal of patient navigation was to address the disparities in cancer care, evident among vulnerable populations. Even before a diagnosis of cancer, underserved populations are known to have lower rates of cancer screening (Freund, 2010). Harold P. Freeman, M.D., a breast surgeon in Harlem, NY, was acutely aware of the disparities in breast cancer among vulnerable populations, particularly among those living in poverty and among racial and ethnic minorities (Freeman & Rodriguez, 2011). He developed a navigation program to address barriers that prevented timely access to care from the point of a suspicious finding identified by screening to diagnosis and treatment. Freeman recognized that these barriers included lack of or inadequate insurance, poor social support, and poor health literacy. Freeman was able to prove a significant benefit of his navigation program by reducing the barriers to timely care, thus increasing the number of patients who were diagnosed at an earlier cancer stage and ultimately improving the overall survival of the patients. Before Freeman's interventions, almost half of patients presented with late-stage disease at diagnosis. The 5-year survival rate was only 39%. After the start of his navigation program, the percentage of women diagnosed at late-stage dropped to 21%, and the 5-year survival rate improved to 70% (Freeman & Rodriguez, 2011).

Freemans's work was recognized nationally and resulted in national legislation, the Patient Navigator Act of 2005. The primary purpose was to establish grants to develop and operate patient navigator programs to improve healthcare outcomes (H.R., 2005). Shortly after the passage of the Patient Navigator Act, the National Cancer Institute began funding the Patient Navigation Research Program at nine sites across the country. The program sites were to develop, implement, and evaluate a patient navigation program that targeted vulnerable populations and could be duplicated at additional sites in the future. Results of the program are still being evaluated, but preliminary results show that patient outcomes improve with increased access to care. However, cost effectiveness must be proven before such programs can be established on a wider scale (Hopkins & Mumber, 2009).

Definition of Navigators

The oncology nurse navigator serves as a single point of contact for patients and their families throughout their entire cancer care experience, and most importantly, is an advocate and personal care coach on the patient's behalf. Patient navigation provided by a layperson, social worker, or nurse refers to the individualized assistance to patients, families, and caregivers to help overcome healthcare system barriers and facilitate timely access to quality medical and psychosocial care from pre-diagnosis through all phases of the cancer experience (National Coalition of Oncology Nurse Navigators, 2010). There are many qualities that make up a navigator, such as a licensed nursing professional, someone who is highly organized, a nurse with extensive knowledge in the oncology field, an educator, a skilled listener, and a communicator. She/he should be committed to being a patient advocate, assisting with important decisions, improving the patient's quality of life, and providing resources to decrease financial costs and psychosocial distress.

Types of Navigators

The title "Navigator" is often used to describe many different professional roles. Some of these roles are clinical and others nonclinical. Examples of nonclinical navigators include lay or patient navigators, financial navigators, and someone who himself/ herself is a survivor. Clinical navigators include nurse navigators, oncology nurse navigators, and social workers. There are several different types of navigation models that have been in practice since the 1990s. Each model is defined by the type of patient navigator who provides the service. The professional model is usually located within a healthcare setting, employs professional patient navigators (e.g., nurses, social workers, or health educators). Professional navigators focus on a wide variety of clinical and support services, including counseling, coordination of care, health education, communication between the patient and the healthcare team, and patient support and management services (Wells et al., 2008; Ell et al., 2002). A second model, lay person navigation, utilizes lay persons from the community as patient navigators. Lay navigators receive training, tend to perform navigation in the community where the patients live, and may be trained and supervised by a social worker or nurse with professional clinical supervision expertise (Wells et al., 2011; Carroll et al., 2010). The third model of navigation, advocated by Dr. Harold Freeman, blends the two previously described navigation models (Petereit et al., 2008; Freeman & Rodriguez, 2011; Willcox & Bruce, 2010). The model is comprised of a team of lay and professional patient navigators that collaboratively assist patients from initial screening through diagnosis, treatment, and follow-up care (Wilcox & Bruce, 2010). The Oncology Nursing Society states that "patient outcomes are optimal when a social worker, nurse, and lay navigator function as a multidisciplinary team" (Oncology Nursing Society, 2010). Patient-centered navigated care is supported by the 2012 release of the American College of Surgeon's Cancer Program Standards, which calls for accredited institutions to have in place "a patient navigation process" to address healthcare disparities (American College of Surgeons, 2012).

Following is an example of a generic nurse navigator job description.

Role and Responsibilities

The Nurse Navigator functions in the multidisciplinary team as an advocate, interpreter, educator, and counselor for oncology patients. She/he is responsible for ensuring that all adult patients with an oncology diagnosis receive quality and comprehensive services. He/she will coordinate patient care throughout the continuum in collaboration with the multidisciplinary team. She/he will serve as a clinical resource with expertise in hematology/oncology care management. He/she will serve as a liaison throughout the facility and in the community regarding services provided for this unique patient population. He/she will provide expert nursing care, which includes direct clinical practice, consultation, education, and research.

Specific Elements and Essential Functions

1. Demonstrates the knowledge, skill, and coordination to provide nursing care and guidance to the cancer patient from screening to survivorship. Systematically and continually performs the functions of assessing, planning, implementing,

and evaluating the care according to the nursing process and Oncology Nursing Society Standards of Practice.*

2. Provides education and information to the patient and family, helping to make the care seamless, continuous, and comprehensive. Initiates and documents patient teaching including family and significant others based on assessment of needs. Responds to patient requests for information regarding the disease process, expected side effects of treatment, and community resources. Responds to patient requests for information regarding the disease process, expected side effects of treatment, and community resources. Uses appropriate patient education documentation modality.*

3. Supports the patient during difficult decision-making periods. Assists in coordination of end-of-life care for patient and family and provides emotional support.*

4. Functions in an organized and time conscious manner. The navigator partners with patients, families, the interdisciplinary team, and community resources to provide well-coordinated, timely, compassionate, exemplary, interdisciplinary care. The navigator communicates with all members of the healthcare team, as appropriate, about patient/family needs and concerns.*

5. Initiates and performs ongoing review of policies related to service provided. Where appropriate, updates or writes new policies to enhance professional practice.

6. Serves as a resource for community educational events, such as health fairs, screenings, symposiums, and lectures as well as staff education along with the Clinical Educator.

*Those specific functions with an asterisk are essential functions considered necessary to accomplish this job.

Navigator Services

Based on the original "Harlem" model, traditional examples of navigator services include:

- Arranging financial support.
- Arranging transportation to, and childcare during, scheduled diagnosis and treatment appointments.
- Identifying and scheduling appointments with culturally sensitive caregivers.

Barriers of Care

A person may face many types of barriers to care when diagnosed with a serious illness. Not everyone will have the same barriers, but we need to be aware of the ones that affect our individual patients. Some of the common ones include: financial and economic, information and education, cultural, spiritual, family and social support, childcare, transportation, and fear. The barriers listed above interfere with access to cancer treatment and also interfere with cancer prevention and control, utilization of available screening, access to and utilization of support services (support groups, palliative care, end-of-life care), and long-term survivorship (National Coalition of Oncology Nurse Navigators, 2010). Navigators can help patients overcome these barriers by promoting one on one contacts to aid patients, families, and caregivers to get through multifaceted health networks; providing education strategies to encourage a sense of empowerment; linking patients to community-based resources; trouble-shooting logistics to and from treatment; and offering psychosocial support.

Navigation Programs

The term "cancer care continuum" encompasses the full spectrum of cancer treatment, which includes primary prevention tasks, such as education and outreach; screening, diagnosis, and staging active treatment; survivorship; and end-of-life care (Hopkins & Mumber, 2009; Wells et al., 2008; Oncology Nursing Society, 2010; Braun et al., 2012).

The primary goal of a cancer screening program is to promote early detection. A navigator's responsibility is to identify and remove barriers that prevent access to screening (Hopkins & Mumber, 2009). Often, these barriers can be cultural. A strong navigation program in a specific community would be able to identify the cultural norm and address ways to remove the barriers within that community.

While the initial tasks involved with education, outreach, and screening are more suited for lay navigators in the community, the other phase of the cancer care continuum require clinical expertise from a navigator in the cancer program. Cancer navigation takes on a much more formal role in most oncology programs within the phases of diagnosis, staging, and active treatment.

A critical role of the navigator at the time of a suspicious screening or the actual diagnosis is to ensure that the patient is not lost to follow-up. An oncology nurse in the role of a navigator can provide the patient with accurate information about the diagnosis, including interpretation of the pathology report and also give the patient an overview of what to anticipate with further evaluation and treatment. The navigator needs to assess patient's literacy and then ensure that any medical information is provided in such a way that the patient can understand (Wilcox & Bruce, 2010). The navigator can explain the various roles within the interprofessional oncology team and may help the patient with referrals and scheduling of consultations with members of that oncology team. The navigator may help guide the patient through the decision-making process since the navigator has a solid knowledge base of the particular diagnosis and treatment. The navigator is often a single point of contact for patients throughout their cancer care, acting as a liaison between patients and their providers. This provides for simpler communication from the patient's perspective and can ensure that the patient's questions and concerns are being addressed promptly.

The navigator also plays a key role at the time of diagnosis by assessing any potential financial or psychosocial barriers that might prevent the patient from receiving care. The navigator can refer patients to oncology social workers for help with financial aid or transportation arrangements.

The oncology nurse navigator is also relevant during active cancer treatment. Many cancer treatments, including chemotherapy and radiation, have a wide range of toxicities. At this point in the cancer care continuum, the navigator has likely established a trusting relationship with patients. Given that, the navigator assesses patients who may be struggling with some of the adverse effects of treatment and can provide symptom management options to help them get through difficult times (Wilcox & Bruce, 2010).

Many patients struggle with long-term effects of their cancer treatment, yet often they are not aware of treatment options or do not seek care to handle these symptoms.

This time can be particularly challenging for cancer survivors in vulnerable populations. Researchers have identified barriers to survivorship care and highlighted ways in which cancer navigators can be valuable in helping patients overcome these obstacles. These barriers included a fragmented medical delivery system in which patients and their providers may not have a clear understanding of who is accepting responsibility for the care and management of certain symptoms, a lack of knowledge about long-term effects of cancer treatment, and how a patient can maximize health outcomes and barriers to communication between patients and providers (Pratt-Chapman et al., 2011). A cancer navigator in a survivorship program can identify barriers that patients may face, help patients coordinate care among their providers, ensure that patients are receiving adequate follow-up care, and connect patients with psychosocial support and community resources (Wilcox & Bruce, 2010).

Successes and Challenges of Patient Navigation Programs

Patient navigation programs have successfully helped patients address and overcome financial barriers (underinsured and uninsured), communication barriers, and systemic barriers (transportation, missed appointments, follow-up calls). Overall, patient navigation programs are bringing about increases in screening and adherence to diagnostic follow-up care after the detection of an abnormality. Many believe patient navigators who act as a bridge between the medical culture and the patient's culture are the most successful (Institute for Alternative Futures, 2007).

A major challenge for many patient navigation programs has been professional role confusion. Depending on the job description, patient navigators are sometimes added to the healthcare team to do a job that the other members of the healthcare team had already been doing (Freeman, 2004; Dohan & Schrag, 2005). As a function, "patient navigation" is not new to the medical field. Helping patients and families "navigate" the healthcare system had been a part of nearly every oncology healthcare professional's daily work for decades. The challenge has become how to define patient navigation as an entity with a job description that is distinctly different from already existing members of the healthcare team (Institute for Alternative Futures, 2007).

When a service-focused definition of patient navigation is used, the services tend to overlap with other positions in cancer care, such as social work, nursing, education, and case management. However, when the focus of a patient navigation program is on assisting patients to overcome barriers to care, less room for role confusion and more room for collaboration exist (Dohan & Schrag, 2005).

Another challenge for patient navigation programs is achieving "buy-in" from all stakeholders on the aim of and need for such a program prior to implementation. For patient navigators to be successful, they must be an integrated part of the healthcare team. The integration is much more likely to happen when each member of the healthcare team understands his or her responsibilities and those other members of the team. After implementation, multidisciplinary meetings (including patient navigators, social work, nursing, outreach, and other team members) that provide education on respective roles and referral processed, as well as serving as arenas for open communication are also helpful. Interdisciplinary communication is a must in setting up a successful program (Warner, 2010).

CASE STUDY

S.W. is a 55-year-old female who has been diagnosed with thyroid cancer, Stage II. She is married with three adult children. Currently she is unemployed but her husband is self-employed as an accountant. After discussing her diagnosis with the endocrinologist she was referred to the oncology nurse navigator. She informs the nurse navigator that she does not understand why surgery is necessary. She is also concerned about how long she will be hospitalized and what she can expect after surgery.

• Critical Thinking **Questions**

1. What role will the oncology nurse navigator have in terms of this patient?
2. What barriers to care may exist for this patient?
3. What interventions can the oncology nurse navigator carry out to meet the needs of this patient?
4. How can the oncology nurse navigator assist the patient in the perioperative period?

References

American College of Surgeons. (2012). *Cancer program standards 2012 version 1.1: Ensuring patient centered care.* Chicago, IL: American College of Surgeons.

Braun, K. L., Kagawa-Singer, M., Holden, A. E., Burhansstipanov, L., Tran, J. H., Seals, B. F., ... Ramirez, A. G. (2012). Cancer patient navigator tasks across the cancer care continuum. *Journal of Health Care Poor Underserved. 23*(1):398–413.

Carroll, J. K., Humiston, S. G., Meldrum, S. C., Salamone, C. M., Jean-Pierre, P., Epstein, R. M., & Fiscella, K. (2010). Patients' experiences with navigation for care. Patient education and counseling. *80*(2):241–247. doi: 10.1016/j.pec.2009.10.024.

Dohan, D., & Schrag, D. (2005). Using navigators to improve care of underserved patients. Current practices and approaches. *Cancer. 104*(4):848–855.

Ell, K., Padgett, D., Vourlekism, B., Nissly, J., Pineda, D., Sarabia, O., ... Lee, P. J. (2002). Abnormal mammograms follow-up: A pilot study women with low income. *Cancer Practice. 10*(3):130–138.

Freeman, H. P. (2004) A model patient navigation program. *Oncology Issues. 19*(5):44–46.

Freeman, H. P., & Reuben, S. H., eds. President's Cancer Panel: Voices of a broken system: Real people, real problems. National Cancer Institute web site. Retrieved January 7, 2013 from http://deainfo.nci.nih.gov/advisory/pcp/archive.pcp00-01rpt/PCPvideo/voices_files/PDFfiles/PCPbook.pdf. Published September 1, 2001.

Freeman. H. P., & Rodriguez, R. L. (2011) History and principles of patient navigation. *Cancer. 117*(15 Suppl):3537–3540.

Freund, K. M. (2010). Patient navigation; The promise to reduce health disparities. *Journal of General Internal Medicine. 26*(2):110–111.

H.R. (2005). 1812: Patient Navigator Outreach and Chronic Disease Prevention Act of 2005. GovTrack. us. Retrieved July 25, 2014 from http://www.govtrack.us./comgress/bills/109/hr1812

Hopkins, J., & Mumber, M. P. (2009). Patient navigation through the cancer care continuum: An overview. *Oncology Practice. 5*(4):150–152.

Institute for Alternative Futures. (2007). Patient Navigation Program Overview: A report for the Disparity Reducing Advances (DRA) Project. Institute for Alternative futures. Retrieved

July 25, 94 from www.altfutures.com/draproject/pdfs/Report_07_02_Patient_Navigator_ProgramOverview.pdf.

National Coalition of Oncology Nurse Navigators. (2010). *NCONN General core competencies for the oncology nurse navigator.* Retrieved July 25, 2014 from http://www.nconn.org.

Oncology Nursing Society. (2010). Oncology Nursing Society, the Association of Oncology Social Work, and the National Association of Social Workers Joint Position on the Role of Oncology Nursing and Oncology Social Work in Patient Navigation. Retrieved July 25, 2014 from http://www.ons.org/publications/positions/navigation.

Petereit, D. G., Molloy, K., Reiner, M. L., Helbig, P., Cina, K., Miner, R., ... Roberts, C. R. (2008). Establishing a patient navigator program to reduce cancer disparities in the American Indian communities of Western South Dakota: Initial observations and results. *Cancer Control. 15*(3):254–259.

Pratt-Chapman, M., Simon, M. A., Patterson, A. K., Risendal, B. C., & Patierno, S. (2011). Survivorship navigation outcome measures: A report from the ACS Patient Navigation Working Group on survivorship navigation. *Cancer. 117*(15 Suppl):3575–3584.

Warner A. (2010). Cancer patient navigation: Where do we go from here? *Oncology Issues.* 50–53.

Wells, K. J., Battaglia, T. A., Dudley, D. J., Garcia, R., Greene, A., Calhoun, E., ... Raich, P. C. (2008). Patient navigation: State of the art or is it science? *Cancer. 113*(8):1999–2010.

Wells, K. J., Meade, C. D., Calcano, E. R., Lee, J.H., Rivers, D., & Roetzheim, R. G. (2011). Innovative approaches to reducing cancer health disparities: The Moffitt Cancer patient navigator research program. *Journal of Cancer Education. 26*(4):649–657. doi: 0.1007/s13187–011–0238–7

Wilcox, B., & Bruce, S. D. (2010) Patient Navigation: A "win-win" for all involved. *Oncology Nursing Forum. 37*(1):21–25. doi: 10.1188/10.ONF.21–25

CHAPTER 14

ONCOLOGY CASE MANAGERS

"As a case manager, I promote a collaborative relationship between the payer community, healthcare providers and other stakeholders to promote a patient's self-care abilities so that health is achieved at the highest level possible. My goal is to assist the patient in managing his/her treatment plan and condition(s) with a primary focus of education and medication adherence."

—A case manager

Key Terms

advocacy • case manager • collaboration • self-care management activities

Upon completing this chapter, you will be able to do the following:

1. Describe how nurse case managers play an integral role on the healthcare team.
2. Describe what the role of the nurse case manager is in cancer survivorship.
3. Describe the interventions that case managers carry out in order to assist patients.
4. Describe the advocacy role of the case manager.
5. Discuss the importance of cultural competency in case management.

Overview

Individuals with significant health issues such as cancer may have difficulty navigating the sometimes-fragmented healthcare system in the United States. One challenge the individual with cancer and family may face is determining what care and services should follow active treatment and how to access those services especially if the necessary support and direction are not available. The case manager is a valuable member of the healthcare team who can provide needed support and guidance to the cancer survivor. The Case Management Society of America (CMSA), the leading member organization for the practice of case management, defines case management as, "a collaborative process

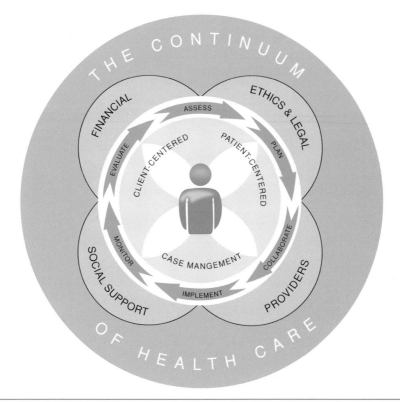

Figure 14.1 • The continuum of health care. (Reprinted with permission from the Case Management Society of America, 6301 Ranch Drive, Little Rock, AR 72223, www.cmsa.org)

of assessment, planning, facilitation, care coordination, evaluation, and advocacy for options and services to meet an individual's and family's comprehensive health needs through communication and available resources to promote quality, cost-effective outcomes (CMSA, 2008–2012)". Figure 14.1 illustrates the CMSA's continuum of health care and depicts the responsibilities and relationships associated with case management.

Case management benefits the individual with cancer as well as individual's support system. The philosophy of case management comes to fruition when an individual achieves the highest level of wellness and function and the individual's support system is no longer burdened with care, fewer resources from the healthcare system are used and therefore, expenditures are reduced as the individual no longer requires costly services (CMSA, 2008–2012).

Case management assists the individual needing care and services through advocacy, facilitation of communication among healthcare providers as well as between the individual and healthcare providers. In addition, disease education, identification of resources to support care not typically covered by traditional insurance, and coordination of care and care transitions are offered. The case manager identifies the care and services needed to bring the individual to an appropriate level of wellness, a process that is accomplished by ensuring that the needed care and services are coordinated timely and in the most cost-effective manner. Appropriate care coordination and cost-effective use of resources result in value for the individual and for reimbursement sources.

Healthcare Settings for Case Managers

- Outpatient clinics
- Medical Homes
- Health plans
- Physician offices
- Accountable Care Organizations
- Hospitals
- Extended Care Facilities
- Long-term Care Facilities
- Postacute Care Facilities
- Skilled Nursing Facilities
- Insurance Companies
- Independent practices

Who Are Case Managers?

Case managers are licensed healthcare professionals or those with advanced health-related degrees which include, but are not limited to, registered nurses, social workers, therapists, licensed counselors, and pharmacists (CMSA-What is a Case Manager, 2008–2012). Physicians and nurse practitioners may practice as case managers; however, the designation of "case manager" according to the CMSA is an individual who is actively involved in the activities of assessing, planning, coordinating, and monitoring the care of individuals ethically, with consideration for preference of culture and religion (CMSA, 2008–2012). Unless a case manager is engaged in the stated activities included in the definition of case management, he or she is not practicing according to the Standards of Practice set forth by the CMSA.

The Standards of Practice were first introduced to the case management community by CMSA in 2002 (CMSA, 2010). The standards are guidelines for case management practice rather than a replacement of relevant legal or professional requirements. The guiding principles of the standards are to clarify and promote the adoption of a patient-centered approach whereby a collaborative partnership is developed with the patient (Case Management Society of America, 2010, Revised).

In this chapter, the standards apply specifically to the role of a case manager working with cancer survivors. In an effort to address care coordination and care transition to improve outcomes, organizations and providers of care have created positions like Care Coordinators or Patient Navigators; however, case management is an established contributor to assist patients with the segmented structure of the healthcare system. Case managers focus on the support of eventual patient self-care management activities so that patients can embrace and adapt healthy behaviors, learn to deal with the burden of illness, and feel comfortable interacting with care providers (Bachmann-Mettler, Steurer-Stey, Wang, Bardheci, & Rosemann, 2011).

A case manager is well prepared to support the patient in developing strategies to improve their health status (Bachmann-Mettler et al., 2011). In order to develop these strategies, the case manager can coach the patient to embrace self-efficacy and can coordinate additional services that will promote the confidence and ability to handle existing and future challenges. The case manager can coordinate counseling services that will assist with the development of skills to better cope with the ups and downs of illness that result in stress and emotional strain. Medication education and promotion of adherence will result in disease management. Promotion of healthier eating habits and physical fitness assist in stress management and result in an overall healthier state. The patient requires support through the continuing adjustment of their place in the family and in a work or professional setting. Promotion of self-management includes learning problem-solving, making decisions, acquiring knowledge of how to locate and utilize resources, developing trusted relationships with providers, and knowing how to implement those strategies into action.

Patient Selection Process

- Age
- Poor pain control
- Cognitive deficits
- Previous home health or durable medical equipment usage
- History of mental illness and/or substance abuse, suicide risk, or crisis intervention
- Chronic, catastrophic, or terminal illness
- Social issues such as a history of abuse, neglect, lack of social support and/or lives alone
- Repeated emergency department visits
- Need for admission or transition to a postacute facility
- Repeated acute care admissions
- Poor nutritional status
- Financial issues

Cancer survivors may meet one or more of these criteria (Nekhlyudov & Snyder, 2013):

Standard: Patient Assessment

- Physical/functional status
- Medical history
- Psychological behavioral history
- Current mental health status
- Cognitive function
- Patient strengths and abilities
- Environment and residential setting
- Family or support system dynamics
- Spiritual preferences
- Financial needs
- Health insurance status
- History of abuse, violence, or trauma
- Vocational and/or educational background
- Recreational and leisure pursuits
- Caregiver availability and capability
- Learning and technology capabilities
- Self-care capabilities
- Health literacy
- Need for a transitional or discharge plan
- Legal concerns
- Transportation capabilities or limitations
- Readiness to change

Patient Assessment

As part of the case management process, the case manager conducts a thorough assessment in order to determine the needs of the cancer survivor. The assessment should further explore and examine resources utilized, primary and secondary diagnoses, past and present care and services, prognosis, short- and long-term goals, and availability and type of health benefits. The data gathered for assessment comes from many sources but should include, at the very least, patient family interviews, reassessments as necessary, providers, physicians, medical records, and claims data.

Cancer survivors can experience delayed and long-term effects of treatment (Nekhlyudov & Snyder, 2013). These effects may be physical, behavioral, social, or financial. They may have chronic medical conditions that require ongoing treatment, depression, fatigue, cognitive deficits, pain, or sleep disturbances (Nekhlyudov & Snyder, 2013). The cost and duration of treatment may have negatively impacted the patient's ability to earn a living, or the cost of treatment may have depleted monetary reserves resulting in financial concerns. If social barriers are present, the patient may not have the ability or the resources to access continued care and treatment. A thorough assessment provides the necessary information to develop a plan for improved access to care and services.

Ideally, once the assessment is completed, the patient, case manager, and caregiver/family members work together on the identified problems and the information should be shared with the patient's healthcare providers. The assessment and problem/opportunity identification processes can assist the primary healthcare provider to be better prepared to manage the patient after cancer treatment is completed since they may not be fully aware of the needs of the cancer survivor. Providing this level of detail will help in the coordination of care for the survivor.

Treatment of cancer results in a significant financial burden long after diagnosis and treatment (Nekhlyudov & Snyder, 2013). The case manager must notify the patient's providers of financial barriers so that expensive or unnecessary services are not ordered in favor of equally effective and less expensive options. Case managers should also make the necessary referrals to community resources and social agencies that may be able to ease the patient's concerns.

Of equal importance is the need to support and encourage wellness strategies once treatment is completed or is at a maintenance level. The patient should to be educated on the importance of regular wellness visits and prevention services with the primary care provider. These services include surveillance for recurrence or other posttreatment complications. All areas that were addressed by the case manager should be included in the case management plan of care.

For the cancer survivor, care planning continues to be important after treatment is completed. The cancer survivor needs to reestablish a relationship with the primary healthcare provider and determine which health-related activities are priorities once treatment is concluded. Wellness activities such as nutrition, exercise, and prevention are important and should also include ongoing surveillance for possible recurrence. The importance of these strategies should be explained to the patient and his/her support system. Short- and long-term goals are developed with the patient and family/caregiver based on the assessment and problem/opportunity identification. Interventions to achieve these goals are then outlined and agreed upon. The interventions should be strategies to remove or eliminate barriers to care, advocacy activities that result in improved care coordination and patient support, and educational activities that result in improved adherence. The patient may also require rehabilitative services to assist with a return to wellness. For example, a patient left debilitated from chemotherapy and radiation may have muscle weakness due to inactivity. Participation in physical therapy to begin to regain strength would be an important intervention before the patient could resume a normal home exercise program.

The case manager should establish a regular communication schedule with the patient so that his/her condition can be monitored for improvement or lack of improvement. The goal is to see improvement with every patient encounter, but this may not always be achievable. Reassessing the patient for complaints, symptoms, and response to current interventions is important so that if changes are needed to the plan of care, they occur timely and with the intention of preventing more severe complications. For a cancer survivor suffering from chemotherapy-related peripheral neuropathy, medication and time are the usual forms of treatment. However, because the neuropathy can be extremely painful and can significantly impact the patient's quality of life, it is important that the case manager monitor the patient's response to the medication. Changes in type and dose of the medications used for neuropathy are often warranted until the right medication(s) and dosage are discovered to improve the patient's discomfort. With each patient encounter, the case manager should ask the patient if they are taking their medication as ordered and how well is it relieving the discomfort. If the patient reports a less than favorable response, the case manager should report this to the ordering physician so that adjustments can be timely and attempts to reduce discomfort are not delayed. Without proper monitoring, the patient may go for an extended period of time in significant discomfort when alternatives could have been implemented.

The goals and interventions that are developed based on assessment should be achievable and measureable. The case manager maximizes the patient's ability to achieve wellness, safety, and self-management by ensuring that the desired outcomes are achieved. For example, if a cancer survivor has a goal of walking up to 10 miles a week over a 6-month period, the care manager has an obligation to ensure the patient has all the encouragement needed to accomplish this goal. If the goal is not achieved, but progress has occurred, the progress toward the goal is documented and the physician is updated on the patient's progress.

Maximizing the patient's outcome potential is the focus of facilitation, communication, coordination, and collaboration. A patient may need to be admitted to an acute care facility due to the effects of cancer treatments and upon discharge from the facility require coordination of services at home such as physical and occupational therapy. The decision process should include both the patient and family member(s).

The ultimate reason to discontinue case management services for the cancer survivor is the determination that the patient has achieved a cure or long-term remission, and has returned to an optimal state of health and wellness. However, there are other occasions when it may become necessary to discontinue case management services such as the patient no longer wishes to work with the case manager, and may or may not choose to adhere to the prescribed treatment program. Every effort should be made to motivate the patient to see the benefits, but ultimately the patient's choice should be respected. Services may be discontinued if the patient loses health coverage or changes to a different health plan, one for which the case manager is not affiliated. Other reasons include achievement of target outcomes or maximum benefit has been reached, change in health setting, patient has opted out of the program or has refused medical/psychosocial services, determination by the case manager that he/she is no longer able to perform or provide appropriate case management services, or death of the patient (Case Management Society of America, 2010, Revised).

Advocacy can sometimes result in conflict between the case manager, patient, and payer source. Patients often seek treatment and services that they believe will impact their conditions; these could be investigational, excluded, or alternative therapies and treatments. These may be legitimate treatment options, or may be options that receive notoriety and publicity but are not based in science or evidence. Regardless of what kind of treatment a patient is seeking or requesting, the case manager has an obligation to help the patient to be well informed. The case manager cannot prescribe or treat, but the case manager can provide everyone involved with information so that well-informed decisions can be made without due influence.

Cultural Competency

The case manager must be aware of and be responsive to the cultural and demographic diversity of the population and specific patient profiles (Case Management Society of America, 2010, Revised, p. 21). This requires the case manager to aware of the preferences and beliefs of the individual's cultural background. If interpreter services are required, the case manager must facilitate this service in order to ensure the patient and family/caregiver has an accurate understanding of care and services. Unless there is no other alternative, family members should not be used as interpreters as they may protect the patient by relaying inaccurate information. After ascertaining the reading ability of the patient, providing printed educational materials in the patient's native language will support the information that is relayed from healthcare providers through the interpreter.

The case manager must also be sensitive to beliefs related to accessing care and services. In many cultures, individuals facing illness prefer to try home remedies before accessing Western medicine; some believe that illness is a result of a spiritual imbalance so will attempt to heal their spirit before accepting treatment; and others may not accept behavioral therapies because this is viewed as a failure of character. While ethically, case managers and all healthcare professionals are bound to do no harm, facilitation of communication between those providing care and services and the patient would be essential so that all parties understand the patient and the patient's preferences. Ultimately, the patient has the power to choose the treatment recommended, but the case manager must do everything possible to ensure that the patient, family/caregiver, and providers of care understand the advantages and consequences of any treatment choices made.

Cancer survivors often have significant financial burdens, especially after lengthy disease treatment. While the acute treatment phase may be complete, continued care and services are typically required. The case manager must be cognizant of any financial burdens the patient may be facing and assist with facilitation of care and services that will meet the patient's needs without causing additional burden. This could mean helping to find pharmacy co-pay assistance, community resources to assist with food, or transportation; these can assist the patient in receiving care and services that would not add to an existing financial burden. If costly services are required, the case manager should monitor these services in order to ensure that the goal of the care is being achieved and the services are appropriate and not overutilized. For example, a patient has a central venous access device that requires flushing and a dressing change and requires a home care nurse for the maintenance of the device since the patient has no transportation resource to travel to the oncology clinic. The patient must pay 20% co-insurance for each visit, but if the care was provided at the clinic, there would be no financial responsibility to the patient. The case manager may be able to arrange transportation to the clinic for the central line maintenance, thereby saving the patient out-of-pocket expenses.

Summary

The functions performed by a case manager include helping patients navigate the healthcare system, find and connect with community resources that will ease financial or social burdens, and facilitate and coordinate with multiple types of care and services (Effectiveness of Outpatient Case Management for Adults With Medical Illness and Complex Care Needs, 2013). Case managers also perform many clinical functions that include assessment, monitoring, medication management, health education and self-management education, and instructions (Effectiveness of Outpatient Case Management for Adults With Medical Illness and Complex Care Needs, 2013). The case manager does not solely focus on disease but is an agent or advocate for the whole person, serving to bridge the patient with the healthcare team, health system, and community resources (Effectiveness of Outpatient Case Management for Adults With Medical Illness and Complex Care Needs, 2013).

Case managers function in multiple healthcare settings and are involved in both acute illness episodes and chronic illness management. While oncology case managers commonly work with the patient during the acute illness phase, we do not see the case manager often continuing past the acute episode. There is little evidence via research that case management of the cancer survivor postacute treatment is beneficial. However, there is a belief that because of the case management approach and evidence of benefit with other chronic illness, working with cancer survivors could improve quality of life and improve coordination of care with the primary care provider and other disciplines (Effectiveness of Outpatient Case Management for Adults With Medical Illness and Complex Care Needs, 2013).

The late effects of cancer treatment and the possibility of recurrence require surveillance. Management of secondary conditions that may or may not be related to the cancer or treatment also requires monitoring and management. A return to primary care may be challenging not just for the patient, but also the primary care provider. Case management can assist in the facilitation of this transition by helping both the patient and primary care provider better understand the needs of the patient through assessment and care planning. The cancer survivor's care plan can serve as a guide and method of communication for the patient and primary care provider. The case manager's skill set and guidance through use of the Standards of Practice will surely be an asset to the survivor as they transition to long-term health.

CASE STUDY

Eleanor is 46-year-old African-American female diagnosed with breast cancer with lymph node involvement. She is the single mother of two sons aged 20 and 13 years. She lives with her elderly mother and is her mother's primary caregiver. Eleanor's mother has early dementia and congestive heart failure. Eleanor works the night shift as a nurse's aide at a nursing home.

Eleanor opted to have a mastectomy with lymph node dissection and 6 months of chemotherapy, which was completed 6 months ago. According to the diagnostics done at treatment completion, there is no evidence of active disease.

Eleanor continued to work during her treatment and missed very few days of work. She still complains of moderate fatigue and has yet to gain back the 20 pounds lost during treatment. Treatment for Eleanor was challenging in that she continued to work, care for her mother, and provide for her sons. It was difficult to find someone to help with her mother and supervise her sons when she was receiving several hours of chemotherapy at the oncology clinic, and then she often was sick and very fatigued after. She would very much like to "just get on" with life and not think about the cancer any more. The co-pays for treatment had depleted her modest savings account. She is scheduled to follow-up with her oncologist for 6 month surveillance testing but she has yet to make the appointment.

• Critical Thinking **Questions**

1. What are the possible barriers keeping Eleanor from scheduling her surveillance testing?
2. How would you encourage Eleanor to schedule her surveillance testing?
3. What strategies could be implemented to alleviate Eleanor's concerns?

References

Bachmann-Mettler, I., Steurer-Stey, C., Wang, M., Bardheci, K., & Rosemann, T. (2011). *National Center for Biotechnology Information/National Library of Medicine/National Institutes of Health.* Retrieved March 20, 2014 from National Center for Biotechnology Information: www.ncbi.nlm.nih.gov/pmc/articles/PMC3113980

Case Management Society of America. (2010). *Standards of practice for case management.* Little Rock, AR: Case Management Society of America.

CMSA-What Is a Case Manager. (2008–2012). Retrieved April 1, 2014 from CMSA: www.cmsa.org/Home?WhatisaCaseManager/tabid/224/Default.aspx

Effectiveness of Outpatient Case Management for Adults With Medical Illness and Complex Care Needs. (2013). Retrieved April 1, 2014 from Agency for Health Care Research and Quality/U.S. Department of Health and Human Services: http://www.effectivehealthcare.ahrq.gov/ehc/index.cfm/search-for-guides-reviews-and-reports/?pageAction=displayProduct&productID=1677

Nekhlyudov, M. M., & Snyder, P. C. (2013). Uptodate. In M. P. Ganz, & M. F. Dison (Eds.), *Overview of cancer survivorship care for primary care and oncology providers.* Retrieved April 1, 2014 from UpToDate: http://www.uptodate.com/contents/overview-of-cancer-survivorship-care-for-primary-care-and-oncology-providers

MENTAL HEALTH NURSES

A hospice nurse in England has expressed concern and sadness over her current patient. She writes, "I have a twenty-three year old patient at the hospice… It's horrible… They want to live." This expression of feelings is one reason why it is important for the oncology nurse to have support from a Psychiatric Clinical Nurse Specialist.

Introduction

The patient diagnosed with cancer has special mental health needs. Although the literature suggests that the prevalence of depression in cancer patients is about the same as the general population, the cancer patient frequently is not treated for depression. The purpose of this chapter is to educate nurses about treatment modalities that nurses and advanced practice nurses can initiate. The supports and suggested readings in this chapter enhance the information presented to educate nurses and fully treat our patients.

Psychiatric–Mental Health Registered Nurse

A Psychiatric–Mental Health Registered Nurse (PMH-RN) has specialized skills and knowledge in mental health issues, psychiatric illness, and substance abuse disorders. The PMH-RN uses the nursing process to treat individuals and promote health and safety; assess dysfunctional behavior; identify strengths of individuals; and foster the patients' personal recovery (American Nurses Association, 2014).

Psychiatric–Mental Health Registered Nurse's Role in a Psychiatric Unit

The Registered Nurse (RN) in a psychiatric unit may need to manage a patient who presents for depression and is being treated for cancer. The RN's role includes monitoring laboratory values, assessing nutritional status, monitoring sleep/wake cycle, promoting ADLs, and assisting when there is a need. The nurse will assess the patient's interaction in the milieu and level of participation in various treatment modalities on the unit. The nurse has 24-hour responsibility for the patient and can get feedback about the patient's performance, needs, and therapies from the multidisciplinary team, which may include activity therapists, social workers, counselors, physicians, and students from all disciplines. The RN is a key person to attend family sessions that may be led by the social worker or nurse practitioner because she has information about the patients functioning on the unit and from each of the shifts when charge nurses are observing the patients.

Psychiatric–Mental Health Advanced Practice Registered Nurse

A Psychiatric–Mental Health Advanced Practice Registered Nurse (PMH-APRN) is a professional nurse who has completed graduate studies in mental health nursing and has attained specialized skills and training with the psychiatric population. PMH-APRNs include Psychiatric Clinical Nurse Specialists (PCNS) and Psychiatric Nurse Practitioners (PNP). PMH-APRNs function in the roles of clinician, educators, consultants, and as treatment providers of medication and various therapies (American Nurses Association, 2014).

Psychiatric–Mental Health Advanced Practice Registered Nurse's Role on a Medical Unit

When a cancer patient presents for treatment on a general medical unit or oncology unit, the nursing staff may assess that the patient is depressed or anxious. The nurse manager can make a recommendation for the PCNS to assess the patient. The PCNS will meet with the patient and provide therapy and intervention as needed for depression or anxiety. According to Sadock, Sadock, and Ruiz (2014), depression typically occurs with medical issues. It is the job of the PNP to determine if medical condition pathology is contributing to the depression, for example, a side effect of a pharmacologic agent could be mood changes. Studies indicate that by treating the depression, one also improves the medical outcome, specifically in the case of cancer (Sadock et al., 2014).

The psychiatric clinical nurse specialist (PCNS) has the key role of providing support for nursing and general staff. An oncology unit in a general medical hospital or hospice center is constantly being confronted with death and dying. The unit nurses are the 24-hour support for their patients and families. This group of providers needs a time and a place to be able to discuss their feelings related to loss and to also support one another. A monthly meeting to address these topics is very therapeutic.

Psychiatric Advanced Practice Nurse and Hospice

The PCNS and hospice nurse can conduct support groups for families and significant others who are caring for their loved ones. These groups should take place weekly and can include all people significant to the patient. The community at a hospice or general medical hospital can post notices to make any interested parties aware of the group. The group needs structure and should begin at the same time each week with chairs in a circle. The members of the group may go around and introduce themselves and later take turns speaking about their experiences. The group members with more experience can share their issues with newer members to provide support.

A hospice nurse in England has expressed concern and sadness over her current patient. She writes "I have a twenty-three year old patient at the hospice… It's horrible… They want to live." This expression of feelings is one reason why it is important for the oncology nurses to have support from a PCNS as well.

Psychiatric Nurse Practitioner

The Psychiatric Nurse Practitioner (PNP) is a leader in providing individual therapy, medication monitoring, and assessment of the patient with cancer. The following are treatment modalities that the PNP can offer to the patient.

Supportive Therapy

In individual therapy, the patient is given the opportunity to vent feelings and express sadness over their illness and loss. The PNP meets with the patient at scheduled intervals. The therapy is a chance for the patient to discuss issues related to the illness, fear, pain, and death. This expression of feelings allows the patient to have relief and support. The patient may want the PNP to conduct sessions with significant others to talk about the issues. It is important to let the patient know that that the PNP is there to listen to the patient and provide support. According to Kübler-Ross (1969), the terminally ill patient has special needs which can be satisfied by sitting and listening and acknowledging their concerns.

Assessment Tools

The PNP is able to use a tool such as the PHQ-9 (Fig. 15.1) to assess the level of depression. This tool can be administered prior to treatment and at intervals throughout therapy to give the clinician an idea about patients functioning. This tool can serve as a guideline to start medications, increase therapy, or make other decisions (Kroenke & Spitzer, 2002).

PATIENT HEALTH QUESTIONNAIRE-9
(PHQ-9)

Over the last 2 weeks, how often have you been bothered by any of the following problems? (Use "✓" to indicate your answer)	Not at all	Several days	More than half the days	Nearly every day
1. Little interest or pleasure in doing things	0	1	2	3
2. Feeling down, depressed, or hopeless	0	1	2	3
3. Trouble falling or staying asleep, or sleeping too much	0	1	2	3
4. Feeling tired or having little energy	0	1	2	3
5. Poor appetite or overeating	0	1	2	3
6. Feeling bad about yourself — or that you are a failure or have let yourself or your family down	0	1	2	3
7. Trouble concentrating on things, such as reading the newspaper or watching television	0	1	2	3
8. Moving or speaking so slowly that other people could have noticed? Or the opposite — being so fidgety or restless that you have been moving around a lot more than usual	0	1	2	3
9. Thoughts that you would be better off dead or of hurting yourself in some way	0	1	2	3

FOR OFFICE CODING ___0___ + _____ + _____ + _____

= Total Score: _____

If you checked off any problems, how difficult have these problems made it for you to do your work, take care of things at home, or get along with other people?

Not difficult at all	Somewhat difficult	Very difficult	Extremely difficult
☐	☐	☐	☐

Developed by Drs. Robert L. Spitzer, Janet B.W. Williams, Kurt Kroenke and colleagues, with an educational grant from Pfizer Inc. No permission required to reproduce, translate, display or distribute.

Figure 15.1 • Patient health questionnaire-9.

Medications

Psychopharmacology can be offered when the patient presents with symptoms of mental illness as defined by the *Diagnostic and Statistical Manual*, 5th edition. Major Depressive Disorder is a common psychiatric disorder seen with the onset of a cancer diagnosis. As the patient is trying to deal with their medical issues and many changes, they become depressed. Symptoms of depression include changes in mood, decrease in pleasure, appetite, and sleep pattern. The patient can also have symptoms of anxiety with depression. According to the Diagnostic and Statistical Manual of Mental Disorder (American Psychiatric Association, 2013) a person with Major Depression has five out of the nine criteria listed below for a 2-week period:

1. Feeling depressed, sad, hopeless for a majority of the day, almost everyday
2. Loss of pleasure
3. Significant weight changes
4. Sleep disturbance
5. Feels restless or very lethargic in a physical sense
6. Low energy
7. Feeling worthless
8. Decrease in functioning, such as ability to work or conduct normal routine
9. Persistent thoughts of dying, harming self, or suicide

Medication Options

The patient can be started on medication for depression. Medications that treat depression and anxiety can be used. Newer antidepressants are more helpful due to decreased side effects. It can take up to a month to see the full effects of these medications. Common antidepressants include paroxetine, fluoxetine, and escitalopram. The patient can be told about expected course of treatment and side effects to watch for. The patient can be given a choice as to which medication they prefer as this seems to put them at ease. It can be explained that if one medication trial is not working there are other antidepressants that can be tried. According to a study funded by the National Institute of Mental Health (2008), in cases with difficulty to treat depression, when one antidepressant does not work, the chances of successful treatment increase with a second antidepressant trial.

If the patient has severe anxiety that requires treatment until the antidepressant works, low-dose antianxiety medications such as clonazepam or lorazepam may be used. The patient should understand that these medications work best when taken as needed and they can be tapered off these medications once the antidepressants seem to be working. The patient needs to be made aware of the potential for addiction and cautious use when driving or operating machinery.

The patient may suffer from insomnia. Antidepressants such as trazodone or mirtazapine can be added to the regimen to promote nighttime rest. Patients may opt to take melatonin to promote sleep, since they may be on many prescribed medications.

The most important issue related to prescribing medication is communication with other medication prescribers. All psychotropic medications should have the approval of the primary care doctor or oncologist. This communication is important to prevent duplication of antianxiety agents. This also lets the patient know that you are working with the team to improve care and provide the best outcome for them.

Support

There are many support services for patients and their families who have cancer. Some of the services available for patients with mental health issues are listed below.

Above C Level Foundation

This is a nonprofit corporation founded by a psychiatric nurse practitioner to allow mental health services to be delivered to individuals and families in need who are being treated for cancer (http://aboveclevelfoundation.org).

National Alliance of Mental Illness

This organization has support groups and information about various mental illnesses on their website. NAMI is the largest grassroots organization for mental illness in the United States. Their volunteers work in communities on the state and across the country to provide support and obtain much needed services for the mentally ill (http://www.nami.org).

National Institute of Mental Health

The National Institute of Mental Health (NIMH) focuses on the prevention and cure of mental illness. Their mission is to disseminate information to the public via basic and clinical research. NIMH has a publication (No. 11–5002) called *Depression and Cancer* which is available on their website and may be reproduced without permission from NIMH (http://www.nimh.nih.gov).

CASE STUDY

A 70-year-old married male, father of three adult children and seven grandchildren, with a 50-plus-year history of smoking tobacco and working with chemicals is diagnosed with pancreatic cancer with multiple nodules in his liver. Two months prior to his diagnosis he experienced "stomach pain" which he gave 10 out of 10 on a pain scale. He asked his daughter, a nurse, if the antibiotic he was on could be causing his stomach pain. The pain persisted after the antibiotic treatment finished. The patient realized his pain was from the growing tumor and started treatment to shrink the tumor.

A Psychiatric Mental-Health Nurse Practitioner, working in the oncologists practice, evaluated this patient for depression and anxiety he experienced. The patient became very depressed because he was aware that he had terminal cancer. The patient scored 23 on the PHQ-9 scale and was placed on Paxil low dose for depression and anxiety. Since the medication made him drowsy, he took it at night. The patient died 12 weeks after initial diagnosis.

• Critical Thinking **Questions**

1. What interventions should the Psychiatric Mental-Health Nurse Practitioner carry out to assist this patient?

2. What do you anticipate the Psychiatric Mental-Health Nurse Practitioner will treat this patient for?

3. How can the Psychiatric Mental-Health Nurse Practitioner assist this patient in terms of diagnosis? What resources do you anticipate being used for this patient? Referrals?

References

American Nurses Association. (2014). *Psychiatric-mental health nursing: Scope and standards of practice* (2nd ed.). Maryland, MD: Nursebooks.

American Psychiatric Association. (2013). *Diagnostic and statistical manual of mental disorders,* (5th ed., pp. 160–161). Arlington, VA: American Psychiatric Association.

Kroenke, K., & Spitzer, R. L. (2002). The PHQ-9: A new depression diagnostic and severity measure. *Psychiatric Annals. 32*:509–521.

Kübler-Ross, E. (1969). *On death and dying.* New York, NY: Simon & Schuster.

National Institute of Mental Health.(2008). U.S. Department of Health and Human Services. *Mental Health Medications.*

Sadock, B., Sadock, V., & Ruiz, P. (2014). *Kaplan & Sadock's: Synopsis of Psychiatry,* (11th ed.). New York, NY: Lippincott, Williams & Wilkins.

Suggested Readings

Jacobsen, P. B., & Jim, H. S.(2008). Psychosocial interventions for anxiety and depression in adult cancer patients. *CA: A Cancer Journal for Clinicians. 58*(4), 214–230.

Kadan-Lottick, N., Vanderwerker, L., Block, S., Zhang, B., & Prigerson, H. G. (2005). Psychiatric disorder and mental health services use in patients with advanced cancer: A report from the coping with cancer study. *Cancer. 104*(12), 2872–2881.

National Institute of Mental Health. (2011). U.S. Department of Health and Human Services. Depression and Cancer, 2011: NIH Publication no. 11–5002.

Rosedale M. (2009). Survivor loneliness of women following breast cancer. *Oncology Nursing Forum. 36*(2), 175–183.

U.S. Department of Health and Human Services.

Williams S, & Dale J. (2006) The effectiveness of treatment for depression/depressive symptoms in adults with cancer. *British Journal of Cancer. 94*(3), 372–390.

COLLABORATION WITH OTHER HEALTH TEAM MEMBERS

CHAPTER 16

ROLE OF THE SOCIAL WORKER

"The social worker who referred me to resources in my community and who provided emotional support and encouragement throughout my cancer diagnosis and treatment was invaluable to me and my family. Without her, we would have felt lost and overwhelmed."

—*A cancer survivor*

Key Terms

biopsychosocial model • person in environment • where the patient is

Upon completing this chapter, you will be able to do the following:

1. Describe the education of a social worker involved in the care of patients with cancer.
2. Describe the role of the social worker who is caring for a patient with cancer.
3. Discuss the importance of including a social worker as part of the health care involved in the care of patients with cancer.
4. Identify at least three modalities that a social worker may employ when caring for a patient with cancer.

The complexity and variability of psychosocial issues associated with cancer survivorship has increased the demand for highly skilled practitioners on the healthcare team, trained to provide multilevel assessments and interventions throughout the illness trajectory. Oncology social workers are primary providers of psychosocial services in many settings, including cancer centers; hospitals; physician's offices; cancer-related agencies; and hospice agencies that facilitate patient family adjustment to a cancer diagnosis, its treatment, and rehabilitation (Smith, Walsh-Burke, & Crusan, 2010). As a member of the interdisciplinary team, the oncology social worker focuses on the psychosocial effects of cancer, cancer treatment, and survivorship.

Medical social work was established early in the 20th century as an essential component of the interdisciplinary healthcare team. Due to the recognition that sources of illness are not exclusively biological, the hospital social work role was initiated to address the social forces that influence disease onset and recovery as well as resumption of function (Smith et al., 2010).

The biopsychosocial model of social work practice creates the need for extensive social work training using a variety of theories that social workers incorporate in their practice. This ecological perspective uniquely equips the social worker to both assess and intervene to assist patients and families with the multiple effects of cancer (Smith et al., 2010). The "person in environment" ecological framework emphasizes both psychological and sociological theories, which prepare the social worker to design and implement interventions aimed at strengthening individual adaptation and environmental responsiveness to the needs of persons affected by cancer (Berkamn, 1981; Tolley, 1994).

Oncology social workers offer comprehensive services through effective screening; sound psychosocial assessment; carefully designed and implemented interventions such as individual, family, and group counseling; use of behavioral techniques; linkage to community resources, and program development (Lauria, Clark, & Hermann, 2001).

Education

A social worker earns a masters degree from a social work program (MSW) accredited by the Council of Social Work Education. This master's level training ensures that social workers are prepared through a broad theoretical foundation in developmental theories, psychodynamic theories, family systems theory, and cultural theories to practice in a wide variety of settings with diverse, vulnerable populations. Most MSW programs are 2 years and 60 credits with at least 600 hours of supervised field practicum. Typical course work includes human behavior and development, social policy, foundations of social work practice, assessment, diagnosis, and research.

In most states, there are two professional licenses with different qualifications. Social workers who wish to work as general practitioners to provide supportive counseling and case management, need only take a state exam upon graduation to become licensed in their state to practice social work. In most states, for social workers who wish to practice psychotherapy, the eligibility requirements include obtaining approximately 3 years of supervised psychotherapy experience and passing the state clinical social work exam. Upon completion of these requirements, the licensed clinical social worker may provide all social work services, including clinical services such as the diagnosis of mental, emotional, behavioral, developmental, and addictive disorders; the development of treatment plans; and the provision of psychotherapy.

Additional training is suggested for oncology social workers to acquire the necessary skills and expertise required to facilitate patient and family adjustment to a cancer diagnosis, its treatment, and rehabilitation. This training can be accomplished through multidisciplinary rounds, professional conferences, continuing education, or professional education provided through the American Cancer Society, The National Cancer Institute, and the Leukemia and Lymphoma Society (Lauria et al., 2001). The oncology social worker must have an understanding of the cancer disease process, and possess an understanding of how illness and treatment can affect an individual's psychosocial well-being. In addition, having the ability to elicit information regarding a patient's coping skills, and sources of support and concerns about treatment, work, insurance, and family issues is critical.

Screening and Assessment

Psychosocial assessment is the process by which the oncology social worker evaluates the needs of the patient and family. Assessment involves a psychosocial history, treatment plan, communication of this plan to an interdisciplinary team member, and screening for distress.

Screening and assessment of individual psychosocial needs are crucial to developing a care plan that is tailored to the concerns and needs of the cancer patient and identify those who are at high risk and require routine assessments (Lauria et al., 2001). Social workers can identify factors in the person's environment that may cause them to be more vulnerable to psychological and social problems.

Interventions

The choice of intervention depends on the particular needs identified in the assessment of the patient. Some interventions may occur only once, for example, referrals to financial assistance programs. Other interventions such as counseling may continue during treatment and survivorship. An intervention that might be appropriate at one stage of the illness might be detrimental at another. Comprehending this fundamental principle is at the core of the oncology social worker's ability to listen and follow the patient's needs. Starting "where the patient is" is a core social work value (Smith et al., 2010). The psychosocial needs of someone with a cancer diagnosis changes over time and are influenced by environmental and life factors. The social work systems perspective allows for the consideration of the effects of these other factors.

Counseling

Oncology social workers spend a considerable amount of time with survivors and their families discussing responses to the cancer diagnosis, treatment, and survivorship. At each stage of the disease, the survivor may struggle with difficult decisions; overwhelming feelings; communication problems at home and work; or personal feelings of helplessness and hopelessness. Injuries to self-esteem, feelings of dependence, fear of pain, and death are common experiences (Lauria et al., 2001). Through individual counseling, the social worker can assist with specific concerns of the survivor and set priorities. Counseling should be tailored to the individual's energy and progression of illness. While the process is therapeutic, the goal of social work intervention is not intrapsychic change but emotional support and guidance; when this is the case, the oncology social worker should be knowledgeable about clinicians who are capable of providing psychotherapy to meet the unique needs of the cancer survivor. In many settings, oncology social workers are clinical social workers trained to provide psychotherapy. Research demonstrates that most survivors and families possess a natural inclination to retain hope (Farran, Herth & Popovich, 1995). Counseling sessions can elicit a survivor's feelings of despair, sadness, and futility. Trying to maintain hope is an important goal of social work counseling.

Social workers have successfully incorporated behavioral techniques into their repertoire of skills and have used these techniques with individual patients and in groups (Beahr, 1999). In this age of shrinking healthcare resources, behavioral methodologies could become a more cost-efficient service delivery. Survivors can be taught techniques to use as coping strategies whenever they experience difficulty with an emotional reaction to the illness.

Mind–Body Therapies

Hypnosis, guided imagery, meditation, relaxation training, and music therapy are all used as interventions by oncology social workers to enhance a sense of control and empowerment over the illness for the survivor. Many cancer centers will offer or refer a cancer survivor to a "mind/body" program that teaches techniques to help the survivor feel more in control over their fears about cancer or to change automatic "negative thinking" into a more positive way of approaching the cancer experience (Lauria et al., 2001).

Resources, Information, and Advocacy

Oncology social worker provides referrals to various community resources to assist the cancer survivor with financial assistance, transportation, homecare, prostheses, insurance coverage, and medical equipment. The referral process is an important component of the psychosocial care provided by oncology social workers. They have a clear understanding of the types of referrals appropriate for patient intervention. Patient and family advocacy is another oncology social work task. Social work training teaches macro skills (community skills) that allow the practitioner to integrate the special needs of survivor and families with larger systems issue; acting as an advocate with religious affiliations, communities, and neighborhoods on behalf of the cancer survivor (Smith et al., 2010).

Discharge Planning

Discharge planning is the process of putting advocacy information programs and direct services together (Lauria et al., 2001). Hospital-based social workers who are responsible for discharge planning assess the patients' needs, identify significant problems, and develop a treatment plan that uses family and community resources. Discharge planning has become extremely intricate. In the case of cancer, the tasks of discharge planning often involve complicated coordination of services with the interdisciplinary team, detailed planning, and a comprehensive environmental assessment (Smith et al., 2010).

Research

Research is a required component of MSW training as it facilitates the development and teaching of professional knowledge and skills required to practice social work (Smith et al., 2010). The interdisciplinary Journal of Psychosocial Oncology, serves as a forum for sharing research and clinical data. Research conducted from the oncology social worker's perspective can include important social and relationship factors, financial and workplace concerns, and by looking at the social context of the cancer experience, can give a much broader understanding of the overall impact of the illness. Oncology social workers are well equipped to conduct qualitative research. They are skillful at interviewing skills, participant observation, case recording, and case analysis (Lauria et al., 2001). Social workers have the capability to look at a social setting and assess various levels from an individual to a society. In addition, oncology social workers can be a participant of the clinical trial team and assist in providing education regarding the benefits of clinical trial participation, may act as advocates in helping individuals enroll, and may help the individual understand their rights regarding continuing or withdrawing from a trial.

CASE STUDY

John, a 59-year-old man brought himself to hospital due to weakness and pain in legs. He was diagnosed with Leukemia and has been given a short life expectancy. John displays a gruff demeanor and can be distrustful of healthcare team. He is divorced and lost his home and business in divorce. John has no children and no social network. The love of his life is his golden retriever. John rents an apartment and does not work. His financial income is from investments which are dwindling. He has no health insurance. John is receiving radiation treatment on an inpatient basis. The palliative care team has consulted on this case for pain management and care of terminal illness. John's hospital stay was for approximately 6 weeks and was discharged to a hospice facility.

• Critical Thinking **Questions**

1. Why would the social work role be important in this case?
2. How could the "person in environment" training a social worker receives be helpful with this patient?
3. Why would a screening and assessment of this patient by the social worker be needed for this patient?
4. What interventions do you think the social worker would apply?

References

Beahr, L. C. (1999). Social work with adult cancer patients: A vote count review of intervention research. *Social Work in Health Care. 29*(2), 39–67.

Berkamn, B. (1981). Knowledge base needs for effective social work practice in health. *Journal of Social Work Education. 17,* 85–90.

Farran, C., Herth, K., & Popovich, J. (1995). *Hope and hopelessness: Critical clinical constructs.* Thousand Oak, CA: Sage Publication.

Lauria, M. M., Clark, E., & Hermann, J. F. (2001). *Social work in oncology: Supporting survivors, families, and caregivers.* Atlanta, GA: American Cancer Society.

Smith, E.D., Walsh-Burke, K., & Crusan, C. (2010). *Principles of training social workers in oncology. Psycho-oncology.* New York, NY: Oxford University Press. Retrieved April 6, 2014 from http://www.socialworkers.org/practice/intl/hungary2008/english/PrinciplesofTraining SocialWorkersinOncology.pdf

Tolley, N. S. (1994) .Oncology social work, family systems theory and workplace consultations. *Health and Social Work. 19,* 227–230.

CHAPTER 17
ROLE OF THE CLERGY

"Once, I received a referral from the nurse manager of the oncology unit for a patient who was nearing death and had requested to see a Unitarian chaplain. Since a Unitarian chaplain was not available, the director instructed me to handle the case. When I arrived at the patient's bedside, she was surprised to see that I was a rabbi. She said, "I specifically asked for a Unitarian Chaplain." I let her know that all chaplains serve in an ecumenical way and we are all the children of God. She asked me to sit down and we had a very meaningful visit. I continued to visit her until she passed away in peace. May her memory be a blessing."

—A chaplain

Key Terms

chaplain · religion · spirituality · pastoral services

Upon completing this chapter, you will be able to do the following:

1. Define what a chaplain is.
2. Differentiate between religion and spirituality.
3. Describe pastoral services in the hospital setting and in the community.

Spiritual Care and Chaplaincy in the Community and in Medical Settings

This chapter will provide nurses with an understanding of the work that clergy and professional chaplains in various settings do to support cancer survivors throughout their journey. Hospitals and other medical institutions are significant parts of the continuum of care for cancer patients but survivors spend most of their time in the community, whether they are receiving treatment or are in the posttreatment phase. It is crucial for nurses to be familiar with the ways in which spiritual care can support their patients, families, and caregivers within and outside of medical settings. The degree to which nurses can collaborate directly or indirectly with spiritual care professionals will vary by the area of nursing practice. For nurses who work in settings where they are part of a multidisciplinary team or have regular access to chaplains and social workers, this chapter will enable them to use their awareness of spiritual resources to involve these specialized professionals within their institutions. For nurses in other settings, in which they may be the professionals who assess how the patient and family are functioning, this chapter will help them to understand what resources for spiritual support may be available in the community and how to guide survivors to those resources.

Religious Identity and the Partnership with Healthcare Institutions

Historically, many hospitals were established and funded by religious orders or community charities to ensure that the needs of both the patients and medical professionals in that religion were met. These roots can be seen in the names of many hospitals around the country, and continue to influence policies in medical systems. Local clergy were, and continue to be, regular visitors when their congregants become patients. In addition, hospitals call on local clergy to meet the needs of unaffiliated patients seeking religious rites. Expressions of faith in public settings, including medical institutions, were and continue to be, an acceptable practice.

As religious and secular institutions merge, tension may arise due to the mandate of separation of church and state in this country. This tension may be due to the joining of diverse origins and the need for public funding such as Medicare, which requires adherence to government regulations.

New Trends in Religious Identity and Spirituality

During the last few decades, religious and spiritual life in the United States has changed in significant ways and nurses need to be aware of these evolving factors as they seek to help their patients in all settings. This country has become more cognizant of its religious and cultural diversity. Recent waves of immigrants have brought multiple expressions of religion in all their national, cultural, and generational varieties. There are now large, organized communities of Hindus, Muslims, and Buddhists. There are hundreds of other smaller religious/ethnic communities as well as syncretistic religions. Some sects have grown due to high birthrates or conversion and have become more visible due to activism or media attention.

While all of these groups provide adherents with meaning and community, the forms of leadership and communal structure may differ from the American model of the recent past. The authority of the religious leadership may not come in the form of "ordination," and their calling to leadership may not require a university degree. The spiritual leader may have another employment in addition to leading the community. The role of women in society in general and as religious leaders in some of these communities may be very different from what has been normative practice in this country. The issues related to religious leadership and gender are important to be aware of and may affect the way that nurses provide direct service as well as advocacy.

American religious expression and diversity is flowering, while simultaneously there is an increase in the number of Americans who do not affiliate with a particular religious group or institution. Nor do they identify themselves as religious although many of those will say they are "spiritual but not religious." This lack of affiliation has implications for the nurse who is trying to connect a cancer survivor to both practical and spiritual resources. Some of those who are unaffiliated may have a strong support system of family and friends. Nurses could guide them to websites such as www.caringbridge.org or www.sharethecare.org, which can help informal networks communicate and manage care. Others who are unaffiliated may be more isolated due to social, psychological, or financial factors and may need assistance in connecting with supportive social services.

Another factor to consider is the increasing number of inter-religious/cultural marriages in which partners do not share religious backgrounds or affiliation. This can have implications at a time of crisis when individuals may seek comfort in spiritual resources or decisions that need to be made about ritual practices. Families may need assistance in negotiating decisions and accepting that not all family members find spiritual meaning in ways that are instinctively understood as sacred.

Individuals who do not identify themselves as religious or believers will still face many of the issues of meaning discussed in the chapter on spirituality or in this chapter. Presently, with the cultural acceptance of the idea that spirituality can be experienced outside of the context of a specific religion, there is a plethora of resources published online or in print on spiritual issues related to illness and other challenges from nonsectarian, humanistic, and/or inter-faith perspectives. There are also organizations offering nonreligious yet spiritually supportive programs of all kinds, from support groups to retreats. Nurses can play an important role by exposing cancer survivors to these resources.

Spiritual Care in the Community: Collaborating with Clergy

No matter where the cancer survivor is along the disease trajectory, isolation is a major spiritual concern. The cancer survivor may be in an unfamiliar environment during treatment, or physically unable to get to those activities in which he/she routinely had social contact. The cancer survivor may be emotionally isolated from family and friends who are unable to "get it" or tolerate his/her feelings. The survivor may feel spiritually isolated from their beliefs, which had been sustaining in the past. Reducing isolation and connecting cancer survivors with the community is a major component of the work of clergy/spiritual caregivers.

Congregations

The most likely setting of spiritual care for those who are religiously affiliated is within the context of the congregation. This can include a variety of services and modalities with care shared by the clergy and laypeople in that congregation. Spiritual care is individualized within the context of the congregation and the member's relationship with other members and the clergy. Usually, at the point that an individual faces cancer, he/she is already a part of the congregation. This means that in contrast to the cancer survivor's primary identity in a medical setting as "the patient with cancer x," in the congregational setting, the individual is Sue or Abdullah or Yitzy or Meera who is now facing a difficult time. An individual's relationship with the community may be temporarily or permanently impacted by a diagnosis of cancer, but the individual still experiences life as a whole person. The congregation is also a natural setting to care for the family in practical ways as well as with companionship. The needs of various family members will be quite different; most congregations already serve families within age appropriate groups and as a unit. Children can receive support from Sunday school teachers, youth group leaders, and others. These congregational settings can offer children, whether survivors or family members, the opportunity to share normal activities with their peers as often as possible over time.

On the other hand, some people facing the challenges of cancer may seek out spiritual and communal support from religion even though previously they were not affiliated with a specific congregation. Congregations and clergy will welcome such individuals into the community and provide spiritual counseling. The goal for the individual, and his/her family, is to eventually integrate into the community. There can be challenges for those who enter a new congregation when they are vulnerable, yet becoming part of a community can be an important element in emotional and perhaps even physical healing.

Congregational Prayer for Healing

There are many approaches to and meanings of prayer. Nurses can be supportive of prayer's importance to many patients, while recognizing that not all patients find prayer meaningful. Congregational prayer may range from being included in weekly communal prayer lists of all those who are ill, to prayer offered privately by fellow congregants on behalf of the ill, prayer recited at the bedside, or special healing services or circles. For believers, prayer is an act that allows them to connect with a higher power and to help in a very real way. Empirical studies about the efficacy of intercessory prayer on the medical status of a patient are inconclusive (Krucoff et al., 2005). Nevertheless, the knowledge that prayer is being offered can keep someone connected to their community even if they cannot be physically present. Prayer and rituals can have special meaning when offered by clergy. In some religions, there are specific rituals and sacraments that only the clergy may perform. Given the significance of prayer, it is appropriate for a nurse to ask if it is important to the cancer survivor.

A significant moment of spiritual transition is when a cancer survivor feels healed enough to ask that prayers on their behalf be stopped. Loved ones and the community may or may not feel it is "safe" to stop those prayers for healing at the time that the survivor requests it. If the illness progresses, worshippers may feel that their prayer has the ability to bring about miraculous cure at a time when medical knowledge suggests that cure is no longer expected and comfort care is most appropriate. Sometimes, education may be necessary to assist individuals who are praying for a miracle to understand that they can continue to do that, while expanding their prayers for strength, love, comfort, inner peace, and so forth. This can facilitate the patient and family in the process of accepting that palliative care is an act of faith; that human hands offer sacred comfort, no matter what the Divine decree will be. A sensitive nurse can play a significant role in this transition by suggesting a conversation with their clergy person to explore how prayer can continue to provide support as the situation changes.

Religious Teaching about Medical Treatments

Most religions have teachings and literature about seeking medical intervention, acceptable treatments, and the withdrawal of treatments. These teachings are derived from particular understandings of the relationship between the Divine and humanity, as well as between the body and that which animates it. Some individuals who are affiliated will give consideration to the teachings of their religion; some will insist on the participation of their clergy in any decision making while others will defer to their physicians or will hold the absolute value of patient autonomy over the teachings of their particular religion. Understanding whether a particular patient will be seeking religious guidance, and from whom, is an important element of assessment by the medical team out in the community as well as in a hospital. There are varying levels of understanding and sophistication among local clergy about the routine as well as cutting-edge teachings on medical treatment. The need for doctors to participate in consultations with a patient's clergy person is beginning to be recognized. Again, advocating for this may be an important task for a nurse, particularly if the illness becomes advanced. However, recognizing the importance of religious teachings for cancer survivors is also relevant at other times. Fertility and reproductive technology are also the subjects of ethical and legal rulings. Survivors of childhood cancer and those diagnosed with cancer during childbearing years may face decisions about preserving fertility or using reproductive technology. They may wish to consult with their religious authorities in making treatment choices.

Pastoral Counseling

A primary role of congregational clergy in many religions is pastoral counseling. This is a process of offering emotional and spiritual support within the context of the theological teachings of that community. At times the cancer survivor, family member, or friend will gain strength, comfort, or meaning from what has always been spiritually sustaining and is able to work with the pastoral counselor to continue to do so. At other times, what has been spiritually meaningful for the cancer survivor in the past, may no longer be meaningful. The pastoral counselor can help the individual find new sources of strength, or other ideas that are helpful based on traditional teachings. It is important to acknowledge that individual clergy have different levels of formal training in pastoral counseling, as well as diverse personalities and strengths and weaknesses as counselors. Some congregational clergy will do all the counseling themselves. Others will refer to outside counselors, while continuing to remain connected in a more practical or ritual way. A nurse who sees a patient or family member in spiritual distress and struggling with meaning can play a critically important role by suggesting that they set up a meeting for pastoral counseling with their own clergy.

Life Cycle Rituals

Congregations are often the setting for major and minor life cycle rituals. Familiarity with the rituals as performed in one's own religious community can be a source of comfort and hope for cancer survivors. Taking part in significant moments as they are marked in the context of sacred community allows one to feel connected to something beyond the boundaries of one's own life. Looking forward to, or even living for, a particular family life cycle event can give meaning and hope to one who is ill. At the same time, this can be a burden on the individual and the family. Whether the beloved grandparent will live long enough to welcome a new grandchild, or the physical arrangements needed so a seriously ill parent can attend a wedding, may distract from the joyful event, even as it lends deeper meaning to it. A nurse who is aware of significant family events can help facilitate a discussion with the doctor about scheduling treatments as well as assessing what is really possible or could make participation feasible.

The rituals associated with the end of life, death, and mourning are some of the most important things that take place in a congregational setting. When shared by the community, individual, and family with the leadership of the clergy, ritual practices can offer structure and guidance for all of those involved as they move through the anticipation of loss, dying, and grief. As medical personnel help a family prepare for the transition to palliative care, knowing that the next steps of care will be shared by and slowly given over to a supportive religious community can ease the anxiety and distress experienced by all involved.

Concerns about Congregational Involvement

There are issues and cautions to keep in mind for nurses who would like to facilitate and support the connection between cancer survivors and a congregation. The first is the issue of privacy and confidentiality. HIPPA is relevant here and a nurse should only share information with the permission of the patient. Equally important is the idea that in order to get help from a congregational community, the cancer survivor has to give up a certain amount of privacy. For example, well-meaning people who have not come home previously may now be bringing food into the kitchen, without checking food preferences. Another example, requesting that one's name be put on a prayer list means having to reveal that something is wrong. As a result, well-meaning discussions may ensue as others try to find out what is going on so they can help.

A second issue is the challenge of accepting help. To be sick or to be a caregiver is to be vulnerable; a status most of us do not accept easily. In addition, when a congregational leader is ill or engaged in intensive caregiving, members may worry for the stability of their community, even as they want to help. Difficult social dynamics and political issues may challenge how help is given and accepted. This can be especially sensitive when the one who is ill or a family member has a strained relationship with the clergy.

A third issue is whether the congregation can support the family in its varied needs, especially over time. The volunteers and clergy must have a realistic sense of what they can do on a practical, service, or financial level, as well as for how long these forms of support can be provided. Congregations must recognize their limits and know when referrals to other programs are appropriate to meet the individual's needs. Stopping support may make the individual resentful. A nurse can be helpful in explaining the medical issues involved, suggesting additional resources for support for the cancer survivor and family members.

Spiritual Support in Community-Based Agencies

Congregations are not the only institutions that provide spiritual support to cancer survivors in the community. Nurses can make referrals to a variety of agencies for spiritual support services to cancer survivors and their families. Until recently, most mental health providers failed to consider the relevancy of spirituality to their assessment or treatment plan. Increasingly the spirituality of the patient is being seen as an important component of culturally sensitive holistic care and viewed as a professional obligation. Many mental health professionals now do a treatment plan based on a "bio-psycho-social-spiritual assessment." This kind of an assessment can be very helpful to cancer survivors and their families who seek support.

Some counseling centers have focused on, or included, a pastoral component in their services. Professionals with degrees or certification in pastoral counseling often staff these centers. Some pastoral counseling centers will provide multifaith services, but most are based in particular religious denominations or theologies. These counselors will be familiar with the spiritual issues that often accompany a diagnosis of cancer and survival.

Family service agencies provide support for individuals and families through all stages of life. However, most are now nonsectarian agencies serving the entire community, with licensed or certified mental health professionals on their staff. Many of their services are covered by private or governmental insurance although often a sliding fee scale is available for individuals with limited income. Family service agencies can be especially effective in serving children because of their knowledge of developmental stages and their expertise in helping parents to raise children in difficult situations. Family service agencies also serve older adults. Their expertise in the issues of aging and caregiving is important as the incidence of cancer increases with age and there are often multiple levels of need (American Cancer Society, 2013). Many family service agencies have come to recognize the importance of integrating religious sensitivity and spiritual awareness into their programs. Some do this by training and encouraging social workers and counselors to make use of spiritual modalities such as meditation in their work. Others include specially trained spiritual care professionals on their staff.

Nurses can also refer cancer survivors to programs that focus on supporting individuals and families such as Cancer Care or Gilda's Club, as well as groups devoted to supporting those with specific cancers. In these groups, professionals, volunteers, and survivors often work together. The programs offer meditation, chanting, and yoga and address spirituality as well as more traditional mental health concerns.

Finally, many survivors prefer to get their support from an individual therapist in private practice. Some therapists are using spirituality in their assessments and helping clients to explore and access spiritual resources as part of their healing process. There are also certified pastoral care counselors in private practice.

Virtual Communities

New technologies, which have led to the creation of virtual communities, will certainly continue to be an increasingly important factor in all kinds of care, including spiritual care. Social media has reshaped the meaning of community and it has become another powerful source of spiritual support and, at times, distress, such as when a request for prayer or treatment related financial support goes viral on Facebook. Confidentiality and privacy may be a concern, yet it can be healing to receive support from friends and strangers around the world. A cancer survivor who is homebound no longer needs to be socially isolated or without support from a spiritual care professional; connection through the internet is possible. Nurses can inquire about the survivor's use of these technologies as part of their daily activities and overall coping.

Spiritual Care in Healthcare Settings

Chaplains

Today, professional chaplains serve in the healthcare system in a way that is very different from the visits or supervision of religious rites done by denominationally based clergy in the past. Spiritual care by professional chaplains is recognized as a necessary component of care for those receiving inpatient care, as well as outpatient services in a hospital or clinic. This is also the case for rehabilitation and long-term care nursing facilities. Many people are unaware of the role of modern chaplains in a medical institution and they may not even recognize when a chaplain enters their room. Traditional clerical garb, such as a collar or a *kipah* (Jewish head covering, also worn by Jews who are not rabbis) may identify some chaplains; most chaplains wear ordinary business dress. Many, but not all chaplains are ordained clergy. Chaplains who are not ordained clergy usually have master's degrees in theology or other advanced studies in religion as a prerequisite for chaplaincy training. Chaplains receive training in a Holistic Care model, which connects the mind, body, and spirit. They emphasize that the spiritual needs of patients are an integral part of the overall treatment plan.

Professional Chaplaincy Standards

Professional chaplains are required to have four units of Clinical Pastoral Education (CPE), which includes 2,000 hours of supervised clinical service. Chaplain interns or chaplains in residence are individuals who are in training. Clergy and others in CPE programs may do this at any point during their seminary studies or careers. There are four major chaplaincy organizations that also offer certification: the Association for Clinical Pastoral Education (ACPE), The Association of Professional Chaplains (APC), the National Association of Catholic Chaplains (NACC), and *Neshama:* Association of Jewish Chaplains (NAJC). APC is the largest of the four. All chaplaincy organizations share the common goals of setting standards and providing a solid educational framework which enables them to minister to the spiritual, religious, and cultural needs of patients, family members, and hospital staff.

How Chaplains Differ from Community Clergy

Clergy are trained to "teach and preach the Word of God" and interpret sacred texts to guide the lives of people within the particular understanding of a religious community or theologically based educational institution. Congregational clergy serve as the spiritual leaders of communities and have a variety of responsibilities to their congregants, to their leadership, to the local and broader religious institutions, and to the community as a whole. They provide support to members of their congregations in times of need or crisis. They do this by inspiring hope in the face of despair, offering reassurance of the connection with community when that is shaken and reinforcing faith in the Divine through prayer, sacrament, teaching, and pastoral counseling. Another role of congregational clergy is to implement and maintain viable community support systems for those who are vulnerable.

Professional chaplains may play the same role as congregational clergy, especially for patients who are unaffiliated, or when the patient is distant from his/her community. The chaplain can bridge the gap between the patient and home congregation by serving as a liaison with community clergy and can supplement the visits made by a patient's own clergy. However, the focus of the professional chaplain is different. The chaplain does not have a responsibility to "teach or preach" in a predefined way or to impose a religious or spiritual agenda in any way. Rather, the chaplain is attuned to the spiritual needs of patients in the context of the medical situation and helps them to explore the spiritual resources that will be helpful. The chaplain's goal is not to inspire unrealistic hope or to reassure the patient that all will be well. The goal is to listen to the patients' expressions of pain and suffering, enabling them to tell their own stories in order to facilitate their ability to cope with the illness. The work of the chaplain is not to foster a particular religious community. Instead, the chaplain strives to create a safe and spiritually supportive space for the patients and families within the medical setting. Therefore, unlike congregational clergy, when the patient is discharged from the medical setting, the chaplain will cease his/her service.

Congregational clergy work largely within the confines of their own religious denominations. Professional chaplains are ecumenically trained to provide spiritual and religious support to individuals of all faiths as well as to those who are without any religious affiliation or faith. This focus on ecumenical training and the spiritual needs of the individual patient is critical to the work of chaplains within medical institutions given the diverse nature of American religious and spiritual identity described at the beginning of this chapter. Professional chaplains may be affiliated with a specific religious tradition such as one of the Protestant denominations, Catholicism, Judaism, Islam, Buddhism, or Hinduism. Sometimes individuals, who are affiliated with a local congregation, prefer to address their religious and spiritual needs with the hospital chaplain rather than with their own clergy. As discussed earlier, patients may find it challenging to show their vulnerability. Some people will feel safer facing their spiritual crisis with the help of a professional chaplain who is not part of their own community. Nurses should remember professional chaplains have the training and resources to be spiritual caregivers to people of all faiths or of no faith by helping all individuals to identify their challenges, sufferings, and strengths, and to tap into their own spiritual and religious resources.

Pastoral care departments vary in their policies regarding visits to patients by chaplains of their own faith since all professional chaplains are able to provide ecumenical support. Some will routinely send chaplains to patients of their own faith, while others will do so only when a rite of passage requires an ordained clergy to perform it.

What Chaplains Do

The main role of the professional chaplain is to make a comprehensive assessment of the spiritual needs and goals of the patient and to create an action plan for addressing them. The format of the assessment may vary, but it should match the requirements of the Joint Commission for Accreditation of Hospitals Organization (Joint Commission, 2005). Training for chaplains includes sensitivity to various religious, cultural, and social issues, and needs of patients and staff. At times, healthcare providers may perceive the religious/cultural needs of a patient as a barrier. The chaplain then becomes an educator, helping to explain the religion/culture of the patient and facilitating discussions, which result in solutions in order to carry out the prescribed medical care. The resourceful chaplain serves as a patient advocate, identifying the sources of conflict and enabling the reduction of tensions.

Chaplains also serve as members of ethics committees and as advisors to institutional review boards, which shape the ethical policies of the medical center. Chaplains lead private and public prayer, both ecumenical and denominational as appropriate, and participate in gatherings such as memorial programs. They offer or facilitate spiritual counseling for patients, families, and staff at times of need. Many chaplains lead spiritual groups for patients and staff on a regular basis. The overarching goal of chaplains is to help people find meaning in suffering and bring some order into chaos.

Spiritual Care in Advanced Illness

Chaplains play a major role in palliative care and end-of-life care. Palliative care and hospice teams often include a dedicated chaplain who works closely with medical and social work professionals in planning treatment and providing end-of-life care. Oncology patients, as well as those facing other life-limiting illnesses, often seek out chaplaincy support. They call on the chaplain to help them resolve personal inner conflicts, conduct life review, seek forgiveness and reconciliation, bring meaning to life and suffering, and, most important, to help them attain inner peace in their transition to the next stage.

The spiritual assessment by the chaplain is a crucial element in the overall treatment plan for a patient. In most cases, it crystallizes the treatment goals and in some cases, it can set the stage to initiate a new treatment plan. For example, the spiritual assessment by the chaplain may reveal the need for improved communication between the patient and family members, among the family members themselves, and between the patient and the healthcare team.

Studies have shown that the provision of spiritual care by medical teams to terminally ill patients is associated with better patient quality of life, greater hospice utilization, and less aggressive medical interventions at End of Life (EOL). A recent study looked at the impact of spiritual care in the community on hospitalized patients with terminal illness (Balboni et al., 2013). It found that patients with high support from religious communities were more likely to receive aggressive EOL care and less likely to use hospice. However, the study concluded that those patients who were well supported by religious communities and who also received spiritual care from the medical team received less aggressive medical care at EOL. While further research in this area is required, it suggests that collaboration between the medical team and the home religious community can benefit patients and their families.

Through the use of a holistic approach, as cultural and religious brokers, leaders in prayers, and facilitators of spiritual counseling, chaplains not only provide healing to the spirit, but also support the medical care being given to the body. As ministers of pastoral care, chaplains can prescribe to the believing patient the most powerful and in some cases only balm remaining, "I, the Lord, am your healer." (Exodus 15:26). However, chaplains can also guide those with no religious tradition, or with no belief in a

Divine Being, along their own paths to find meaning in crisis as they approach moments of transition.

Getting to Know Your Chaplain

In order to address the spiritual needs of their patients, nurses and other healthcare members should take the time to become familiar with the pastoral care department and chaplains in their healthcare setting including knowing the backgrounds, resources, and availability of the chaplains. Some hospitals have a large budget, which allows them to sustain a staff of professional chaplains of many faiths, chaplains in residence, and chaplaincy interns. One common practice in large hospitals is to assign chaplains to particular floors or medical units. Other hospitals have smaller budgets and more limited chaplaincy staff. They may depend on community clergy to supplement their spiritual services. Nurses should be aware of the department's regular hours and be aware that most hospitals do have an on-call chaplain around the clock. Nurses should contact chaplains regarding spiritual and religious resources as well as consultation for individual patient needs. As members of the professional staff, chaplains are subject to patient confidentiality in accordance with HIPAA. Many pastoral care departments also have trained volunteers who assist the chaplains in screening patients, visiting, and bringing ritual objects and books. In order to provide information to clergy, the clergy must be identified as a staff chaplain. If a member of the community clergy requests information, permission from the patient is necessary.

As stated previously, the role of the chaplain is not limited to providing pastoral and spiritual care to patients and their families. The chaplain is there to provide spiritual care to the staff as well. Staff members may consult the chaplain on any personal or work-related issues; the chaplain will maintain confidentiality and respect of personal faith. Contact information for the on-call chaplain should be easily accessible.

Nurses should be aware how often chaplains conduct rounds. In addition, nurses should be familiar with how to notify the chaplain when there is a pastoral need such as in times of spiritual crisis or in the case of a patient who has just received a new diagnosis. Nurses should routinely ask patients if they would like to see a chaplain or if they have any spiritual, religious, or cultural needs. If the patient asks for a prayer, be aware that the chaplain will usually offer a nondenominational prayer unless the patient makes a request for prayer from a specific religious tradition.

When making referrals, be as specific as possible about why you are making the referral and how you feel the patient might benefit from the chaplain's visit. Be clear about any special spiritual or religious requests. After the visit, the chaplain may make an entry into the patient's medical record.

Consider inviting chaplains to participate in patient rounds and to attend any multidisciplinary team meetings. Involving the chaplain will benefit not only the patients but also the healthcare team. The chaplain has special expertise and can play a critical role in helping the healthcare team and the patient. These situations include the removal of ventilator support, feeding tubes, and any end-of-life decisions, as well as when the patient refuses treatment on religious grounds. Chaplains should be included on ethics committees to advocate for the patients' spiritual and moral desires and to facilitate the decision-making processes in patient care.

A rabbi working in a social service agency offers some examples of the spiritual support work she does with cancer survivors. "The client and I may discuss what it means to be 'created in the image of God' when one has lost a body part to cancer. I have shared holiday treats while acknowledging the loss involved in no longer being able to cook for and host a holiday meal. We discuss how to retain some part of that role and identity. We have studied Psalms together which enables survivors to see their varied emotions and spiritual struggles expressed in sacred language. I have helped couples negotiate where they will purchase cemetery plots based on teachings about burial and visiting the dead. I have taught chants and prayers which can be used to calm one's self during scans and radiation. Finally, I offer prayers and sing spiritual melodies when words are no longer possible."

Conclusion

Spirituality may be an important part of the journey of the cancer survivor. Spiritual care can be provided in many settings and can be individualized to the needs of the patient. Congregational clergy offer varying levels of practical help, companionship, and spiritual support in partnership with the members of their congregation. Many agencies now include spiritual care as part of their overall treatment plan and program; some have specially trained clergy as part of their staff. Professional chaplains work within medical institutions supporting patients, family, and healthcare team members and work with people of all religions as well as those without any religious affiliation or faith. By being aware of the spiritual needs of the survivor and the resources that are available, nurses can help cancer survivors connect with sources of spiritual support.

CASE STUDY

The nurse enters the room of B.C., female, 32 years old, who has just been told by her healthcare practitioner that she has stage 3 breast cancer. From previous discussions, the nurse is aware that the patient is married and has three children all under 10 years. The nurse was aware of the diagnosis prior to going to the patient. Upon entering the room, the patient is on the phone, clutching a rosary, and ends the call, crying: "God what am I going to do now?"

• Critical Thinking Questions

1. Give an example of a therapeutic response that the nurse should state to the patient at this point.
2. What additional information should the nurse ascertain in order to develop a plan of care in order to address the psychosocial needs of the patient?
3. Based on the interactions with this patient, which member of the interdisciplinary team would be appropriate for the nurse to contact? Give your rationale(s).
4. If the same patient were in an outpatient facility, what differences (if any) would there be in terms of the assessment and/or referrals that the nurse would make?

References

American Cancer Society. (2013). Retrieved on July 11, 2014 from Cancer Facts and Figures: http://www.cancer.org/research/cancerfactsfigures/cancerfactsfigures/cancer-facts-figures-2013.

Balboni, T., Balboni, M., Enzinger, A., Gallivan, K., Paulk, M. E., Wright, A., ... Prigerson, H. G. (2013). Provision of spiritual support to patients with advanced cancer by religious communities and associations with medical care at the end of life. *JAMA Internal Medicine. 173*(12), 1109–1117.

Joint Commission. (2005) "Evaluating Your Spiritual Assessment Process." The Source 3 no 2, 6–7; Retrieved from http://www.professionalchaplains.org/uploadedFiles/pdf/JCAHO-evaluating-your-spiritual-assessment-process.pdf

Krucoff, M., Crater, S., Gallup, D., Blankenship, J. C., Cuffe, M., Guarneri, M., ... Lee, K. L. (2005) Music, imagery, touch, and prayer as adjuncts to interventional cardiac care: The monitoring and actualisation of Noetic trainings (Mantra) II randomized study. *The Lancet. 366*,(9481), 211–217.

Additional Readings

Dykstra, R. (2005). *Images of pastoral care.* Chalice Press.

Koenig, H. (2007). *Spirituality in patient care.* Templeton Foundation Press.

Roberts, S. ed. (2013). *Professional spiritual and pastoral care.* Woodstock, VT: Skylight Paths.

Professional Chaplaincy Websites

The Association for Clinical Pastoral Education—www.acpe.org
The Association of Professional Chaplains—www.professionalchaplains.org
The National Association of Catholic Chaplains—www.nacc.org
Neshama: Association of Jewish Chaplains—www.najc.org

A Sampling of Other Resources on Spirituality and Health

Health Care Chaplaincy; www.healthcarechaplaincy.org
www.Chaplainsonhand.org and www.cantbelieveihavecncer.org are two initiatives of HCC for direct service to patients and caregivers. 844–242–7524.
George Washington Institute for Spirituality and Health. www.Gwish.org
Kalsman Institute on Judaism and Health. www.huc.edu/Kalsman
The Shira Ruskay Center/Jewish Board of Family and Children's Services offers an integrated model of spiritual and social work support in the community for those who have been diagnosed with a life limiting illness as well as consultation to professionals. 135 West 50th Street, New York, NY 10020. 212–632–4608. www.jbfcs.org/jcs. A connected program is the National Center for Jewish Healing which also offers print and on-line resources and consultations.
New York Chaplaincy Services and its crisis response unit, New York State Chaplain Task Force provides interfaith chaplains to help bring order in the midst of chaos and hope in the midst of despair. www.newyorkchaplaincyservices.org

CHAPTER **18**
PAIN AND PALLIATIVE CARE TEAM

"To me, the palliative care my wife received as she battled a devastating disease meant, aside from the obvious benefits of alleviating excruciating pain and discomfort, giving her a quality of life that she would not have had without such care. It gave us the precious time to be more loving and intimate and to interact with friends and family in a way that would not have otherwise been possible."

—*Spouse of patient who died of breast cancer*

Key Terms

hospice • palliative care • palliative services

Upon completing this chapter, you will be able to do the following:

1. Define hospice and palliative care.
2. Discuss the history and emergence of pain and palliative care as a specialty.
3. Describe the benefits of palliative services.
4. Discuss the role of nursing in pain and palliative care services.

History of Hospice

There was a time in the not too distant past that the word *hospice* referred only to the historical definition. *Hospice* was derived from the Latin meaning hospitality. Hostels were resting places for returning Crusaders from the "holy wars" in "the East" and they were tended to by orders of nuns who cared for them until these travelers were either well enough to continue on their journey home or died. The late physician Dame Cecily Saunders who worked with the dying since the late 1940s created one of the first modern hospices, St. Christopher's Hospice in London, England in 1967 (Saunders, 1975). Dame Saunders visited the United States (US) in 1963; her lectures at Yale University inspired the then Dean of the Yale School of Nursing, Florence Wald, to begin her own journey leading to the founding of the first official hospice in the United States in 1974 (Clark, 2000; Wald, 1999). This was succeeded soon by other hospices throughout the country.

Following the groundbreaking foundation by Dame Saunders, the grass-roots beginnings of care for the dying continued in North America. It seems a logical extension of the "do-it-yourself world" in the latter 1960s and 1970s which included car maintenance, garden growing, and childbirth which arose. This was the time to reintroduce the concept of de-medicalizing death and dying.

In time, the United States Federal government acknowledged the value of this philosophy and in 1982 added the *hospice* benefit to the Medicare program (a federal program for those over 65 or who otherwise qualify) (Department of Health and Human Services, 1983). This provided reimbursement for the care which until that point was a combination of volunteers and paid professionals in agencies throughout the United States. Hospice has defined eligibility criteria which include two physicians certifying life expectancy of 6 months or less, and that individuals forego curative treatments (e.g., chemotherapy or radiation) for purely comfort measures (Department of Health and Human Services, 1983). A reliance on symptom management in the home was the backbone of hospice, which is increasingly a more common type of care given at the end-of-life. In 2012, according to the National Hospice and Palliative Care Organization (NHPCO), almost 38% of all expected deaths in the United States took place under the auspices of hospice (National Hospice and Palliative Care Organization, 2013).

Growth of Palliative Care as a Specialty

As the hospice movement grew, additional needs were recognized. The supportive type of care individuals received in hospice was defined as *palliative*, taken from the Latin *pallium* meaning "to cloak." Furthermore, members of the hospice movement realized there were patients in need of support and care who were not eligible for the hospice program. Approaching this type of care became the purview of in-hospital physicians as well as hospice care providers who embraced the concept of easing suffering regardless of where patients were on their illness continuum. For example, patients receiving chemotherapy, or pulmonary or cardiac interventions in the hospital have the same right to symptom relief as those patients who had forgone aggressive curative treatment and were dying on hospice.

Pioneers in symptom management began researching and publishing information on symptom management which led to recognition of a palliative care subspecialty. The goal of palliative care is to provide symptomatic support at any stage of serious life-limiting disease including management of pain and nonpain symptoms such as anxiety, dyspnea, nausea, constipation, and emotional stressors (World Health Organization, 2014). Unlike hospice care, palliative care can be provided in conjunction with potentially curative treatments.

The National Consensus Project for Palliative Care originally developed in 2003, set out a framework for quality in palliative care nation-wide (National Consensus Project for Quality Palliative Care, 2004). The collaborating agencies have expanded but the goal remains the same: provide national guidelines for the care of people with life-threatening illnesses from the time of diagnosis through the patient's death.

Unfortunately, all too often, there is confusion on what palliative care actually means. Some of this confusion is because of the Medicare insurance guidelines which limit hospice-based symptom management to the last 6 months of life. Many people including healthcare providers incorrectly equate palliative care with hospice, and as a result, symptom management is postponed. Too often people and their caregivers accept suffering as a natural part of cancer treatment. In reality, patients can benefit from symptom management at all stages of diagnosis and regardless of treatment goals.

Hospice care means that patients and their families are supported by a team of experts delineated by Medicare: a physician hospice medical director, a registered nurse (RN), certified personal care aide, social worker and/or chaplain, and a volunteer. Sometimes there are additional team members such as a nurse practitioner, music/art/ pet therapists, and massage therapists. While on hospice, the patient's medications related to their terminal illness and any durable medical equipment (DME), such as oxygen or a hospital bed, are included in the daily (per diem) payment the hospice receives. The Center for Medicare & Medicaid Services (CMS) requires that all hospice benefits through Medicaid or private insurance are comparable to the Medicare Hospice benefit in terms of eligibility criteria, services provided, and per diem payment schedules.

In contrast, nonhospice palliative care is reimbursed as fee-for-service similar to other specialty consultations. The team for palliative care may include all of the team members listed above. Unlike hospice, DME and medications are paid for separately by insurance. The fundamental difference between hospice and palliative care is that hospice care is solely for end-of-life noncurative care while palliative can be at any stage of illness and be given concurrently with curative treatments.

Benefits of Palliative Care

Patients receiving palliative care truly are the center of the palliative team focus. Recent research has demonstrated that cancer patients can benefit from palliative symptom management including better quality *and quantity* of life (Temel et al., 2010). Sometimes the benefits are more qualitative as opposed to quantitative: Does the patient feel supported? Does the family feel equipped? Is there sufficient rapport with healthcare providers and/or palliative team members to address concerns and add to comfort during treatment?

There has been a push from palliative care providers for other medical providers involved in patient's care to share in providing a palliative approach. Keeping patients informed of their prognosis, monitoring patients during treatments, as well as easing any discomfort from treatment, can aid in a patient's well-being. Sometimes primary healthcare providers are not comfortable with discussions about goals of care and treatment options, or may not have knowledge about managing symptoms. Working to bridge the gap between patient, caregivers, and the other healthcare providers is a large focus of palliative care.

Palliative care specialists are often consulted when there is a knowledge or communication gap between the team and the patient or family. The goal of any palliative team is to collaborate with the primary care team, not to uproot it. Care plan meetings with patient and/or family should include the primary team as the best way to bridge the gap and keep the primary team engaged and included. If the primary team cannot attend when the patient and/or family are present, then a meeting between the palliative and the patient's primary teams is compulsory, not optional.

Resources such as EPERC's *Fast Facts* (www.eperc.mcw.edu) provide medical providers with information about symptom management and communication tools. With the assistance of a palliative care approach, all providers can assist in delivering comprehensive patient care no matter what the ultimate patient outcome is.

Palliative Care Certification

Although palliative care has been provided by clinicians for decades, in 2006 the American Board of Medical Specialties formally declared a new subspecialty certificate in Hospice and Palliative Medicine for physicians. Unlike other specialties, this is the first and only physician specialty which is available through ten medical fields. After obtaining certification in a primary medical field such as Anesthesiology, Emergency Medicine, Family Medicine, Internal Medicine, Obstetrics and Gynecology, Pediatrics, Physical Medicine and Rehabilitation, Psychiatry and Neurology, Radiology, or Surgery, physicians can complete a 1-year Hospice and Palliative Medicine fellowship training and take the certification exam. From 2008 to 2012, physicians with sufficient clinical experience were able to apply to take the certification exam without a year of formal palliative fellowship training. Certification is renewable every 10 years, pending successful completion of certain education, training, and examination requirements.

Physicians are not the only healthcare providers who can earn certification in palliative care. Beginning in 1994, registered nurses could attain hospice certification. Currently, the National Board for Certification of Hospice and Palliative Nurses (NBCHPN) offers specialty certification for all levels of the hospice and palliative nursing care team including nurses, nurses assistants, advanced practice nurses, and nursing home administrators with a certification valid for a 4-year period which is renewable. Social workers with a bachelor's degree can attain a Certified Hospice and Palliative Social Worker (CHP-SW) title. In addition, palliative care specialty certification is available for chaplains through the Board of Chaplaincy Certification Incorporated (BCCI).

Similarly, hospitals can attain palliative certified status through The Joint Commission which is an independent, not-for-profit organization which accredits and certifies more than 20,500 healthcare organizations and programs in the United States. Joint Commission accreditation and certification is recognized nationwide as a symbol of quality that reflects an organization's commitment to meeting certain performance standards (The Joint Commission, 2014a). In 2011, The Joint Commission developed an Advanced Certification Program for Palliative Care which recognizes hospital inpatient programs that demonstrate exceptional patient- and family-centered care and optimize the quality of life for patients (both adult and pediatric) with serious illness (The Joint Commission, 2014b). This too demonstrates the growing recognition of the additional benefits which palliative care provides.

Palliative Care Legislation

Lawmakers, in recognition of the value of palliative care, have passed legislation to increase access to palliative care. In New York State, the need for greater incorporation of palliative care for patients with serious, life-limiting illness was recognized and formalized into law. Effective February 9, 2011, the Palliative Care Information Act amended the Public Health Law, by requiring "physicians and nurse practitioners to offer terminally ill patients information and counseling concerning palliative care and end-of-life options" (New York State Department of Health, 2014). As such, information and counseling concerning palliative care and end-of-life options must be offered to patients with an illness or condition that is reasonably expected to cause death within 6 months. According to the state's webpage, the law is not intended to discourage conversations about palliative care with patients whose life expectancy exceeds 6 months, as it is often appropriate to discuss palliative care with patients earlier in the disease process (New York State Department of Health, 2014).

Subsequently in 2013, Rhode Island, Maryland, Connecticut, and New Hampshire all passed palliative care-specific legislation. Generally, the bills seek to establish one (or more) of four policies: the creation of a palliative care advisory council to assist in state palliative care initiatives (CT, MA, NH, RI), the development of educational web resources (MA, RI), the requirement that all licensed facilities facilitate access to palliative care or provide information about palliative care services (MA, RI), or the development of palliative care pilot programs for data collection (MD) (Palliative In Practice, 2013). This growing legislative support clearly demonstrates the growing recognition of palliative care as a valuable part of management of serious medical conditions including cancer.

Does Palliative Care Mean Less Care or Dying Sooner?

A research study about the impact of palliative care was published in the *New England Journal of Medicine* in 2010. People who were recently diagnosed with metastatic non-small cell lung cancer were divided into two groups: standard care versus standard care in combination with early palliative care. The study found that early palliative care led to significant improvements in both quality of life and mood (less depression). In addition, the people who received early palliative care had less aggressive interventions at the end of life but actually lived longer by 2.7 months (Temel et al., 2010). Other studies have shown that early addition of specialty palliative care improves quality of life and helps clarify treatment preferences and goals of care for patients with advanced cancer (Parikh, Kirch, Smith, & Temel, 2013).

Though many consider these studies to have debunked the presumption that palliative care = end of life = less care = dying sooner, there are many healthcare providers who care for people with cancer who still believe that "it's too soon for palliative" and wait until the patient's disease is very advanced and symptom burden is great. This actually is a disservice to patients who likely would benefit earlier in their care from specialized symptom management, emotional support (for themselves and their loved ones), and honest discussions about treatment options and planning for the future.

Finding Palliative Services

Palliative care is available in a variety of healthcare settings. Many hospitals have a Palliative Care Consult team, which may include physicians, nurse practitioners, nurses, social workers, and pastoral care. Generally, in the hospital setting calling for a palliative consult must be approved by one of the physicians currently caring for the patient. In such cases, if a patient would like to be seen by the palliative team in the hospital, please ask the primary physician caring for the patient to make a referral. There are online directories such as the "Palliative Care Provider Directory" to locate a hospital that provides palliative care (http://www.getpalliativecare.org/howtoget) (Get Palliative Care, 2014).

Outpatient (office-based) palliative consultation is also available for people living at home or in an assisted living facility. Many hospitals which have palliative care consult programs for their hospitalized patients also provide palliative consultation services in the outpatient setting. Depending on the insurance, a referral from the primary or treating physician (e.g., oncologist) for palliative care may not be needed. An insurance company may have provider listing for palliative specialists. If they do not list any, a hospital with a palliative care program may provide outpatient services as well. Some home healthcare agencies may also be able to provide a more palliative focused home care. In addition, some cancer care programs are including palliative consultation automatically or based on screening tools for their patients. There are some oncology offices, and/or chemotherapy infusion centers which have palliative care consultants on-site to assist patients at this critical time of their treatment.

Nursing homes generally can provide two types of care: subacute rehabilitation (SAR) and long-term care (LTC). SAR is paid for by Medicare (a federal program for those over 65 or who otherwise qualify) or private insurance and is generally for a 3- to 4-week stay to improve physical functioning, for intravenous antibiotics, or for wound care treatment with the anticipation that the individual will return home. LTC is custodial care paid for by private pay, LTC insurance or Medicaid (a combined state and federal program usually for lower income individuals) for those who live in the nursing home long term. Often nursing homes can offer hospice care, comfort care, or palliative care programs. Hospice can be provided to patients on LTC, but not for SAR (Medicare benefit will not pay for rehabilitation *and* hospice at the same time). Palliative or comfort care programs can be provided in LTC or SAR; however, not all nursing homes have certified or trained palliative healthcare providers, so it is important to inquire about who is providing the palliative or comfort care services and what they entail. Often, comfort care in the nursing home means "comfort measures only" whereas palliative care can mean symptomatic support with ongoing curative interventions. Medicare will *not* pay for both SAR and hospice concurrently, so palliative care in the nursing facility allows people to receive rehabilitation while simultaneously getting symptom management and support from palliative care. Neither hospice nor palliative care will pay for the daily rate for a long term or subacute nursing home stay.

Conclusion

Physicians and nurses will often consider palliative care to be the same as hospice care and end-of-life care, which, is *not true*. As such, individuals with cancer and their caregivers (including nurses) often need to be an advocate and trigger a palliative care evaluation themselves. One of the roles of a nurse when caring for a patient with cancer, is explaining the difference between hospice and palliative care. It *is never* "too soon" for palliative care, especially for people with cancer!

CASE STUDY

Ms. C is a 60-year-old woman with end-stage recurrent colon cancer who went to the hospital with generalized pain, debility, severe anasarca, and malignant bowel obstruction. Her husband (and proxy) provides much of the history and because Ms. C is quite weak. She was initially diagnosed 8 years earlier and was in remission until a year ago. She recently had a feeding tube placed to provide nutrition. During this hospitalization, the oncologists told the spouse that they are waiting for the swelling in her legs to get better to restart chemotherapy.

He reports that his wife told him that she "had enough" of all these medical treatments, but he persuaded her to accept TPN (total parenteral nutrition) since she is unable to take any food by mouth or feeding tube. She is receiving IV fluids as well. Ms. C is groaning and unable to answer questions. Vitals are: RR 26, HR 110, BP 90/60. She has diffuse severe swelling of all extremities with distant heart sounds, lungs with fair air entry, and a firm, distended abdomen with no bowel sounds audible.

Questions (Select the Best Answer)

1. The earliest moment of palliative consultation appropriate for this patient is?
   a. At time of cancer recurrence 1 year ago
   b. Upon admission to the hospital
   c. Once her heart rate went above 100 bpm
2. Who is able to recognize that a palliative consultation would be appropriate?
   a. Patient
   b. Spouse
   c. Primary medical doctor
   d. Oncology specialist
   e. Nurse
   f. All of the above
3. Which of the following is true about hospice?
   a. Patients can receive hospice care while at a subacute rehabilitation nursing home facility
   b. Patients can receive hospice care while at a long-term care nursing home facility
   c. To qualify, two physicians (one of whom is a hospice medical director) certify patient has less than 6-month life expectancy if disease takes expected course
   d. Patients can continue curative treatments such as chemotherapy or radiation
   e. All of the above are true
   f. Only a, c, and d are true
   g. Only b and c are true
   h. Only b, c, and d are true

ANSWERS: 1-a; 2-f; 3-g

References

Clark, D. (2000). Total pain: The work of Cicely Saunders and the hospice movement. *American Pain Society Bulletin. 10*(4), 13–15.

Department of Health and Human Services. (1983). Medicare Fee for Service Payment: Hospice. [Online] December 16, 1983. [Cited: July 22, 2014.] Retrieved from https://www.cms.gov/Medicare/Medicare-Fee-for-Service-Payment/Hospice/Downloads/1983-Final-Rule.pdf

Get Palliative Care (2014). Center to Advance Palliative Care. [Online] [Cited: May 6, 2014.] Retrieved from http://getpalliativecare.org/howtoget/

National Consensus Project for Quality Palliative Care. (2004). Clinical Practice Quality Guidelines for Palliative Care. [Online] May 2004. [Cited: July 22, 2014.] Retrieved from http://www.nationalconsensusproject.org/guideline1.pdf

National Hospice and Palliative Care Organization. (2013). NHPCO Facts and Figures: Hospice Care in America. [Online] October 2013. [Cited: May 25, 2014.] Retrieved from http://www.nhpco.org/sites/default/files/public/Statistics_Research/2013_Facts_Figures.pdf

New York State Department of Health. (2014). Palliative Care Information Act. [Online] [Cited: May 6, 2014.] Retrieved from http://www.health.ny.gov/professionals/patients/patient_rights/palliative_care/information_act.htm

Palliative in Practice. (2013). Rhode Island Passes Palliative Legislation. [Online] [Cited July 23, 2014] Retrieved from http://palliativeinpractice.org/2013/07/03/rhode-island-passes-palliative-care-legislation/

Parikh, A. B., Kirch, R. A., Smith, T. J., & Temel, J. S. (2013). Early specialty palliative care translating data in oncology into practice. *New England Journal of Medicine. 369*(24), 2347–2351.

Saunders, C. (1975). *The care of the dying patient and his family; documentation in medical ethics.* London: London Medical Group.

Temel, J. S., Greer, J. A., Muzikansky, A., Gallagher, E. R., Admane, S., Jackson, V. A., … Lynch, T. J. (2010). Early palliative care for patients with metastatic non–small-cell lung cancer. *New England Journal of Medicine. 363*(8), 733–742.

The Joint Commission. (2014a). About The Joint Commission. [Online] [Cited: May 30, 2014.] Retrieved from http://www.jointcommission.org/about_us/about_the_joint_commission_main.aspx

The Joint Commission. (2014b). Advanced Certification for Palliative Care Programs. [Online] [Cited: May 30, 2014.] Retrieved from http://www.jointcommission.org/certification/palliative_care.aspx

Wald, F. S. (1999) Hospice Care in the United States: A Conversation With Florence S. Wald. Interview by M. J. Friedrich. *Journal of the American Medical Association. 281*(18), 1683–1685.

World Health Organization. (2014). WHO Definition of Palliative Care. [Online] [Cited: July 22, 2014.] Retrieved from http://www.who.int/cancer/palliative/definition/en/#.U3w3npDXWKM.email

LIFE AFTER CANCER TREATMENT

CHAPTER **19**

WHEN THE CLOUD RETURNS

Key Terms

cancer survivor · cancer survivorship · transitional survivorship · fear of cancer recurrence (FCR)

Americans are living longer with cancer as a result of early detection, medical advances in treatment modalities, and supportive care. The number of cancer survivors is expected to rise in the United States from the current 14.5 to nearly 19 million by 2024. People are living longer after a primary cancer diagnosis extending the trajectory of living with cancer that impacts the quality of life, mental health, after-care, and finances of survivors. Most recent estimates indicate that among cancer survivors 64% were diagnosed 5 or more years ago and 15% were diagnosed 20 or more years ago with 5% of cancer survivors younger than 40 years; while 46% are 70 years or older (National Cancer Institute, NIH, DHHS, 2011/2012). Cancer survivors exhibit increased distress associated with the physical and psychological cancer experience often fearing that the cancer may return.

Research has repeatedly evidenced that the diagnosis with cancer has a tremendous psychological impact on the person and their families increasing distress levels that impair psychological functioning. The most important psychological factors associated with cancer are: depression, hopelessness, helplessness, loss of autonomy, lack of control, inappropriate social support, spiritual and existential concerns (Pessin, Amakawa, & Breitbart, 2010). In this context, factors affecting the cancer survivors' quality of life, physical and psychological functioning are an imperative of nurses caring for cancer survivors.

Hou, Law, Yin, and Fu, (2010) assert that cancer stressors are complex and compounded, subtle and ambiguous. Stressors are threats encompassing the past as well as future dynamics for survivors beginning with diagnosis, implications for treatment, changes in family dynamics, impaired functioning, uncertainly of illness progress and treatment efficacy. The coping ability and adaptation of cancer survivors requires managing expectations and reorganization of his/her self-view that includes: facing mortality, making good treatment decisions, fostering personal resolve, and maintaining hope and optimism while living healthy for long-term gains.

Life after Cancer Treatment

Transition from cancer patient to survivor poses challenges for individuals and a range of problems when primary cancer treatment ends. Persistent fatigue, physical changes, fears of a reoccurrence, and the expectations to "get back to normal" add stress to the daily functioning at the end of treatment. During cancer treatment individuals and families are enveloped in supportive and nurturing healthcare providers navigating them through the cancer treatment maze that suddenly ends with the completion of treatment. The shift from active treatment to follow-up care has been associated with distress due to a lack of support and loss of frequent medical monitoring. The responsibility of self-care can be overwhelming to the survivor resulting in feelings of abandonment, vulnerability, and the loss of a "safety net" (Ward, Viergutz, Tormey, DeMuln, & Paillen, 1992). Individual fears may include the ineffectiveness of curative treatment, survival disability and disfigurement, and cancer reoccurrence over the long-term survival trajectory. Anecdotally, survivors narrate this timeframe as "living under a cloud."

Many cancer survivors experience ongoing fears of cancer recurrence (FCR) and the chronic uncertainty of his/her health status during and after cancer treatment can be a significant psychological burden (Thewes, Butow, Zachariae, Christensen, SImard, & Gotay, 2012; Lebell et al., 2014). A study by Simard et al. (2013) found that FCR was among the most commonly reported problems in adult cancer survivors. FCR was found to be one of the primary concerns and the most frequently unmet need for cancer survivors and their caregivers. Additional results yielded that although FCR remained stable over the survivorship trajectory, younger age, presence and severity of physical symptoms, psychological distress, and lower quality of life were associated with higher FCR. Fear of reoccurrence is a predominant worry for cancer survivors and warrants interventions that evidence the efficacy in decreasing FCR.

Cancer survivorship has been described using numerous metaphors and frameworks. The seminal work of Dr. Fitzhugh Mullan (1983; 1985), a cancer survivor, proposed that cancer survivorship included three seasons: acute survivorship, extended survivorship, and permanent survivorship. It was within the extended survivorship season, that recovery, coping, and fear were dominant. It was a time of watchful waiting with celebration, uncertainty, and transition. In his 1985 article Dr. Muller notes that "for better or worse physically and emotionally the experience leaves an impression." This would indicate that there is a gradual sense that the risk of recurrence is low and that the chance of survival is great. Miller, Merry, and Miller (2008) assert that since Dr. Muller wrote "Seasons of Survival," the subsequent decades of cancer research and treatment have contributed to the increase in survivorship. People are living longer, with cancer or are cancer-free increasing the risk of a second or subsequent malignancy because of side effects of high-dose therapy, or in remission that is dependent on the use of targeted agents such as radiation or Imatinib for patients with chronic myelogenous leukemia.

Miller, Merry, and Miller's proposed framework for "Seasons of Survival" incorporated an updated model of survivorship that reflects the dynamics of current cancer survivors that include acute survivorship, transitional survivorship, three categories of extended survivorship, and four categories of permanent survivorship. The needs of cancer survivors during each of the seasons are specific to cancer survivors living with various adverse health results of the cancer experience that include disruptions in quality of life, emotional health, physical ability, sexuality, interpersonal relationships, career, finances, and uninsurability (Miller, Merry, & Miller, 2008).

Klimmek and Wenzel (2012) attempted to clarify the concept of cancer survivorship. Utilizing a theory derivation process, a descriptive framework involving the work of transitional cancer survivorship emerged making explicit the many types of work that survivors and the people who support them contribute to the survivorship process. Transitional cancer survivorship, defined as survivor tasks, engaged in three reciprocally interactive lines of work. The first was *illness-related* that included numerous tasks related to maintain secondary and adjuvant therapies, treatment of functional losses, and physical changes posttreatment. Cancer survivors engage in the management of treatment-related illness and late symptoms. It is within the second line of work entitled *biographical work* where the survivor puts the cancer experience into context and comes to accept the implications of cancer and cancer survivorship by restructuring his/her past and present perspective, then looking forward to the future. Within the restructuring of his/her biography the survivor gives new direction to a life plan including managing fear and uncertainty and growing as a survivor.

Some survivors describe ambivalence between cancer fatalism and cancer activism. Cancer fatalism is defined as "a belief that death is inevitable when cancer is present, whereby cancer activism is describe as "strong action and motivation to overcome negative view of cancer and to achieved the goal of addressing cancer issues" (Morgan, Tyler, & Fogel, 2008; p.238). The third type of work addresses *everyday life work* that represents the activities of daily living such as eating, dressing, bathing, toileting, cooking, and shopping. Integration of everyday work into survivorship requires refinement of these tasks based on individual physical, mental, and environmental abilities and limitations. *Every day life work also* encompasses emotional responses that include coping and putting on a "game face" and psychological work managing daily and prolonged stress and depression. Survivor work includes social engagement to overcome the sense of social isolation that accompanies cancer treatment (Beatty, Oxlad, Koczwara, & Wade, 2008). Survivors may become involved with cancer activism in the form of volunteer work with cancer organizations and survivorship communities in an effort to remain close to others with shared experiences and an informal support network.

Cancer survivors exhibit psychological distress following a cancer diagnosis that includes uncertainty about the future (Dunkel-Schetter, Feinstein, Taylor & Falke, 1992; Ashing-Giwa et al., 2004), fear of death and reoccurrence not only during treatments but also years after completion of cancer treatments (Leake, Gurrrin, & Hammond, 2001; Saleh & Brockopp, 2001). Current research by Kim, Carver, Spillers, Love-Ghaffari, and Kaw (2012) studied the dyadic effect between severity of the cancer and fear of recurrence on the quality of life 2 years post diagnosis on cancer survivors and their caregivers. The researchers identified that the level of fear of recurrence on reported quality of life for survivors and caregivers were directly related and suggest that subgroups of survivors and caregivers will benefit from interventions designed to help them manage their FCR. Similar results were reported by Lambert, Jones, Girgis, and Lecathelinais (2012) who examined the trajectories of anxiety and depression among partners and caregivers of cancer survivors within the first 2 years postdiagnosis and suggested interventions may have the greatest impact if implemented early in survivorship, particularly for caregivers experiencing chronic anxiety and depression.

The development of nursing models for cancer care that focus on the recovery of health and well-being following cancer diagnosis and treatment should incorporate extended strategies aimed at bolstering cancer individuals and their caregivers' self-efficacy, coping, and support. Oncology nurses are poised to manage the sense of uncertainty and fear associated with cancer reoccurrence tempered with optimism and hope along the survivorship trajectory.

References

Ashing-Giwa, K. T., Padilla, G., Tejero, J., Kraemer, J., Wright, K., Coscarelli, A., … Hills, D. (2004). Understanding the breast cancer experience of women: A qualitative study of African American, Asian American, Latina and Caucasian cancer survivors. *Psycho-Oncology.* 13, 408–428.

Beatty, L., Oxlad, M., Koczwara, B., & Wade, T. D. (2008). The psychological concerns and needs of women recently diagnosed with breast cancer: A qualitative study of patient, nurse and volunteer perspectives. *Health Expectations.* 11, 331–342. doi: 10:1111/j1369-7625.2008.00512.x.

Dunkel-Schetter, C., Feinstein, L. G., Taylor, S. E., & Falke, R. L. (1992). Patterns of coping with cancer. *Health Psychology.* 11, 79–87.

Hou, W. K., Law, C. C., Yin, J., & Fu, Y. T. (2010). Resource loss, resource gain, and psychological resilience and dysfunction following cancer diagnosis: A growth mixture modeling approach. *Health Psychology.* 29(5), 484–495.

Kim, Y., Carver, C.S., Spillers, R.L., Love-Ghaffari, M, & Kaw, C. (2012). Dyadic effects of fear of recurrence on the quality of life of cancer survivors and their caregivers. *Quality of Life Research.* 21(3), 517–525. doi: 10.1007/s11136–011–9953–0.

Klimmek, R., & Wenzel, J. (2012). Adaptation of the illness trajectory framework to describe the work of traditional cancer survivorship. *Oncology Nursing Forum.* 39(6), E499–E510.

Lambert, S.D., Jones, B.L. Girgis, A., & Lecathelinais, C. (2012). Distressed partners and caregivers who not recover easily: Adjustment trajectories among partners and caregivers. *Annals of Behavioral Medicine.* 44, 225–235.

Leake, R. L., Gurrin, L. C., & Hammond, I. G. (2001). Quality of life in patients attending a low-risk gynecological oncology follow-up clinic. *Psycho-Oncology.* 10, 428–435.

Lebell, S., Maheu, C., Lafebvre, M., Secord, S., Courbasson, C., Singh, M., … Catton, P. (2014). Addressing fear of cancer recurrence among women with cancer: A feasibility and preliminary outcome study. *Journal of Cancer Survival.* 8(3), 485–496.

Miller, K., Merry, B.A., & Miller, J. (2008). Seasons of survivorship revisited. *Cancer Journal.* 14(6), 369–374. doi: 10.1097/PPO.0b013e31818edf60.

Morgan, P. D., Tyler, I. D., & Fogel, J. (2008). Fatalism revisited. *Seminars in Oncology Nursing.* 24, 237–245. doi: 10.1016/j.soncn.2008.08.003.

Mullan F. (1983). *Vital signs: A young doctor's struggle with cancer.* Boston, MA: Farrar, Straus and Giroux.

Mullan F. (1985). Seasons of survival: Reflections of a physician with cancer. *New England Journal of Medicine.* 313, 270–273.

National Cancer Institute, NIH, DHHS. (2011/2012). *Cancer trends progress report–update.* Bethesda, MD, August 2012, Retrieved from http://progressreport.cancer.gov

Pessin, H., Amakawa, L., & Breitbart, W. S. (2010). Suicide. In J. C. Holland, W. S. Breitbart, P. B. Jacobsen, M. S. Lederberg, M. J. Loscalzo, R. S. McCorkle (Eds.), *Psycho-oncology* (2nd ed., pp. 319–323). Oxford: Oxford University Press.

Saleh, U. S., & Brockopp, D. Y. (2001). Quality of life 1 year following bone marrow transplantation: Psychometric evaluation of the quality of life in bone marrow transplant survivors' tool. *Oncology Nursing Forum.* 28, 1457–1464.

Simard, S., Thewes, B., Humphris, G., Dixon, M., Hayden, C., Mireskandari, S., & Ozakinci, G. (2013). Fear of cancer recurrence in adult cancer survivors: A systematic review of quantitative studies. *Journal of Cancer Survival.* 7(3), 300–322. doi: 10.1007/s11764–013-0272z.

Thewes, B., Butow, P., Zachariae, R., Christensen, S., Simard, S., & Gotay, C. (2012). Fear of recurrence: A systematic literature review of self-report measures. *Psycho-Oncology.* 21, 571–587. doi: 10. 1002/pon.2070.

Ward, S., Viergutz, G., Tormey, D., DeMuln, J., & Paillen, A. (1992). Patients reactions to completion of adjuvant breast cancer therapy. *Nursing Research.* 42(6), 362–366.

NURSING DIAGNOSIS

As survivorship becomes more of reality for an increasing number of individuals diagnosed with cancer, the nurse's role in addressing psychosocial issues becomes increasingly important. The nursing process is one tool available to nurses to provide support to the patient/family by correctly identifying areas of needed intervention. The nursing process is a problem-solving tool and is the traditional methodological approach that nurses are taught in order to assess, analyze, plan, intervene, and evaluate outcomes of patient responses across the health continuum.

After reviewing the data collected (assessment), the nurse should identify the relevant data that can indicate patient/family strengths, potential problems in which the nurse needs to take preventive measures, and/or any actual problem(s) that exist. This analysis of data, the nursing diagnosis segment of nursing process, equates to the identification of the area(s) that the nurse needs to address with a patient/family after which the plan of care can be developed. Collaborative problems will also occur that the nurse should be cognizant. There is a need to know which members of the healthcare team may best address these potential problems, actual problems, and strengths to be promoted. Communication is an essential component of the collaborative process.

The following are possible examples of the analysis portion of nursing process that may relate to the cancer survivorship continuum. The specific defining characteristic(s)/patient or family clinical manifestations are not included in these statements. In addition, the physiological problems occurring with different types of cancer have been excluded (NANDA, 2014).

Early in the cancer diagnosis trajectory:

- Deficient Community Health related to lack of accessibility to resources
- Risk-Prone Health Behavior related to lack of social support
- Risk for Compromised Human Dignity related to loss of control
- Disturbed Personal Identity related to the crisis of a new diagnosis of cancer
- Caregiver Role Strain related to changes in family relationships
- Impaired Parenting related to caregiver's statement of not feeling able to care for child
- Interrupted Family Processes related to changes in family functional roles
- Parental Role Conflict related to disruption of normal family function
- Anxiety related to change in patient's health status
- Ineffective Coping related to an uncertain outcome of the cancer diagnosis

Mid to late in the continuum of care:

- Ineffective Protection related to the side effects of cancer treatments
- Readiness for Enhanced Self-Health Management related to the patient's expressed desire to learn how to

- Ineffective Family Therapeutic Regimen Management related to the family's inability to manage the complex therapeutic course of therapy
- Readiness for Enhanced Self-Concept related to patient's acceptance of their limitations
- Readiness for Enhanced Self-Care related to the patient's expressed desire to strengthen their level of independence
- Hopelessness related to patient's declaration of feeling alone
- Compromised Family Coping related to the withdrawal of the significant other's support
- Ineffective Denial related to the patient's inability to acknowledge cancer's impact on their life
- Grieving related to the spouse's loss of a life partner
- Powerlessness related to reported lack of control over the outcome of the disease
- Readiness for Enhanced Resilience related to patient's self-report of improved feelings of control
- Moral Distress related to patient and/or family's need to make end-of-life decisions
- Spiritual Distress related to patient's statement of absent self-forgiveness
- Readiness for Enhanced Coping related to patient's use of spiritual resources as a support

GLOSSARY

Activities of Daily Living: Age-appropriate physical and cognitive activities.

Adaptation: Occurs when an individual's physical or behavioral responses to any change in his or her internal or external environment result in preservation of individual integrity or timely return to equilibrium.

Advocacy: Any beneficial activity, such as actively defining and supporting their rights, decisions, choices, privacy, and autonomy or promoting access to the most effective and timely healthcare services, resources, and support that is performed on behalf of patients who are not able to speak for themselves.

Affect-control strategies: Strategies undertaken by the person with an illness to manage the emotional responses to illness.

Anxiety: An uneasy feeling of discomfort or dread accompanied by an automatic response; a feeling of apprehension caused by anticipation or danger.

Assessment of readiness: Assessment through multidisciplinary endeavor to obtain a comprehensive understanding of the patient that requires assessment of each of the transition conditions in order to create an individual profile of client readiness and to enable clinicians and researchers to identify various patterns of the transition experience.

Assessment tool-PHQ-9: Depression scale designed to make a rapid assessment of areas affected by the diagnosis. The scale has a score with proposed treatment actions.

Awareness (as a property of transitions): Perception, knowledge, and recognition of a transition experience.

Barriers to improvement: Clinical and nonclinical health and life circumstance factors that are associated with impairment of a person's ability to adhere to healthy behaviors or follow through on activities that lead to stabilized health and maximal function.

Cancer survivor: A patient with cancer from diagnosis and for the balance of life.

Biopsychosocial model: A method of understanding health and illness through biological, psychological, and social factors. The principle of this model states that all issues relating to health are products of a complex interplay of these three factors.

Care coordination: The deliberate organization of patient care activities between two or more participants (including the patient) involved in a patient's care to facilitate the appropriate delivery of healthcare services. Organizing care involves the marshaling of personnel and other resources needed to carry out all required patient care activities, and is often managed by the exchange of information among participants responsible for different aspects of care.

Care management: The targeted role of assisting clients/patients initiate and/or follow through on health-improving activities by individuals with sufficient background and/or specific training to accomplish desired health-related program outcomes. ("Care management" is an encompassing term that includes the full range of management activities from wellness coaching to complex case management. Case management is a subset of care management.)

Case management: A collaborative process of assessment, planning, facilitation, care coordination, evaluation, and advocacy for options and services to meet an individual's and family's comprehensive health needs through communication and available resources to promote quality cost-effective outcomes (CMSA Standards of Practice for Case Management.)

Case managers: Licensed health professionals, usually nurses and social workers, with backgrounds and specific training that allow them to disentangle and assist with overcoming targeted barriers to health improvement in clients/patients with health conditions through implementation of a care plan.

Changes (as a property of transitions): Changes in identities, roles, relationships, abilities, and patterns of behavior, and transitional changes are supposed to bring a sense of movement or direction to internal processes as well as external processes.

Chaplain: A clergy or lay representative of a religious tradition who is attached to a secular, often residential, institution, such as a hospital, the military, university, prison, police department, and so forth. Professional Chaplains are trained and accredited by chaplaincy organizations and they are not necessarily members of the clergy. Certified chaplains are trained through Clinical Pastoral Education (CPE), a method of learning ministry by means of pastoral functioning under supervision.

Chaplaincy care: It is provided by a board-certified chaplain or student in a training program. Such care may include emotional, spiritual, religious, pastoral, ethical, and/or existential care.

Chemotherapy: The treatment of disease by means of chemicals that have a specific toxic effect upon the disease-producing microorganisms or that selectively destroy cancerous tissue; used to treat infections, cancers, and other diseases and conditions.

Clergy: One category of formal leaders within certain religions. Their roles and functions vary in different religious traditions, but these usually involve presiding over specific rituals and teaching religious doctrines. In some religions clergy are ordained. Ordination is a process by which individuals are consecrated, set apart as clergy, in order to be able to perform certain rites and ceremonies. In other religions, clergy have achieved a certain level of education and/or have a calling to serve in this role but are not consecrated.

Community conditions (as transition conditions): Conditions of specific communities (e.g., community resources, community environments) that facilitate or inhibit transitions.

Complementary and Alternative Medicine (CAM): Any therapies designed to promote and improve health and well-being that are usually considered to be outside the scope of Western, allopathic, medical practice.

Congregation: A gathering of people for the purpose of worship and community within a particular shared religious practice/faith tradition. A congregation may have a formal meeting place, such as a church, temple, mosque, synagogue, and so forth. Affiliation is a formal connection between an individual and a specific congregation. This connection is, in practice, voluntary on the part of the individual, although some denominations may consider all of the individuals of their faith within a catchment area to be members of a particular congregation.

Constipation: A decrease in a person's normal frequency of defecation accompanied by difficult or incomplete passage of stool and/or passage of excessively hard, dry stool.

Damocles syndrome: A nagging and disabling fear that cancer will reappear at some point.

Depression: One of several mood disorders marked by loss of interest or pleasure in living.

Developmental transitions: Transitions due to developmental processes such as birth, adolescence, menopause, elderly, and death.

Critical points and events: Identifiable marker events, such as birth, death, the cessation of menstruation, or the diagnosis of an illness.

Diarrhea: The passage of fluid or unformed stools.

Differences (as a property of transitions): Unmet or divergent expectations, feeling different, being perceived as different, or seeing the world and others in different ways.

Dimension: The degree by which the symptom(s) bother the individual.

Distress dimension: The degree by which the symptom(s) bother the individual.

Ecumenical (in the context of professional chaplaincy): Describes interfaith pluralism which involves respect, toleration, cooperation, and understanding of and among various religious faiths. The original definition refers to unity among various Christian churches and denominations.

Endoprosthetic devices: Prosthetic limbs that are implanted into remaining bone and remain permanently in place.

Engagement (as a property of transitions): The degree to which a person demonstrates involvement in the process inherent in the transition.

Event congruence: A match between expected and actual illness-related events.

Event familiarity: An illness situation is familiar or contains recognized cues that enables the person to associate it with some earlier illness-related event or condition.

Family/child/geriatric/social service agencies: Government and/or nonprofit organizations designed to better the well-being of individuals and/or families facing challenging situations which may be social, psychological, or biological in origin and current presentation. These organizations are also often concerned about the well-being of communities in order to strengthen and support the members of those communities.

Family relationships: The relationships that exist between an individual and a spouse or partner, and children.

Fatigue: An overwhelming sustained sense of exhaustion and decreased capacity for physical and mental work at the usual level.

Grand nursing theories: Broad-scoped conceptual frameworks designed as blueprints for the discipline—not easily used as free-standing guides to practice or as bases for research.

Health and illness transitions: Transitions due to recovery process, hospital discharge, and diagnosis of chronic illness.

Health coach (wellness counselor): Personnel that assist clients in understanding (and implementing) habits of healthy behavior who are at risk for development of health conditions or complications from existing conditions.

Hospice: A healthcare program and philosophy for the terminally ill that emphasizes pain control and emotional support for the patient and family, typically refraining from taking extraordinary measures to prolong life which may be provided in various settings.

Illusion: The process of positively evaluating an illness related experience to see it as an opportunity.

Inference: The process of negatively evaluating an illness experience resulting in heightened uncertainty levels and the perception of the illness as dangerous. The process is influenced by personality, knowledge, and contextual cues.

Influencing factors: The three categories that influence the symptom experience identified in TOUS—physiologic factors, psychological factors, and situational factors.

Insomnia: The subjective experience of insufficient sleep or sleep that is not refreshing.

Late-effects: Effects from treatments for cancer that occur in survivors after treatment has been completed.

Major depressive disorder: Psychiatric illness involving mood dysregulation.

Malabsorption: Disordered or inadequate absorption of nutrients from the intestinal tract resulting from surgery; disease including the intestinal mucosa, infections, celiac, and pancreatic diseases; or treatments such as chemotherapy and antibiotics.

Maladaptation: Occurs when an individual's physical or behavioral responses to any change in his or her internal or external environment result in disruption or individual Medicaid (a US government program, financed by federal, state, and local funds, of hospitalization and medical insurance for persons of all ages within certain income limits).

Medical treatments: Diagnosis and staging, surgical treatment, adjuvant or definitive chemotherapy and/or, radiotherapy and ongoing management of co-morbid problems.

Medicare: A US government program of hospitalization insurance and voluntary medical insurance for persons aged 65 and over and for certain disabled persons under 65.

Middle-range nursing theories: Theories that lie between working hypotheses necessary to conduct research and the "all-inclusive" grand theories that unify a discipline.

Miracle: An event not explicable by natural or scientific laws and may be attributed to a supernatural being. The word is often used to characterize any beneficial event which is statistically unlikely but not contrary to the laws of nature, including surviving a life-threatening situation such as an illness diagnosed as terminal. It may also be used to describe a wondrous natural occurrence such as birth.

Mobilizing strategies: Strategies including direct action, vigilance, and information seeking, undertaken by the person with an illness to reduce perceived uncertainty.

Mucositis: Inflammation of a mucous membrane.

Nausea: An unpleasant, queasy, or wave-like sensation in the back of the throat, epigastrum, or abdomen that may or may not lead to the urge or need to vomit.

Nursing therapeutics: Nursing measures that are widely applicable to therapeutic intervention during transitions.

Oncology clinical nurse specialist (OCNS): An expert clinician who provides direct care for patients with cancer. The role extends beyond clinical expertise, making a significant impact on nursing practice. The OCNS is involved with advancing nursing practice by utilizing evidence-based practice to influence nursing practice changes within an organization.

Oncology nurse navigator: A nurse with extensive knowledge in the oncology field, an educator, skilled listener, and a communicator-committed patient advocate. Assists with important decisions, improving the patient's quality of life, providing resources to decrease financial costs and psychosocial distress.

Organization transitions: Transitions in institutions/organizations that influence their members' and their clients' lives.

Outcome, measured health: During the process of care/case management assistance, this is a documentation of defined changes in targeted health status (BP change, ROM change, PHQ-9 change, etc.), function (exercise tolerance, employment, return to hobbies, sexual activity, etc.), cost (pre–post change in healthcare service use, in healthcare spend, in hospitalizations, etc.), quality of life (pre–post analogue scale, etc.), and satisfaction with care (availability of services during care process, etc.; generally not with provider).

Outcome indicators: The indicators of whether a transition is a healthy one or not.

Pain: An unpleasant sensory and emotional experience arising from actual or potential tissue damage or describe in terms of such damage. Pain includes not only the perception of an uncomfortable stimulus but also the response to that perception.

Palliative care: Care to relieve or lessen symptoms without goal of curing (synonyms for palliate: mitigate; alleviate).

Paraneoplastic syndromes: Indirect effects of cancers such as metabolic disturbances or hormonal excesses produced by chemicals released by tumor cells.

Pastoral care: Developed within the socially contracted context of a religious or faith community wherein the pastor is the community's designated leader who oversees the faith and welfare of the community. The faith they shared is a mutually received and agreed upon system of beliefs, actions, and values. The pastor's care for the community is worked out within a dialectical relationship between the person's unique needs on one hand and the established norms of the faith community on the other.

Patient navigators (health related): Individuals with sufficient background and/or the specific training to understand client/patient needs, the health system, and client/patient's personal and living situation sufficiently that they can help clients/patients find providers; services; and personal, social, financial, and living situation supports.

Performance outcome: Represents the consequence of the symptom experiences; must be able to be measureable.

Personal concerns: The specific concerns related to the diagnosis of cancer. These include fear of recurrence, self-perception of body image, financial concerns, side effects of treatments, and sustaining the day-to-day routines and role expectations.

Personal conditions (as transition conditions): Meanings, cultural beliefs and attitudes, socioeconomic status, preparation, and knowledge.

"Person in environment": This perspective is based on the notion that an individual and his/her behavior cannot be understood adequately without consideration of the various aspects of that individual's environment (social, political, familial, temporal, spiritual, economic, and physical).

Pharmacotherapy: The use of medicine in the treatment of disease.

Physiological factors: The anatomical, physiological, genetic, and treatment-related variables that contribute to symptom the experience.

Plan of care (case management): Mutually defined case manager and client/patient goals linked to a written timeline of prioritized assist activities designed to reverse assessment-based and targeted barriers to improvement. (The "plan of care" is often an iterative, dynamic longitudinal document in which adjustments to assist activities are made when goals are not being reached. Clients/patients graduate to self-management when goals are achieved.)

Preparation of transition: Education as the primary modality for creating optimal conditions in preparation for transition.

Probabilistic thinking: A changed view of the expectation of certainty in the presence of a chronic illness.

Process indicators: Indicators of moving clients either in the direction of healthy or toward vulnerability and risk that could allow early assessment and interventions by nurse to facilitate healthy outcomes.

Professional support: Professional healthcare providers and other professionals who provide assistance to individuals diagnosed with cancer.

Psychological distress: A multifactorial unpleasant emotional experience of a psychological (cognitive, behavioral, emotional), social, and/or spiritual nature that may interfere with the ability to cope effectively with cancer, its physical symptoms, and its treatment.

Psychological factors: The affective and cognitive state of the patient prior to and during the symptom experience.

Psychopharmacology: Medication used to treat mental health conditions.

Psychosocial interventions: Therapeutic techniques, usually classed as nonpharmacological (not involving medication), that address the psychological aspects of an individual or group and consider the person's or group's situation from a societal, familial perspective.

Physiological factors: The anatomical, physiological, genetic, and treatment-related variables that contribute to symptom the experience.

Quality dimension: What it feels like to have the symptom(s).

Quality of Life (QOL): The degree of satisfaction an individual has regarding a particular style of life, a general sense of well-being or satisfaction with one's life. (Miller-Keane, 1992).

Recurrence anxiety: Worry focused on the possibility that the cancer will return.

Religion: An organized collection of beliefs, cultural symbols, and a worldview related to the sacred. Many religions have narrative, symbols, and a sacred history, which are intended to explain the meaning of life and/or explain the origin of life or the universe. Denomination or sect is a subgroup within a particular religion that operates under a common name, tradition, and identity.

Religious/religiousness: A set of organized expectations, behaviors, and attitudes supporting a particular belief system. (Refer to previous term and definition.)

Resilience: The ability to become strong or successful again after something bad happens; a phenomenon of positive adjustment in the face of adversity.

Ritual: A familiar action or pattern of action that works to connect individuals with their larger community. There are many types, including religious, cultural, familial, and individual rituals. Lifecycle rituals/rites are used to mark defined moments of transition in the life of an individual and/or family. Religious communities often designate who can provide a ritual or officiate at a rite.

Role supplementation: Any deliberative process whereby role insufficiency or potential role insufficiency is identified by role incumbent and significant others, and the conditions and strategies of role clarification and role taking are used to develop a preventive or therapeutic intervention to decrease, ameliorate, or prevent role insufficiency.

Secondary malignant neoplasm: A secondary cancerous growth located in a site different from the original cancer.

Secondary survivors: Family members of those who are cancer survivors.

Self-organization: The process undertaken in the presence of continuous uncertainty, such as that seen in chronic illness.

Situational factors: The environment, both physical and social, of the individual prior to and during the symptom experience.

Social support: The relationships that an individual has with family, friends, and the community. This support may be socioeconomic, and/or psychosocial in nature and is deemed instrumental by the individual.

Social worker: An individual who possesses a baccalaureate or master's degree in social work from a school or program accredited by the Council on Social Work Education. Each social worker should be licensed or certified, as applicable and required, at the level appropriate to her or his scope of practice, in the practitioner's jurisdiction(s).

Societal conditions (as transition conditions): Conditions of specific society (e.g., sociopolitical issues, societal expectations) that facilitate or inhibit transitions.

Spiritual care: The interventions, individual or communal, that facilitate the ability to express the integration of the body, mind, and spirit to achieve wholeness, health, and a sense of connection to self, others, and/or a Higher Power.

Spirituality: Experiences, beliefs, and phenomena that pertain to the transcendent and existential aspects of life; the aspect of humanity that refers to the way individuals seek and express meaning and purpose and the way they experience their connectedness to the moment, to self, to others, to nature, and to the significant or sacred. The concept of spirituality is found in all cultures and societies. It is expressed in an individual search for ultimate meaning through participation in a religion and/or belief in a Higher Power, family, naturalism, rationalism, humanism, and the arts.

"Starting where the patient is": A social work value of addressing the issues most important to the client based on their perspective.

Stimuli frame: The nature of the stimuli or symptoms that a person with an illness perceives. These influence uncertainty.

Stomatitis: Inflammation of the mouth including the lips, tongue, and mucous membranes.

Stress: Pressure or tension on a material object or on emotions. The source of the stress, the demanding situation, is known as a stressor.

Stressor: A biological, psychological, social, or chemical factor that causes physical or emotional tension and may be a factor in etiology of certain illnesses.

Structure providers: Credible people or education that reduces uncertainty in illness by assisting with interpretation of illness-related events.

Supportive therapy: Treatment modality of individual, group, or family sessions designed to provide assistance for client and significant others.

Survive: To continue to live; to continue to exist.

Survivorship care plan: A comprehensive summary of a patient's diagnosis, treatments, prevention, and detection of recurrent and new cancers, surveillance for cancer spread, relapse, or second cancers, interventions for short and long treatment effects, and the basis for coordination of care between the oncologist and primary care providers.

Symptom pattern: The consistency of a set of symptoms that enables a person to determine that an illness is present and determine the meaning of the symptoms.

Symptoms: Any change in the body or its function as perceived by the patient; a symptom represents the patient's subjective experience of disease.

Theistic/nontheistic worldview: A person's core belief about whether God exists or not. Secondarily, if God exists, who is their God? A singular, holy God? A higher being/spirit/energy? A vague distant deity?

Time dimension: How the symptom(s) vary in duration and frequency.

Time spans: Time periods with an identifiable end point, extending from the first signs of anticipation, perception, or demonstration of change; through a period of instability, confusion, and distress; and to an eventual 'ending' with a new beginning or period of stability.

Transition conditions: The conditions that influence the way a person moves through a transition and that facilitate or hinder progress toward achieving a healthy transition.

Uncertainty: Difficulty with determining the meaning of an illness-related event.

Vomit: Material that is ejected from the stomach through the mouth.

Xerostomia: Dry mouth.

SUGGESTED RESOURCES

Internet Resources

Academy of Nurse Navigators: www.aonnonline.org
American Cancer Society: www.acs.org
American College of Surgeons Commission on Cancer: www.facs.org
Association of Clinical Professional Chaplains: www.acpe.org
Case Management Society of America: www.cmsa.org
Institute of Medicine: www.iom.edu
NANDA International: www.nanda.org
National Association of Clinical Nurse Specialists: www.nacns.org
National Association of Social Workers: www.naswdc.org
National Cancer Institute: www.cancer.gov
National Coalition of Oncology Nurse Navigators: www.nconn.org
National Comprehensive Cancer Network: www.nccn.org
National Institute of Nursing Research: www.ninr.nih.gov
Oncology Nursing Society: www.ons.org

Books

Herdman, T. H., & Kamitsuru, S. (Eds.). (2014). *Nursing Diagnoses Definitions and Classification. 2015–2017.* Oxford: Wiley Blackwell.
Petersen, S. J., & Bredow, T. S. (Eds.). (2009). *Middle Range Theories.* Philadelphia: Wolters Kluwer.

INDEX

Note: The letters f or t following page numbers indicate figure or table.